45

MANUAL AND COLOR ATLAS

OF THE

OCULAR FUNDUS

SCANDINAVIAN UNIVERSITY BOOKS

DENMARK MUNKSGAARD *Copenhagen*
NORWAY UNIVERSITETSFORLAGET *Oslo, Bergen*
SWEDEN LÄROMEDELSFÖRLAGEN *Stockholm, Gothenburg, Lund*

Published by
MUNKSGAARD, Copenhagen

Distributors in North and South America
W. B. SAUNDERS COMPANY

MANUAL AND COLOR ATLAS

OF THE

OCULAR FUNDUS

BY

HANS-WALTHER LARSEN, M.D.
DEPARTMENT OF OPHTHALMOLOGY
COPENHAGEN COUNTY HOSPITAL

523 color photographs
illustrating common and rare fundus diseases
with clinical notes and descriptive text
including considerations
of differential diagnosis

W. B. SAUNDERS COMPANY

PHILADELPHIA · LONDON · TORONTO

MANUAL AND COLOR ATLAS OF THE OCULAR FUNDUS has been designed by the author and the publishers, Munksgaard, in collaboration with the printers C. Hamburger. The type-face used is French Antiqua. The text is printed on paper from Munkedal AB and the illustrations on paper from Papierfabrik Scheufelen. Photographic processing by Brdr. Jacobsen. Blocks by Rotogravure A/S.

© 1969 by Munksgaard, Copenhagen, Denmark

Published simultaneously in the U.S.A. by W. B. Saunders Company, Philadelphia.

Library of Congress Catalog Card Number: 76-97055

Printed in Denmark by C. Hamburgers Bogtrykkeri, Copenhagen.

Preface

Since the publication of my "Atlas of Diabetic Retinopathy" in 1959 and "Atlas of the Fundus of the Eye" in 1964 it has become evident that a great demand exists for such photographic color atlases.

During the last few years, however, there has been a growing desire for a more detailed color atlas of the ocular fundus.

The present book, which is quite different from the previous atlases mentioned, should satisfy this need.

The first part, the Manual, contains a description of the various diseases of the fundus illustrated in the second part. It includes discussions of diagnoses and differential diagnoses, and is accompanied by references mainly chosen from the recent literature, enabling the reader to explore the different subjects in greater detail. This part of the book is printed on mat paper to prevent the inconvenient reflex which is produced by coated art paper.

The second part, the Color Atlas, contains not only typical pictures of the most common fundus changes in ocular and systemic diseases, but also includes various rare fundus lesions, different stages of the diseases in the same and different patients, and details of variant fundus diseases, information valuable in diagnosis and differential diagnosis. It also contains several montage photographs which illustrate more completely the fundus lesions.

The pictures are placed on the right-hand pages and accompanied by descriptive text and clinical notes on the corresponding left-hand pages.

The Atlas is intended especially for ophthalmologists and residents in ophthalmology, but should also give other clinicians—internists, neurologists, neurosurgeons, doctors in general practice, students, etc., who wish to perform an ophthalmoscopy themselves or interpret the observations of the ophthalmologist— the possibility of studying these changes by means of fundus photographs in color. For technical reasons, the second part of the book is printed on heavy coated art paper.

All photographs were taken by the author with a Zeiss Fundus Camera or a Nikon Hand Fundus Camera on Agfacolor Reversal Film CT 18 or Kodachrome II Daylight Film K 135. The pictures are reproduced from color copies as near as possible to the original diapositives. The montage photographs are enlarged 1.75 times and the other photographs 2.5 times.

In addition to the ordinary objectives with which 30° of the fundus can be photographed, a special objective was used in connection with the Zeiss Fundus Camera, permitting only 15° of the fundus to be photographed. In the text, the term "15°" refers to pictures taken with this special objective.

The pictures are a selection of fundus photographs from in-patients and out-patients at the Steno Memorial Hospital (Niels Steensens Hospital, Gentofte, Denmark), the Eye Clinic and Eye Department, Copenhagen University Hospital (Rigshospitalet), the Eye Clinic and Eye Department, Copenhagen Municipal Hospital (Kommunehospitalet), the Eye Department, Copenhagen County Hospital (Amtssygehuset, Gentofte, Denmark) and my own private practice, during the period 1957—1968.

Histopathological examination of the enucleated eyes was made by S. Ry Andersen, M.D., Ophthalmic Pathology Laboratory, Rigshospitalet, Copenhagen.

I am very grateful to Holger Ehlers, M.D., Professor and Chairman, Department of Ophthalmology, Copenhagen University Hospital, for his encouragement and never-failing interest during the preparation of this Manual and Atlas.

I am also indebted to H. C. Hagedorn, M.D., Jac. E. Poulsen, M.D., Professor P. Brændstrup, M.D., and Victor Larsen, M.D., Heads of the various departments mentioned, for giving me the opportunity to publish these cases, and to all my colleagues who referred their patients to the above mentioned clinics for further study and fundus photography.

Last but not least, I am grateful to all those patients who made this extensive study possible.

My thanks are also due to Messrs. Jacobsen Brothers, who made the color copies and the montage pictures, to Messrs. Rotogravure Ltd., Blockmakers, and to Messrs. C. Hamburger, Printers, for their excellent cooperation. To Messrs. Munksgaard Ltd., Publishers, I would like to express my deep indebtedness for giving me the opportunity to publish this Manual and Atlas in its present form.

Copenhagen, May 1969.

HANS-WALTHER LARSEN

CONTENTS

MANUAL

OF THE

OCULAR FUNDUS

The Normal Fundus
(Figures 1—11)

The appearance of the normal fundus varies within wide limits.

The optic disc is the most obvious feature in the ophthalmoscopic view of the fundus. It measures about 1.5 mm in diameter and corresponds in position with the entrance of the optic nerve into the bulb. It is seen as a pale, round or oval, well-defined structure, with a pink or yellowish-red tint, which contrasts notably with the color of the fundus.

The central retinal artery and vein normally appear close to each other at the nasal side of the center of the optic disc. Within the disc margin, they usually divide into a large superior and inferior branch and soon after into temporal and nasal branches. The four principal divisions supply the four quadrants of the fundus and take a slightly sinuous course as they proceed into their respective quadrants, dividing dichotomously into innumerable branches (Fig. 1). In addition to these main divisions, one or more small nasal arteries are often seen to run from the nasal side of the optic disc into the retina, and one or two small macular arteries may run temporally towards the macula (Figs. 1 and 3). In the macular area, there is a capillary-free zone of about 0.5 mm corresponding to the fovea centralis (Figs. 1—2 and 4—8).

The arteries appear lighter red and narrower than the dark-red or purplish veins, and normally the arteriovenous ratio is about 2:3. The retinal vessels have a continuous yellow-white axial light re-flex, and the arterial reflex is more brilliant than the venous reflex (Fig. 1).

The macula is situated about two disc diameters temporal to and slightly below the optic disc (Figs. 1—2 and 4—8). It is a horizontally oval area about the same size as the disc, appearing slightly deeper red or darker in color than the adjacent fundus and surrounded by an annular light reflex (Figs. 2, 4, 5, 7). At the center of the macula, there is a small depression, the fovea, indicated by a deep-red or red-brown color and a small brilliant reflex, the foveal reflex (Fig. 2).

As the light from the ophthalmoscope is moved, shimmering reflexes frequently become apparent. The fundus reflexes are most prominent in children and young individuals (Figs. 2 and 7) and show a gradual decrease as age advances (Fig. 6).

The color of the fundus varies considerably, depending on the amount and distribution of pigment in the individual retina and choroid.

In lightly pigmented subjects the fundus assumes an orange-red color and sometimes the choroidal vessels are seen plainly (Fig. 3). In medium pigmented subjects the color is more red (Figs. 1—2), while in heavily pigmented subjects it is dark-red (Figs. 8—9), red-brown (Fig. 4) or even brownish-green (Figs. 5—7). If the choroidal pigmentation is heavier than the retinal pigmentation, it may give rise to the appearance of a tessellated or tigroid fundus (Figs. 8—9).

In very lightly pigmented subjects with
extensive exposure of the choroidal vessels (Fig. 11), the ophthalmoscopic appearance may resemble that in albinism,
but in the former condition, pseudoalbinism, the macula and fovea remain
normal (Fig. 10) in contrast to true albinism (Fig. 12).

The retinal and partly also the choroidal blood circulation can be visualized
by fluorescein angiography.

After injection of a solution of sodium
fluorescein into the cubital vein, the dye
normally appears in the retinal arteries
after 10 to 15 seconds. The arterial phase
is followed by arteriovenous and venous
phases. Normally the retinal vessels show
no leakage of dye, and fluorescein has
left the retinal circulation after 40—60
seconds.

In the choroidal vascular system and
cilioretinal arteries, fluorescein shows up
shortly before or simultaneously with the
early retinal arterial phase. Normally,
the dye has disappeared from the choroidal vascular system in the retinal venous phase, while some fluorescence
usually persists from the choroidal tissue
for about 10 minutes.

In pathological conditions, fluorescein
angiography may reveal changes in the
retinal blood circulation, demonstrate
leakage of dye from the vessels or may
show characteristic fluorescein patterns,
some of which may be of value in the
differential diagnosis of various fundus
diseases.

REFERENCES:
Ballantyne, A. J. & I. C. Michaelson: Textbook
    of the fundus of the eye. Livingstone, Edin-
    burgh. 31, 1962.
Duke-Elder, S. & K. C. Wybar: System of oph-
    thalmology. *Vol. II.* Kimpton, London. 223,
    286, 363, 1961.
Rutnin, U. & C. L. Schepens: Fundus appear-
    ance in normal eyes. II. The standard peri-
    pheral fundus and developmental variations.
    Amer. J. Ophthal. *64:* 840—852, 1967.
Shikano, S. & K. Shimizu: Atlas of fluorescence
    fundus angiography. Saunders, Philadelphia.
    11, 1968.
Wessing, A.: Fluoreszenzangiographie der Re-
    tina. Lehrbuch und Atlas. Thieme, Stuttgart.
    31, 1968.

Albinism
(Figures 12—13)

Albinism is a congenital and hereditary defect, due to an inhibition of pigment development. It may involve all pigmented structures including the hair, skin or eyes, but this is rare. More often the condition is incomplete, showing a deficiency of pigment in various structures or involving the eyes alone. In the last condition, called ocular albinism, the rest of the body is normally or lightly pigmented.

General albinism is inherited as an autosomal, recessive trait, while ocular albinism is usually sex-linked, affecting the males through female carriers.

Albinism is frequently accompanied by photophobia, nystagmus, amblyopia and considerable errors of refraction. The irides are pink-gray and translucent and the pupil is red.

OPHTHALMOSCOPICALLY, the fundus is orange-yellow (Fig. 13) and the macular area has a pink tint (Fig. 12). The foveal and macular reflexes are absent (Fig. 12). The choroidal vessels are seen plainly. The retinal vessels and the disc are normal (Fig. 13).

The condition is very characteristic and should not be confused with pseudoalbinism.

HISTOPATHOLOGICALLY, the retina and the choroid show no or only small amounts of pigment, and a real fovea is often lacking.

REFERENCES:
Duke-Elder, S.: System of ophthalmology. *Vol. III.* Kimpton, London. 803, 1964.
Falls, H. F.: Albinism. Trans. Amer. Acad. Ophthal. Otolaryng. *57:* 324—331, 1953.
Krill, A. E. & G. B. Lee: The electroretinogram in albinos and carriers of the ocular albino trait. A.M.A. Arch. Ophthal. *69:* 32—38, 1963.
Norn, M. S.: Ocular albinism. Incidence and occupational prognosis. Acta ophthal. (Kbh.). *44:* 20—24, 1966.
Scialfa, A.: Albinisme oculaire et dyschromatopsie. Arch. Ophtal. (Paris). *27:* 483—494, 1967.

Carriers of Albinism
(Figures 14—15)

In ocular albinism, which is usually sex-linked, female carriers frequently show characteristic morphological fundus changes. However, visual disturbances are not present.

OPHTHALMOSCOPICALLY, the fundus periphery shows coarse pigmentation and depigmentation (Figs. 14—15), in some places assuming a salt-and-pepper appearance. The pigmentation diminishes in the macular direction. The disc and the retinal vessels are normal.

REFERENCES:

Falls, H. F.: Sex-linked ocular albinism displaying typical fundus changes in the female heterozygote. Amer. J. Ophthal. *34* (May Pt. II): 41—50, 1951.

François, J. & J. P. Deweer: Albinisme oculaire lié ou sexe et altérations caractéristiques du fond d'oeil chez les femmes hétérozygotes. Ophthalmologica. *126:* 209—221, 1953.

Ohrt, V.: Ocular albinism with changes typical of carriers. Brit. J. Ophthal. *40:* 721—729, 1956.

Medullated Nerve Fibers
(Figures 16—21)

The normal centrifugal myelinization of the optic nerve fibers usually stops at the lamina cribrosa. Sometimes, however, myelinization continues into the retina for a variable distance. Medullated nerve fibers are never present at birth, but may develop during the first few months of postnatal life. Once developed, the medullated nerve fibers remain unchanged throughout life, except in cases where an atrophic process of the optic nerve supervenes, in which case they gradually disappear.

Vision is seldom affected in this condition unless the macula is involved. However, macular involvement is rare. There is usually a scotoma which is slightly smaller than the corresponding opaque area in the fundus.

The condition is rather common. It is usually unilateral, but may occur bilaterally.

OPHTHALMOSCOPICALLY, medullated nerve fibers are seen as whitish, brilliant-white or yellowish-white, opaque, silky patches with a finely striated surface and a feathered margin (Figs. 16—19). Most frequently, the patches are tongue-shaped or flame-shaped and situated at the upper or lower margin of the disc (Fig. 16), but size and shape vary widely (Figs. 16, 18—21). Occasionally, the medullated fibers surround the disc (Figs. 18 and 20) or the macular area (Fig. 19). Rarely, they involve the macular area (Fig. 21) or lie as isolated patches in the fundus periphery (Fig. 17). The retinal vessels are partly or completely obscured by the medullated fibers in the opaque area.

The ophthalmoscopic picture of medullated nerve fibers is very characteristic, and should not be confused with woolly exudates, acute juxtapapillary choroiditis, optic atrophy or retinal branch artery occlusion.

HISTOPATHOLOGICALLY, myelinated nerve fibers are found corresponding to the opaque patches.

REFERENCES:
Bonamour, G., M. Bonnet, P. Brégeat & P. Juge: La papille optique. Masson, Paris. 104, 1968.
Duke-Elder, S.: System of ophthalmology. *Vol. III.* Kimpton, London. 646, 1964.
Lorentzen, S. E.: Incidences of medullated nerve fibres in retina and of epipapillary membrane. Acta ophthal. (Kbh.). *41:* 279—284, 1963.

Pits in the Optic Disc

(Figures 22—23 and 377)

Pits or holes in the optic disc are not uncommon. The condition is generally considered to be a minimal, atypical coloboma and the defect is usually unilateral.

Pits in the optic disc are frequently present in cases of central serous retinopathy (Fig. 377).

The anomaly usually causes no visual disturbances, but if the papillomacular bundle is involved, central vision may be gravely affected. The visual field usually shows enlargement of the blind spot or sector-shaped defects, sometimes producing a partial or complete paracentral or central scotoma.

Ophthalmoscopically, the pit is usually seen as a small vertically oval, sharply defined depression at the temporal side of the disc (Figs. 22—23). The base of the pit may be seen clearly or may be covered by grayish-white tissue. Some pigment accumulation may also be present.

Histopathologically, the lamina cribrosa is defective, corresponding to the pit, and the defective area is partially filled with glial tissue.

References:

Andersen, O. C.: Grubenbildungen auf der Papille mit Gesichtsfeldausfällen. Klin. Monatsbl. Augenh. *122:* 159—168, 1953.

Bonamour, G., M. Bonnet, P. Brégeat & P. Juge: La papille optique. Masson, Paris. 89, 1968.

Farpour, H. & J. Babel: Les fossettes papillaires; Diagnostic différentiel, anomalies vasculaires et cas limites. Ann. Oculist. (Paris). *201:* 1—17, 1968.

Kranenburg, E. W.: Crater-like holes in the optic disc and central serous retinopathy. A.M.A. Arch. Ophthal. *64:* 912—924, 1960.

Sugar, H. S.: Congenital pits in the optic disc. Amer. J. Ophthal. *63:* 298—307, 1967.

Colobomas of the Fundus
(Figures 24—27)

Colobomas may involve the eyelid, iris, ciliary body, lens, choroid, retina, and the optic nerve head. Typical bulbar colobomas are the result of imperfect closure of the fetal ocular cleft. They may be complete, involving all the bulbar structures associated with the embryonic cleft, or partial, when the defect is less extensive. Typical colobomas are situated in the lower nasal region of the eye, atypical elsewhere. Typical colobomas are often bilateral, while atypical are usually unilateral.

Central vision is frequently reduced, although the macula may appear normal ophthalmoscopically. In the visual field there is a scotoma corresponding to the coloboma, although usually smaller than the defective area. Strabismus and nystagmus are common in this condition.

OPHTHALMOSCOPICALLY, a fundus coloboma is seen as a sharply defined, whitish or grayish-white area of variable extension, and usually situated below the disc (Figs. 26—27).

It is frequently bridged by a few retinal and some choroidal vessels (Fig. 26) and bordered by some pigment deposits (Figs. 25—27). In the colobomatous area the sclera may appear ectatic (Fig. 27). Colobomas are usually single, but several colobomas may be present in the same fundus. The defect may also involve the disc (Fig. 24). In these cases, the disc is seen as a shallow or deep grayish-white cavity, and the cavity is filled with varying amounts of whitish glial tissue.

Fundus colobomas, even the small ones, are very typical and should not be confused with chorioretinal scars, which sometimes may assume an appearance resembling small isolated colobomas.

HISTOPATHOLOGICALLY, typical fundal colobomas are characterized by localized defects in the retina and choroid. The defective retina may be represented by a thin membrane containing scattered retinal elements and the choroid by some mesodermal remnants, while Bruch's membrane is absent. The sclera is often abnormally thin and somewhat ectatic. If the optic disc is involved, the coloboma may be represented by a mass of poorly developed glial and neural tissue at the disc.

REFERENCES:

Bonamour, G., M. Bonnet, P. Brégeat & P. Juge: La papille optique. Masson, Paris. 95, 1968.

Duke-Elder, S.: System of ophthalmology. *Vol. III*. Kimpton, London. 465, 1964.

Klien, B. A.: The pathogenesis of some atypical colobomas of the choroid. Amer. J. Ophthal. *48 (1)*: 597—607, 1959.

Congenital Macular Cyst
(Figures 28—29)

A congenital macular cyst is a rare condition, but constitutes a well-defined clinical entity. It may occur sporadically, affecting one or both eyes, or be transmitted hereditarily. In the latter case, the condition is possibly identical with the infantile type of heredomacular degeneration (Best's type).

In early stages vision is only slightly affected, and much less than should be expected from the fundal lesion. During middle age, however, visual disturbances usually develop and eventually central vision is lost.

OPHTHALMOSCOPICALLY, the congenital macular cyst, also named vitelliform macular cyst, is seen as a pale, rounded, slightly elevated patch in the macular area (Figs. 28 and 29). The evolution of the lesion is exceedingly slow. Finally, however, the lesion is converted into an atrophic scar with or without pigmentation.

REFERENCES:

Biró, J.: Die Umbildung der zentralen Netzhaut-degenerationen und die "Cysta vitelliformis". Klin. Monatsbl. Augenh. *153:* 363—370, 1968.

Braley, A. E. & B. E. Spivey: Hereditary vitelline macular degeneration (possibly of vitelliform origin): A clinical and functional evaluation of a new pedigree with variable expressivity and dominant inheritance. Trans. Amer. ophthal. Soc. *61:* 339—371, 1963.

François, J.: Vitelliform degeneration of the macula. Bull. N.Y. Acad. Med. *44:* 18—27, 1968.

Krill, A. E., P. A. Morse, A. M. Potts & B. A. Klien: Hereditary vitelliruptive macular degeneration. Amer. J. Ophthal. *61:* 1405—1415, 1966.

Remky, H., J. Rix & K. F. Klier: Dominant-autosomale Maculadegeneration (Best, Sorsby) mit zystischen und vitelliformen Stadien (Huysmans, Zanen). Klin. Monatsbl. Augenh. *146:* 473—497, 1965.

Epipapillary Membrane and Bergmeister's Papilla
(Figures 30—31)

Throughout the greater part of embryonic life the hyaloid artery and some of the major retinal vessels are sheathed by cells originating from the primitive epithelial papilla of Bergmeister. Shortly before birth, the hyaloid artery and its sheaths atrophy.

Sometimes, however, remnants of the sheath may remain on the disc, either sheathing the retinal vessels for a short distance (Fig. 30) or persisting as a well-defined membrane or web of opaque tissue, the epipapillary membrane, stretching over the optic disc (Fig. 30) or even presenting a more solid, prominent mass of tissue in front of the disc (Fig. 31), known as Bergmeister's papilla. This mass, which may be very prominent at birth and during infancy, often projects several diopters into the vitreous, and frequently has a tendency to reduce in size while the child is growing up.

In the differential diagnosis persistent primary vitreous, retinoblastoma and angiomatosis of the retina have to be considered.

REFERENCES:

Bonamour, G., M. Bonnet, P. Brégeat & P. Juge: La papille optique. Masson, Paris. 102, 1968.

Lorentzen, S. E.: Incidences of medullated nerve fibres in retina and of epipapillary membrane. Acta ophthal. (Kbh.). *41:* 279—284, 1963.

Petersen, H. P.: Persistence of the Bergmeister papilla with glial overgrowth. Acta ophthal. (Kbh.). *46:* 430—440, 1968.

Persistent Hyperplastic Primary Vitreous
(Figures 32—36)

Persistent hyperplastic primary vitreous is rare. It is usually characterized by a hyperplastic membrane covering a smaller or larger part of the posterior surface of the lens, but at times the preretinal changes may be more obvious than those behind the lens. In these cases, prepapillary (Figs. 32—33) or preretinal veils or masses of whitish tissue (Figs. 34—35) are present together with remnants of the hyaloid artery (Fig. 36).

The condition may also be related to congenital retinal detachment with falciform retinal folds.

REFERENCES:

François, J. & E. de Vos: Persistance du vitré primaire. Bull. Soc. Belge Ophtal. *122:* 457—474, 1959.

Jensen, O. A.: Persistent hyperplastic primary vitreous. Cases in Denmark 1942—1966. A mainly histopathological study. Acta ophthal. (Kbh.). *46:* 418—429, 1968.

Olsen, J. & P. M. Møller: Persistent primary hyperplastic vitreous. Acta ophthal. (Kbh.). *46:* 413—417, 1968.

Reese, A. B.: Persistent hyperplastic primary vitreous. Amer. J. Ophthal. *40:* 317—331, 1955.

Retrolental Fibroplasia
(Figures 37—39)

Retrolental fibroplasia is a condition occurring especially in premature infants, but it may also occur, although rarely, in full-term children.

The condition is usually seen in premature infants who have been placed in a highly oxygenated incubator or who have received oxygen in high concentration by other methods.

The condition becomes evident ophthalmoscopically usually five to ten weeks after removal from the high oxygen level, and is nearly always bilateral.

In cases of retrolental fibroplasia, vision is almost invariably decreased and blindness often occurs in the cicatricial phase. In addition to the ocular symptoms, neurological symptoms and mental retardation occur in a high percentage of cases.

OPHTHALMOSCOPIC APPEARANCE: When the premature infant with his immature retinal vascular system is exposed to a high oxygen level, the retinal vessels and especially the arteries become narrowed or even obliterated. When the infant is later exposed to a normal oxygen level which means that the retina is now suffering from relative anoxia, the retinal vessels may react with venous fullness (Fig. 39) and later with a disorganized new vessel formation, especially in the fundus periphery. Together with this new vessel formation, a certain amount of fibrous tissue is developed. If not too extensive, these fibrous formations may remain as isolated patches, but the fibrous

tissue formation usually continues, leading to traction in the retina within the first year of life. This causes retinal detachment (Figs. 37—39) and eventually the formation of a retrolental fibrous membrane, resulting in microphthalmos or phthisis of the globe.

In the differential diagnosis, retinoblastoma and congenital malformations of the eye have to be considered. At a late stage congenital falciform detachment is often impossible to distinguish from a not fully developed retrolental fibroplasia.

HISTOPATHOLOGICALLY, the condition is characterized by the formation of newformed vessels, which at the early stage are limited to the retinal surface, but later are present together with fibrous tissue formation in the vitreous. Later still, the condition shows detachment of the retina due to traction and eventually the formation of a dense sheath of retrolental fibrous tissue, producing a retrolental membrane.

REFERENCES:

Cohen, J., J. E. Alfano, L. D. Boshes & C. Palmgren: Clinical evaluation of school-age children with retrolental fibroplasia. Amer. J. Ophthal. 57: 41—57, 1964.

Holtermann, W. & M. Schmidt: Die retrolentale Fibroplasie. Klin. Monatsbl. Augenh. 144: 704—710, 1964.

Patz, A.: New role of the ophthalmologist in prevention of retrolental fibroplasia. A.M.A. Arch. Ophthal. 78: 565—568, 1967.

Reese, A. B. & F. C. Blodi: Retrolental fibroplasia. Amer. J. Ophthal. 34: 1—24, 1951.

Seedorff, H. H. & H. Andersen: Oxygen problems in incubator-treated prematures. Acta ophthal. (Kbh.). *46:* 506—512, 1968.

Seedorff, T.: Retrolental fibroplasia. Incidence of irreversible cases. Role of oxygen. Diagnosis. Extraocular diseases. Acta ophthal. (Kbh.). *46:* 500—505, 1968.

Tassman, W. & W. Annesley: Retinal detachment in the retinopathy of prematurity. A.M.A. Arch. Ophthal. *75:* 608—614, 1966.

Falciform Retinal Detachment

(Figures 40—41)

Falciform retinal detachment is frequently bilateral, and is typically associated with the persistance of remnants of the hyaloid artery. In most cases the condition is due to developmental arrest, but in some cases it must be regarded as an abortive form of retrolental fibroplasia.

Visual acuity may be reduced or even damaged severely as the process usually occurs in the lower temporal quadrant and may show some extension into the macular area.

OPHTHALMOSCOPICALLY, the falciform detachment is usually seen as a broad retinal fold extending from the disc into the far fundus periphery (Figs. 40—41), but folds may also commence elsewhere in the fundus. In most cases the fundus appears quite normal apart from the retinal fold (Fig. 41), but sometimes the retina appears very thin or absent, giving the impression of looking straight into the choroid (Fig. 40). In these cases, only few retinal vessels may be encountered. Remnants of the hyaloid artery are usually present, and the condition is usually stationary.

HISTOPATHOLOGICALLY, the retina is pulled inwards and the whole retina may show some dysplasia, suggesting a disturbance of growth of the inner layer of the optic cup. Retinal rosettes may be present, but the retinal pigment epithelium is unaffected.

REFERENCES:

Badtke, G.: Über seltene Duplikaturenbildungen in der embryonalen Netzhaut. Graefes Arch. Ophth. *155:* 266—283, 1954.

Badtke, G.: Zur Frage des entwicklungsphysiologischen Zusammenhangs zwischen der Ablatio falciformis congenita und pathologischen Entwicklungsschritten der Netzhaut im Bereich der embryonalen Augenbecherspalte, insbesondere den typischen Funduskolobomen. Klin. Monatsbl. Augenh. *136:* 806—815, 1960.

Thiel, H.-J.: Beitrag zur Klinik und Genese der Ablatio falciformis congenita. Klin. Monatsbl. Augenh. *152:* 46—50, 1968.

Fundus Changes in Myopia
(Figures 42—53)

Clinically, cases of myopia may be divided into two groups, simple myopia and excessive or malignant myopia.

Simple myopia is a physiological variation in refraction, usually appearing in children of school-age. When demonstrated it seldom exceeds a few diopters. Although the myopia may increase half a diopter or more annually over a period of years, progression always stops at adolescence, and good vision is maintained with suitable correction throughout life.

The fundus may be normal, tessellated or show a myopic crescent at the temporal side of the disc, or it may be lightly pigmented, or even pseudoalbinotic.

OPHTHALMOSCOPICALLY, early cases of simple myopia may show no fundus changes, but later myopic crescent or conus formation usually becomes apparent as a whitish crescent outside the scleral ring at the temporal side of the disc (Figs. 43—45). The crescent is frequently bordered temporally by some pigment. The fundus color is frequently uniform, but tessellation or lightly pigmented areas may occur (Fig. 42), except in the macular area, and the retinal vessels appear normal.

Excessive or malignant myopia occurs at all ages and may be present even at birth. In this condition there is usually progressive elongation of the posterior segment of the eye, excessive increase in the myopia and a development of degenerative changes in the fundus. Visual acuity is reduced in spite of correction of the error of refraction.

The fundus changes include myopic crescent, disseminated choroidal atrophies, macular degeneration and cystoid degeneration in the fundus periphery, and the changes may occur singly or together.

OPHTHALMOSCOPICALLY, excessive or malignant myopia almost always shows a myopic crescent of varying size (Fig. 45) or more extensive peripapillary atrophy (Figs. 46—47). The fundus color may vary widely, ranging from the normal red color (Figs. 48—50) to an orange color (Fig. 53). The latter is seen in quasi-albinotic cases where the choroidal vessels are seen plainly and the choroidal intervascular spaces appear enlarged. The retinal vessels appear slightly narrower than in the normal fundus.

In the course of time, disseminated choroidal atrophies may occur (Figs. 51—52). They are seen as sharply defined, more or less confluent white or yellowish-white patches of variable size and shape, often accompanied by some irregular, patchy pigmentation.

At times, macular changes develop. They often start quite suddenly with subretinal or deep retinal hemorrhages (Figs. 48—50) accompanied by some macular edema. The hemorrhages and the edema are absorbed slowly and may ultimately be replaced by organized exudate, an atrophic chorioretinal scar (Fig. 52) or a mass of nearly black pigment (Fig. 51). The latter is known as Fuchs' spot.

In the fundus periphery, besides small pigmented spots and depigmented patches, cystoid degeneration often appears in girdles which run concentrically or lie in irregular nests. The cystoid degeneration gives the fundus periphery a fine, honeycombed appearance. In time, the cystic spaces enlarge. Vitreous adhesions, together with increased mobility of the vitreous due to liquefaction and perhaps trauma, may convert the cystic spaces into holes; in some cases this may be a factor in the development of retinal detachment.

HISTOPATHOLOGICALLY, a myopic crescent is formed at the temporal side of the disc by the lack of retinal pigment epithelium, Bruch's membrane and choroid, the latter defect being usually the smallest. The myopic atrophy in the fundus is characterized by changes in the choroid and the retina. The choroid is thinned, stroma pigment is reduced and the choroidal vessels diminished in number, especially in the choriocapillaris, which is atrophic. The elastic part of Bruch's membrane is thinned and holes develop. The retina shows varying degrees of atrophy and cystoid degeneration.

REFERENCES:
Blatt, N.: Augenhintergrundveränderungen bei hochgradiger Myopie. Klin. Monatsbl. Augenh. *146:* 391—411, 1965.
Busacca, A., H. Goldmann & S. Schiff-Wertheimer: Biomicroscopie du corps vitré et du fond de l'oeil. Masson, Paris. 357, 1957.
Franceschetti, A., J. François & J. Babel: Les hérédo-dégénérescences chorio-rétiniennes. Masson, Paris. 677, 1963.
Goldschmidt, E.: On the etiology of myopia. An epidemiological study. Acta ophthal. (Kbh.). *Suppl. 98,* 1968.
Sachsenweger, R.: Pathologie und Klinik der Refraktionsanomalien. In Velhagen, K. (Ed.): Der Augenarzt. *Band II.* Thieme, Leipzig. 259—298, 1959.
Weigelin, E., A. Apollonio, W. Marx & A. Pilke: Zum Verlauf der hochgradigen Myopie. Statistische Untersuchungen. Adv. ophthal. *16:* 1—62, 1965.

The Optic Disc

Physiological Variations and Congenital Abnormalities.
(Figures 54—78)

The optic disc is the most obvious feature in the ophthalmoscopic view of the fundus. It measures about 1.5 mm in diameter and corresponds in position with the entrance of the optic nerve into the bulb.

OPHTHALMOSCOPICALLY, the optic disc is seen as a pale, well-defined, round (Fig. 54) or vertically slightly oval disc (Figs. 55—59) with a pink or yellowish-red tint which contrasts notably with the color of the fundus. The nasal part of the disc is often slightly redder than the temporal part (Fig. 54). The retinal vessels usually make their appearance at the nasal side of the center of the optic disc. At the temporal side of the entering vessels, the disc usually shows a central depression. This physiological excavation may be shallow (Fig. 58) or deep (Fig. 59), small (Figs. 54—55) or large (Fig. 60), but it never occupies the full extent of the optic disc. The central excavation is lighter than the surrounding part of the disc, and when deep, the lamina cribrosa may be visible in its base. Although the optic disc usually measures about 1.5 mm in diameter, it may show wide variations from very small (Figs. 61—62) to very large (Figs. 63—64). In old people, a large disc may be simulated by the occurrence of massive peripapillary atrophy (senile peripapillary atrophy) (Fig. 65).

The optic disc is frequently bordered by two more or less complete rings. The outer, the choroidal ring, is pigmented (Figs. 67—69) and the inner, the scleral ring, is whitish (Figs. 60, 70—71).

In rare instances, the disc may assume a grayish-red color due to pigment accumulation on the disc (Fig. 66), or it may even appear slate-gray or nearly black (papilla grisea).

Conus formation is a rather common occurrence, especially in myopic eyes. The condition may be divided into temporal conus, which is the most frequent, nasal conus and inferior conus.

Temporal conus or crescent is seen as a whitish crescent outside the scleral ring at the temporal side of the disc, and is most often found in association with myopia (Figs. 43—45).

Nasal conus or crescent is seen as a whitish crescent at the nasal side of the disc (Figs. 72—74) and the condition is often accompanied by some deformity of the disc. The disc is often slightly elevated temporally and shallowed nasally. The retinal vessels emerge from the temporal side of the disc, at first running nasally and then bending sharply when passing into the retina. This condition is often associated with myopia and a notable degree of astigmatism.

Inferior conus or crescent is a whitish

crescent situated just below the disc (Figs. 75—77) and often accompanied by some deformity of the disc. It is most often seen in myopic eyes and especially in those exhibiting a notable degree of astigmatism. Inferior conus is considered to be a developmental defect, a kind of incomplete coloboma.

In rare instances, the physiological optic cup and the whole surface of the disc may be covered by a delicate web of glial tissue (Fig. 78), which may give the disc an appearance of swelling, but just as in pseudopapilledema, venous engorgement, hemorrhages and exudates are never present.

The condition Membrana epipapillaris and Bergmeister's papilla are discussed elsewhere.

REFERENCES:

Aichmair, H.: Ein Knabe mit Hypoplasie der rechten Papille. Klin. Monatsbl. Augenh. *153:* 523—526, 1968.

Bonamour, G., M. Bonnet, P. Brégeat & P. Juge: La papille optique. Masson, Paris. 57, 76, 83, 1968.

Duke-Elder, S.: System of ophthalmology. *Vol. III.* Kimpton, London. 668, 1964.

Smith, H. E.: Aplasia of the optic nerve. Amer. J. Ophthal. *37:* 498—504, 1954.

Somerville, F.: Uniocular aplasia of the optic nerve. Brit. J. Ophthal. *46:* 51—55, 1962.

Streiff, B.: Über Megalopapille. Klin. Monatsbl. Augenh. *139:* 824—827, 1961.

Pseudopapilledema
(Figures 79—83)

Pseudopapilledema or pseudoneuritis is a rare congenital variation most often observed in small, hypermetropic eyes or in eyes with hypermetropic astigmatism.

The condition is stationary and visual disturbances are seldom present.

OPHTHALMOSCOPICALLY, it is characterized by swelling of the disc, which is slightly reddened, the margin having a blurred appearance and the disc projecting forward, but seldom more than a few diopters (Fig. 79). The retinal vessels are of normal caliber. Venous engorgement, hemorrhages and exudates are never present. The condition is sometimes associated with drusen of the optic disc, which will be discussed separately (Figs. 80—83).

The condition is of importance as it may be confused with papilledema. In the differential diagnosis, fluorescein angiography may be of value. In papilledema, there is usually a leakage of dye from the disc. In pseudopapilledema the angiogram is always normal. In the earliest stages of papilledema, however, the angiogram may also be normal. Normal fluorescein angiography therefore does not exclude papilledema, and repeated angiography may be necessary to exclude papilledema. The conditions can also be differentiated by observation over a period of the non-progressive nature and absence of vascular changes in pseudopapilledema.

REFERENCES:

Hoyt, W. F. & D. Beeston: The ocular fundus in neurologic disease. Mosby, St. Louis. 26, 1966.

Hoyt, W. F. & M. E. Pont: Pseudopapilledema: Anomalous elevation of optic disk. J.A.M.A. *181:* 191—196, 1962.

Jütte, A. & L. Lemke: Intravitalfärbung am Augenhintergrund mit Fluoreszein-Natrium. Klin. Monatsbl. Augenh. *Suppl. 49:* 57, 1968.

Marquart, G.: Pseudostauungspapille. Klin. Monatsbl. Augenh. *127:* 546—558, 1955.

Miller, S. J. H., M. D. Sanders & T. J. Ffytche: Fluorescein fundus photography in the detection of early papilloedema and its differentiation from pseudo-papilloedema. Lancet. *2:* 651—654, 1965.

Drusen of the Optic Disc
(Figures 80—83)

Drusen of the optic disc is a rare hereditary condition inherited as an irregular dominant trait and unrelated to colloid bodies in Bruch's membrane. Drusen of the optic disc may be observed at any age and the condition is frequently bilateral.

There are usually no or only slight visual disturbances, but the blind spot may be enlarged, and sectorial or irregular scotomas may result from nerve fiber degeneration. In rare instances, the visual field shows a concentric constriction.

OPHTHALMOSCOPICALLY, drusen of the optic disc are seen as small white or yellowish-white, glistening, spherical or grain-like depositis, situated superficially (Figs. 80—81) or deeply (Figs. 82—83) in the optic disc tissue. They often lie in groups either at the periphery of the disc or centrally. The disc margin is more or less blurred and the disc often shows an apparent increase in size, especially if the drusen are situated deep in the optic nerve head. They may also cause prominence of the optic disc and mimic papilledema.

In cases with blurred margins and elevation of the optic disc, the condition has to be distinguished from papilledema and papillitis. Occasionally, the condition may mimic an optic atrophy.

In the differential diagnosis, fluorescein angiography is valuable because drusen of the optic disc often show a characteristic fluorescein pattern.

HISTOPATHOLOGICALLY, drusen of the optic disc are seen as laminated, homogeneous, acellular masses, usually containing calcareous concretions and situated within the substance of the optic disc.

REFERENCES:
Bonamour, G., M. Bonnet, P. Brégeat & P. Juge: La papille optique. Masson, Paris. 485, 1968.
Lorentzen, S. E.: Drusen of the optic disk, An irregularly dominant hereditary affection. Acta ophthal. (Kbh.). *39:* 626—643, 1961.
Lorentzen, S. E.: Drusen of the optic disk. A clinical and genetic study. Acta ophthal. (Kbh.). *Suppl. 90,* 1966.
Marquart, G.: Pseudostauungspapille. Klin. Monatsbl. Augenh. *127:* 546—558, 1955.
Petersen, H. P.: Colloid bodies with defects in the field of vision. Acta ophthal. (Kbh.). *35:* 243—272, 1957.
Sanders, M. D. & T. J. Ffytche: Fluorescein angiography in the diagnosis of drusen of the disc. Trans. ophthal. Soc. U.K. *87:* 457—468, 1967.
Wessing, A.: Fluoreszenzangiographie der Retina. Lehrbuch und Atlas. Thieme, Stuttgart. 171, 1968.

Papilledema
(Figures 84—102, 136, 185—188, 192 and 222—225)

Papilledema is a non-inflammatory swelling of the optic nerve head or disc. It is an important ophthalmoscopic sign in different intracranial, ocular, neural and orbital conditions, as well as in some systemic diseases.

In the vast majority of cases, papilledema or choked disc is due to brain tumors. Papilledema is more frequently present in subtentorial than supratentorial conditions. Tumors localized to the region of the corpora quadrigemina, pineal body, fourth ventricle and cerebellum often produce papilledema. Pituitary tumors, however, rarely produce papilledema. Occasionally, tumors of the olfactory or frontal lobe, or the sphenoidal ridge may cause optic atrophy on the same side and papilledema on the opposite side (Foster-Kennedy syndrome). Chiasma arachnoiditis may sometimes give rise to a similar ophthalmoscopic picture (Pseudo Foster-Kennedy syndrome—Figs. 102—103).

Papilledema may also be observed in such conditions as brain abcesses, cerebral metastases (Figs. 90—91), meningitis, sinus thrombosis (Fig. 93), intracranial hemorrhage (Fig. 92), hydrocephalus, premature cranial synostosis, cerebral syphilis (Fig. 100) and tuberculosis; in tumors of the optic nerve, in orbital tumors (Fig. 101), cysts and vascular abnormalities; in central retinal venous thrombosis (Figs. 222—225); in congenital heart disease (Fig. 136); in leukemia (Fig. 97), severe anemia, polycythemia, dysproteinemia (Figs. 98—99),

and malignant hypertension (Figs. 96, 185—188, 192).

Papilledema or choked disc usually occurs bilaterally, although the degree of swelling may differ on the two sides. In ocular, orbital and neural conditions, however, papilledema is usually unilateral.

Papilledema usually develops slowly in the course of weeks or months. Occasionally, for example in traumatic intracranial hemorrhage, it may develop in the course of a few hours.

For a long period there may be no symptoms at all or only short attacks of hazy vision or even momentary blindness (obscurations) lasting from to 10 to 30 seconds. At this stage, the blind spot is enlarged, but the vision and the peripheral visual field are intact unless the basic disorder causes field defects.

Long-standing papilledema sooner or later leads to optic atrophy. When atrophy develops, there is progressive contraction of the visual field and reduction of vision even to blindness.

OPHTHALMOSCOPICALLY, the disc in the early stages of papilledema is slightly redder than normal (compare Figs. 84 and 85) owing to a dilatation of the capillaries within the substance of the optic disc. The disc margin is slightly blurred, at first above and below, then nasally and finally temporally. The veins become congested (Fig. 89) and venous pulsation is almost always absent. The small vessels at the disc are dilated and seen more plainly than in the normal disc, and slight edema may fill the normal disc cup (Figs. 86—87).

When papilledema progresses into the fully developed stage, the increasing edema causes swelling and some pallor of the disc (Figs. 88, 90). The disc gradually projects forward from one (Figs. 86—89) to several diopters (Figs. 92, 98, 100), and may sometimes resemble a mushroom. The veins become engorged (Fig. 89), small splinter or flame-shaped hemorrhages and cotton-wool exudates appear at and around the disc (Figs. 91—93, 96, 97), fine light streaks indicating retinal edema radiate from the disc into the surrounding retina (Figs. 86—87), and sometimes a macular star may develop. If the papilledema persists for some months glial proliferation may occur at the disc (Figs. 93—95).

If the basic disorder is removed or disappears, papilledema subsides, leaving no or only slight ophthalmoscopic traces.

In long-standing papilledema and in cases with persistent papilledema, chronic atrophic papilledema with optic atrophy develops. The edema gradually decreases and the disc becomes paler as a result of glial proliferation (Figs. 94—95). Finally, the disc appears grayish-white or white, flat or slightly cupped, the lamina cribrosa obscured by glial tissue, and the disc margin slightly ill-defined (Figs. 106—107, 111). Venous fullness disappears and the arteries become narrow.

The degree of pallor of the disc, however, often does not correspond with the degree of the functional loss.

It is not possible ophthalmoscopically to differentiate papilledema from acute optic neuritis (papillitis). Clinically, the two conditions are distinguished by early loss of vision and presence of a central scotoma in optic neuritis.

Early stages of papilledema have to be distinguished from pseudopapilledema or pseudoneuritis. The distinction is almost impossible in a single ophthalmoscopy so that the patient has to be followed at short intervals. At times, fluorescein angiography may be of value in the differential diagnosis. A normal angiogram, however, does not exclude papilledema, while leakage of dye from the disc is characteristic of papilledema. Ophthalmoscopically, the conditions are differentiated by the continuous lack of venous engorgement, hemorrhages and exudates in pseudopapilledema. In the differential diagnosis, drusen of the optic disc has also to be considered. Papilledema should never be confused with occlusion of the central retinal vein or hypertensive neuroretinopathy.

HISTOPATHOLOGICALLY, papilledema is characterized by edema of the disc and the adjacent retina, swelling of the nerve fibers, engorgement of the veins, and frequently by hemorrhages and exudates.

REFERENCES:
Bonamour, G., M. Bonnet, P. Brégeat & P. Juge. La papille optique. Masson, Paris. 167, 1968.
Brégeat, P.: L'oedème papillaire. Masson, Paris. 1956.
Haining, W. M.: Diagnostic value of intravenous fluorescein studies. Brit. J. Ophthal. 50: 587—591, 1966.
Hayreh, S. S.: Pathogenesis of oedema of the optic disc. Docum. ophthal. 24: 289—411, 1968.
Hogan, M. J. & L. E. Zimmerman (Ed.): Ophthalmic pathology. 2nd ed. Saunders, Philadelphia. 587, 1962.
Hoyt, W. F. & D. Beeston: The ocular fundus in neurologic disease. Mosby, St. Louis. 1966.
Huber, A.: Augensymptome bei Hirntumoren. Huber, Bern. 1956.
Miller, S. J. H., M. D. Sanders & T. J. Ffytche: Fluorescein fundus photography in the detection of early papilloedema and its differentiation from pseudo-papilloedema. Lancet. 2: 651—654, 1965.
Scott, G. I.: Optic disc oedema. Trans. ophthal. Soc. U.K. 87: 733—753, 1967.
Walsh, F. B.: Clinical neuro-ophthalmology.

2nd ed. Williams & Wilkins, Baltimore. 276, 1957.

Wessing, A.: Fluoreszenzangiographie der Retina. Lehrbuch und Atlas. Thieme, Stuttgart. 166, 1968.

Witmer, R.: Differentialdiagnostische Aspekte bei retinalen Gefässstörungen und Papillenoedem. Ophthalmologica. *156:* 313—321, 1968.

Atrophy of the Optic Nerve
(Figures 103—113, 115—125, 301 and 435)

Optic atrophy is an irreversible degeneration of the optic nerve, and can be divided into the following three types: descending, ascending and post-inflammatory atrophy.

Descending optic atrophy is usually referred to as simple or "primary" atrophy, as there is no evidence of fundal disease, preceding papilledema or papillitis, but it also includes conditions such as tabetic (Fig. 435) and hereditary optic atrophy (Figs. 112—113), where the pathogenesis of the atrophy is not entirely clear. Descending or simple atrophy may follow retrobulbar neuritis in multiple sclerosis (Fig. 119), other demyelinating diseases (Fig. 110), intoxications, severe anemia, vascular disease (Figs. 108—109) including giant-cell arteritis, tumors in the optic nerve, tumors or hemorrhages compressing the optic nerve, traumatic lesions of the optic nerve, chiasma arachnoiditis (Fig. 103), and pituitary tumors (Fig. 107) or craniopharyngiomas (Figs. 104—105).

Ascending optic atrophy is secondary to retinal degeneration and inflammation. It occurs in conditions such as retinitis pigmentosa (Fig. 301) and glaucoma (Figs. 120—125, 161).

Post-inflammatory optic atrophy, usually referred to as "secondary" atrophy, may follow papilledema (Figs. 106, 111) or papillitis (Figs. 115—118).

In optic atrophy, vision is diminished and the visual field contracted to a varying degree. The diagnosis of optic atrophy, however, is more dependent on the loss of function than on the color of the disc, as we encounter cases with pallor of the disc in which no functional defect is present, and cases with functional defect but only slight pallor.

OPHTHALMOSCOPICALLY, the disc in descending or simple optic atrophy (Figs. 103, 105, 107—110, 112—113, 435) is sharply defined, pale, whitish or yellowish-white and shows a shallow saucer-shaped cupping. The lamina cribrosa is often seen plainly and without retraction of the base of the disc cup. The retinal vessels are narrow.

Following retrobulbar neuritis, there is usually only temporal sector-formed pallor of the disc (Fig. 119), with or without functional loss.

In ascending optic atrophy (Figs. 120—125, 161, 301), the disc is usually well-defined, pale, waxy-yellow or dirty-pink and slightly cupped, and the retinal vessels are narrow.

In post-inflammatory optic atrophy (Figs. 106, 111, 115—118), the disc is also pale, whitish or yellowish-white, but the margin is slightly irregular and there is no or only slight cupping of the disc, as glial tissue may fill the cup and sometimes continue along the retinal vessels for a short distance. The retinal vessels are narrow and peripapillary atrophy is usually present together with some pigmentation.

However, the ophthalmoscopic appearance of descending, ascending and post-inflammatory optic atrophy is often very similar, and it may be difficult or impossible to distinguish these conditions ophthalmoscopically.

It is, however, of importance to distinguish glaucomatous optic atrophy from other kinds of optic atrophy. Drusen of the optic disc should not be confused with optic atrophy.

HISTOPATHOLOGICALLY, descending, ascending and post-inflammatory optic atrophy are characterized by degeneration of the nerve fibers, glial proliferation and increase of the collagenous tissue in the pial septa.

REFERENCES:

Bettelheim, H.: Beiträge zur Klinik und Diagnostik der Arteriitis cranialis. Klin. Monatsbl. Augenh. *152:* 805—813, 1968.

Bonamour, G., M. Bonnet, P. Brégeat & P. Juge: La papille optique. Masson, Paris. 348, 1968.

Cullen, J. F.: Occult temporal arteritis. A common cause of blindness in old age. Brit. J. Ophthal. *51:* 513—525, 1967.

Hogan M. J. & L. E. Zimmerman (Ed.): Ophthalmic pathology. *2nd ed.* Saunders, Philadelphia. 623, 1962.

Hoyt, W. F. & D. Beeston: The ocular fundus in neurologic disease. Mosby, St. Louis. 1966.

Huber, A.: Augensymptome bei Hirntumoren. Huber, Bern. 1956.

Kjer, P.: Infantile optic atrophy with dominant mode of inheritance. A clinical and genetic study of 19 danish families. Acta ophthal. (Kbh.). *Suppl. 54,* 1959.

O'Day, D., G. Crock, J. E. K. Galbraith, J. M. Parel & A. Wigley: Fluorescein angiography of normal and atrophic optic discs. Lancet. *2:* 224—226, 1967.

Walsh, F. B.: Clinical neuro-ophthalmology. *2nd ed.* Williams & Wilkins, Baltimore. 324, 1957.

Optic Neuritis
(Figures 114—119)

Acute optic neuritis is an inflammatory affection of the optic nerve. If the nerve head or disc is involved, the term papillitis is used. If the lesion lies in the optic nerve behind the lamina cribrosa, the term retrobulbar neuritis is applied.

Optic neuritis may occur in such conditions as intraocular and orbital inflammations, inflammation of the nasal sinuses, in syphilis, diabetes, encephalitis and meningitis. In multiple (disseminated) sclerosis, the neuritis is nearly always retrobulbar. In many cases, however, the cause of neuritis is unknown.

Optic neuritis most often develops in young adults. It is usually unilateral, but may occur bilaterally.

The symptoms usually start quite suddenly with hazy vision, and vision may be reduced to counting of fingers or even light perception. Sometimes, the patient also complains of some retrobulbar pain on movement of or pressure upon the bulb. The visual field shows a central or paracentral scotoma with absolute or relative loss to colors, but rarely sector-formed or peripheral field defects. The blind spot is enlarged.

Neuritis often disappears within a few weeks, leaving no or only slight reduction of vision or defects in the visual fields, although the optic disc may show permanent pallor of the temporal part of the disc or the whole disc.

OPHTHALMOSCOPICALLY, papillitis (Fig. 114) is often indistinguishable from papilledema. Fully developed, however, papillitis may be less strictly limited to the disc, and prepapillary there is often some vitreous haze. The prominence of the swelling of the disc is usually less, and the color of the disc usually more red than in papilledema. Hemorrhages often occur as splinter or flame-shaped hemorrhages on or around the optic disc, and the retinal veins are usually congested. When papillitis subsides, the optic disc may regain its normal appearance. Most often, however, papillitis is followed by a varying degree of pallor of the optic disc (Figs. 115—118).

In the differential diagnosis, papilledema, pseudopapilledema and drusen of the optic disc have to be considered.

In acute retrobulbar neuritis the disc has a normal appearance. Weeks or months later, a sector-formed pallor may develop at the temporal side of the optic disc (Fig. 119).

HISTOPATHOLOGICALLY, papillitis is characterized by edema of the optic nerve head and the adjacent retina, accumulation of inflammatory cells, proliferation of the interstitial tissue and degeneration of the neural tissue, fullness of the veins and sometimes hemorrhages and exudates. Retrobulbar neuritis shows inflammatory and degenerative changes in the optic nerve behind the lamina cribrosa.

REFERENCES:

Bonamour, G., M. Bonnet, P. Brégeat & P. Juge: La papille optique. Masson, Paris. 292, 1968.

Bradley, W. G. & C. W. M. Whitty: Acute optic neuritis: Prognosis for development of multiple sclerosis. J. Neurol. Neurosurg. Psychiat. *31:* 10—18, 1968.

Brégeat, P.: L'oedème papillaire. Masson, Paris. 1956.

Hoyt, W. F. & D. Beeston: The ocular fundus in neurologic disease. Mosby, St. Louis. 1966.

Huber, A.: Augensymptome bei Hirntumoren. Huber, Bern. 1956.

Leibowitz, U. & M. Alter: Optic nerve involvement and diplopia as initial manifestations of multiple sclerosis. Acta neurol. scandinav. *44:* 70—80, 1968.

Walsh, F. B.: Clinical neuro-ophthalmology. *2nd ed.* Williams & Wilkins, Baltimore. 299, 1957.

Glaucomatous Optic Disc Changes
(Figures 120—125 and 161)

Glaucoma is a condition due to various mechanisms, and characterized by elevation of the intraocular pressure.

Glaucoma may be primary or secondary. Cases of primary glaucoma are usually bilateral and can be divided into closed-angle, chronic simple, juvenile, congenital and absolute glaucoma. The most common form is chronic simple glaucoma. Secondary glaucoma is usually unilateral and a result of inflammatory, vascular, traumatic or neoplastic diseases of the eye.

In all kinds of long-standing ocular hypertension, vision may decrease and characteristic changes develop in the visual field and the optic disc.

The two principal types of glaucoma, closed-angle glaucoma and chronic simple glaucoma which is open-angled, will be discussed in the following.

Closed-angle glaucoma is usually bilateral, although the acute attack often involves one eye only. In the majority of cases, acute closed-angle glaucoma is preceded by prodromal attacks which arise suddenly and subside spontaneously within a few hours. The prodromal attack is similar to the acute attack, but milder. During the acute attack, the intraocular pressure is much increased and colored halos are observed around lights. Vision is blurred and reduced in varying degrees, and may be diminished even to light perception. There is intense pain in the ocular region, radiating into the temporal region. The eyelids may show some edema, there is considerable lacrimation, intense congestion of the bulbar conjunctiva, edema of the cornea—which loses its transparency—and shallow anterior chamber. The pupil is moderately dilated and rigid, and the chamber angle closed.

If normal or approximately normal intraocular tension is re-established within twenty-four to forty-eight hours, useful vision is usually restored. If not, vision is seriously damaged or lost.

OPHTHALMOSCOPIC EXAMINATION is seldom possible during the acute attack. When it is possible, the disc appears somewhat hyperemic (Fig. 124), pulsation may be observed in the central retinal artery and the retinal veins are engorged, but the disc is never pathologically cupped during the first attack.

Chronic simple glaucoma is usually bilateral, but often affects the eyes unequally. It starts insidiously with increased intraocular pressure and progresses very slowly, giving no symptoms until the advanced stage, where characteristic visual defects and reduction in visual acuity develop. The anterior chamber is of normal depth and the chamber angle is open.

OPHTHALMOSCOPICALLY, the early stages of chronic simple glaucoma show no visible fundus changes. In long-standing cases, however, the disc becomes paler and the central retinal vessels are displaced nasally. The pathological cupping of the disc starts temporally (Fig. 120) and proceeds until it occupies the full extent of the disc (Figs. 121—125, 161). Fully developed, the glaucomatous optic disc is atrophic, whitish, yellowish-white or grayish-white and deeply cupped, and the lamina cribrosa, displaced backwards, is seen plainly at the base. At the disc margin the cup shows an abrupt step down from the retinal level. If the margin becomes undermined, the retinal vessels disappear from ophthalmoscopic view when running under the overhanging edge of the cupped disc, and bend sharply as they reappear at the edge. The retinal vessels, therefore, appear as if broken off at the disc margin. Peripapillary, the disc is often surrounded by a whitish or yellowish-white atrophic zone known as glaucomatous halo (Figs. 124—125). The retinal vessels show no characteristic changes.

In the differential diagnosis, other kinds of optic atrophy, senile peripapillary atrophy and pronounced physiological excavation of the disc have to be considered.

HISTOPATHOLOGICALLY, long-standing glaucoma is characterized by backwards displacement of the lamina cribrosa, cupping of the optic disc and cavernous atrophy of the optic nerve. The retina shows degeneration of the nerve fiber, ganglion cell and internal nuclear layers, while the outer retinal layers usually remain normal. Choroidal atrophy occurs, principally in the peripapillary region.

REFERENCES:
Becker, B. & R. N. Shaffer: Diagnosis and therapy of the glaucomas. *2nd ed*. Mosby, St. Louis. 1965.
Hogan, M. J. & L. E. Zimmerman (Ed.): Ophthalmic pathology. *2nd ed*. Saunders Philadelphia. 714, 1962.
Leydhecker, W.: Glaukom. Ein Handbuch. Springer, Berlin. 151, 1960.

The Retinal Vessels

Physiological Variations and Congenital Abnormalities.
(Figures 1—9, 72—77 and 126—143)

The retinal vessels are usually termed arteries and veins, but from a histological point of view, these vessels are correctly described as arterioles and venules.

The central retinal artery and vein normally appear close to each other at the nasal side of the center of the optic disc (Figs. 1—9). Within the disc margin, they usually divide into a large superior and inferior branch and soon after into a large temporal and nasal branch. Four principal divisions are thereby formed, supplying the four quadrants of the fundus. At the disc, small vessels also leave the main trunks in a temporal and nasal direction. From the disc, the four principal divisions of the retinal vessels take a slightly sinuous course as they proceed into their respective quadrants and divide dichotomously into innumerable branches. Passing through the fundus, the retinal arteries and veins cross each other at many points, and as a rule the vein dips below the artery at the crossing. In the periphery, the vascular system stops about one mm behind the ciliary body. In the macular area there is a capillary-free zone of about 0.5 mm corresponding to the fovea centralis.

HISTOLOGICALLY, those parts of the central retinal artery and vein running in the optic nerve are true artery and vein, corresponding to those of comparable size in other situations. After piercing the lamina cribrosa and entering the retina, the arteries soon lose their internal elastic lamina and their multi-layered muscular coat, and in the retina, therefore, are correctly described as arterioles and venules. A single layer of muscle fibers is usually found in the wall of the arteriole, for a considerable part of its way in the retina. In the fundal periphery, however, the arterioles contain no muscle fibers.

The retinal arteries are end-arteries. The arteries appear lighter red and narrower than the dark-red or purplish veins, and normally the arteriovenous ratio is about 2:3. The retinal vessels have a continuous yellow-white light reflex axially. The arterial reflex is more brilliant than the venous, and covers about one third of the arterial and one fourth to one fifth of the venous blood column.

At the disc, pulsation is often found as a physiological condition in the vein, while pulsation in the arteries is only observed in pathological conditions. Arterial pulsation may be observed as locomotion pulse or volume pulse. The first may occur in coarctation of the aorta, and the second in glaucoma, in incomplete occlusion of the central retinal artery or in aortic insufficiency.

However, the arrangement of the retinal vessels as described is subject to many minor or major physiological variations, and a few will be mentioned below.

A cilioretinal artery (Fig. 126), a branch from the short posterior ciliary arteries, appears separately in about 10 per cent of the cases, usually in the temporal part of the disc, and supplies a smaller or larger part of the macular area. More than one cilioretinal artery may occasionally be present (Figs. 127—128). The cilioretinal arteries may become important in cases of occlusion of the central retinal artery, since the area supplied by the cilioretinal artery is left intact (Fig. 210). On the other hand, occlusion of a cilioretinal artery, which is a rare condition, may damage central vision severely (Fig. 211).

At times, the retinal vessels divide behind the lamina cribrosa and then make their appearance on the disc as two or four branches (Fig. 129). They may also emerge from the upper (Figs. 75—77) or temporal (Figs. 72—74) part of the disc, being accompanied by some deformity of the disc and, respectively, an inferior and nasal crescent.

Occasionally, remnants of the hyaloid artery are seen as a grayish-white cord extending forwards from the optic disc into the vitreous and often ending in a disc-like manner at the posterior lens capsule (Fig. 36).

The retinal vessels may show abnormalities in their course, including vascular tortuousity (Figs. 131—133), and the retinal artery and vein may even be twisted around each other (Fig. 130). The retinal vessels may show abnormal dilatations, abnormal crossings, abnormal directions, abnormal vascular loops and finally abnormal vascular communications.

In congenital tortuousity of the retinal vessels (Figs. 131—133), the arteries or veins, or both arteries and veins appear tortuous and lengthened, but their size and color are normal and the disc is normal.

In coarctation of the aorta (Figs. 134—135), the retinal vessels often show some tortuosity and a locomotion pulse may be present.

In congenital heart disease with cyanosis (Figs. 136—137), the retinal vessels are more or less tortuous and also dilated. The arteries are dark-red or purplish and the veins cyanotic. The disc is reddened and the disc margin often blurred. Fully developed, papilledema may occasionally be present.

Abnormal vascular communications may occur as a simple communication between an artery and a vein (Fig. 138) or between two arteries. In this rare congenital abnormality the retinal vessels often show racemose dilatations. The condition is therefore often referred to as racemose hemangioma or arteriovenous aneurysm of the retina (Fig. 139). This abnormality is often confined to the retina. Sometimes, however, vascular abnormalities may coexist in the orbit and in the midbrain, as in the Wyburn-Mason syndrome. The affected retinal vessels are congested and tortuous, sometimes forming loops or coils in which arteries are difficult or impossible to differentiate from veins. Occasionally, gross dilatation of the retinal vessels may occur without obvious angioma or aneurysm formation. The condition may sometimes be associated with facial and orbital hemangioma (Fig. 140).

Another rare congenital abnormality is retinal cavernous hemangioma which is characterized by telangiectasia of the retinal vessels, resembling miliary aneurysms. Some hemorrhage may also be present. The condition is located in a circumscribed, elevated area with some pigmentation in the fundus periphery, usually in the lower nasal quadrant (Figs. 141—143). The condition may be associated with retinal or preretinal veils of connective tissue.

The lesion gives no visual disturbances unless a hemorrhage develops and bursts into the vitreous. The condition which is usually non-progressive and shows no exudates, must not be confused with early stages of Coats' syndrome or angiomatosis of the retina.

REFERENCES:

Ballantyne, A. J. & I. C. Michaelson: Textbook of the fundus of the eye. Livingstone, Edinburgh. 48, 1962.

Baurmann, H., F. Meyer & P. Oberhoff: Komplikationen bei der arteriovenösen Anastomose der Netzhaut. Klin. Monatsbl. Augenh. *153:* 562—571, 1968.

Bech, K. & O. A. Jensen: Racemose haemangioma of the retina. Acta ophthal. (Kbh.). *36:* 769—781, 1958.

Bonnet, M.: Le fond d'oeil dans la sténose de l'isthme de l'aorte. Presse méd. *75:* 2791—2794, 1967.

Cagianut, B.: Das arterio-venöse Aneurysma der Netzhaut. Klin. Monatsbl. Augenh. *140:* 180—191, 1962.

Duke-Elder, S. & K. C. Wybar: System of ophthalmology. *Vol. II.* Kimpton, London. 363, 1961.

Frenkel, M. & H. P. Russe: Retinal telangiectasia associated with hypogammaglobulinemia. Amer. J. Ophthal. *63:* 215—220, 1967.

Piper, H. F.: Über cavernöse Angiome in der Netzhaut. Ophthalmologica. *128:* 99—107, 1954.

Reese, A. B.: Telangiectasis of the retina and Coats' disease. Amer. J. Ophthal. *42:* 1—8, 1956.

Reese, A. B.: Tumors of the eye. *2nd ed.* Hoeber, New York. 383, 1963.

Schwab, F.: Die Tumoren der Netzhaut und der Aderhaut mit Ausnahme des Retinoblastoms und des bösartigen Melanoms der Aderhaut. Ophthalmologica. *151:* 231—259, 1966.

Seitz, R.: Klinik und Pathologie der Netzhautgefässe. Enke, Stuttgart. 1968.

Unger, H.-H. & W. Umbach: Kongenitales okulozerebrales Rankenangiom. Klin. Monatsbl. Augenh. *148:* 672—682, 1966.

Phacomatoses or Hamarthomas Affecting the Eye
(Figures 144—161)

Under this heading four syndromes are classed together because they all show tumor-like malformations particularly in the central nervous system and the retina, they are congenital in origin, and the heredity is dominant. The syndromes are: Angiomatosis of the retina (von Hippel's disease or von Hippel-Lindau's syndrome), Tuberous sclerosis (Bourneville's disease), neurofibromatosis (von Recklinghausen's disease), and encephalofacial angiomatosis (Sturge-Weber's syndrome).

Angiomatosis of the Retina
(Figures 144—157)

Angiomatosis of the retina is a rare, congenital and frequently familial angioblastic retinal malformation. When confined to the retina it is known as von Hippel's disease. Associated with cerebellar cysts or visceral lesions it is known as von Hippel-Lindau's syndrome.

Angiomatosis may be observed at all ages, but most frequently it is discovered in the twenties or the thirties. The lesion is bilateral in about 50 per cent of the cases.

In early stages vision remains unaltered. Later, however, visual field defects develop in the presence of massive retinal exudates. Gross intraocular hemorrhage may occur at any stage. In the advanced stages the tumor often produces retinal detachment and finally painful secondary glaucoma. In these stages vision is severely impaired.

Angiomatous tumors are frequently situated in the peripheral part of the fundus (Figs. 147, 150—153, 157), but angiomatous tumors may occur at the disc (Figs. 144—145) or even in the macular area. They are usually single but multiple tumors may occur in the same eye.

General symptoms usually start later than the eye symptoms, but may occur even before those symptoms have developed. The most frequent general symptom is evidence of intracranial hemorrhage from an angiomatous tumor in the cerebellum, and such hemorrhages are frequently the cause of the patient's death.

OPHTHALMOSCOPICALLY, the fundus lesion may start in one of two ways. In some cases it commences with enlargement and tortuosity of a major retinal vein, which is soon followed by enlargement of the accompanying artery, but not until later is a retinal tumor visible. In other cases the condition commences as a small vascular tumor in the fundus, followed by enlargement and tortuousity of the vessels supplying the tumor. Characteristically, an angiomatous tumor is supplied by a single dilated and tortuous artery and vein, and it is often difficult to distinguish which is the artery and which is the vein. An angiomatous tumor is seen as a yellowish or whitish (Figs. 144—145, 157) or as a reddish (Figs. 147, 150—153) mass in the retina, measuring from about half a disc diameter to about four disc diameters and projecting forward for a variable distance. In the early stage, there are no or only sparsely scattered exudates (Figs. 150—154), but later, massive whitish or yellowish-white deeply situated exudates develop, at first in the areas neighboring the tumor (Figs. 155—156). Later, the exudate becomes more widespread (Figs. 146—147). Finally, retinal detachment develops (Figs. 148—149). Vitreous hemorrhage is not infrequent and may obscure the ophthalmoscopic picture at any stage.

Angiomatosis of the retina is easy to diagnose in fully developed cases.

In early stages with dilation and tortuosity of retinal vessels but without visible angioma, the condition may be confused with racemose hemangioma of the retina or a condition with similar changes in the retina and vascular lesions in the midbrain, the Wyburn-Mason syndrome. Also Coats' syndrome and Eales' disease must be considered in the differential diagnosis. Coats' syndrome is characterized by massive, deep retinal and subretinal exudates and miliary aneurysms, or by miliary aneurysms together with some deeply situated exudate. It is differentiated from angiomatosis of the retina by the lack of angiomatous tumors. Eales' disease is characterized by sheathing of the retinal vessels, new vessel formation and recurrent vitreous hemorrhage. It is differentiated from angiomatosis of the retina by the lack of massive exudate and angiomatous tumor.

HISTOPATHOLOGICALLY, the tumor consists of new-formed capillary vessels and solid cords of endothelial cells, both arising from angioblasts and lying in a cellular matrix with an abundance of glial cells. Secondary changes are often present, such as cystic cavities, gliosis, lipid-laden macrophages and accumulations of exudative material between the choroid and the retina.

REFERENCES:

Goldberg, M. F. & J. R. Duke: Von Hippel-Lindau disease. Histopathologic findings in a treated and an untreated eye. Amer. J. Ophthal. *66:* 693—705, 1968.

Haining, W. M. & P. H. Zweifach: Fluorescein angiography in von Hippel-Lindau disease. A.M.A. Arch. Ophthal. *78:* 475—479, 1967.

Reese, A. B.: Tumors of the eye. *2nd ed.* Hoeber, New York. 368, 1963.

Schwab, F.: Die Tumoren der Netzhaut und der Aderhaut mit Ausnahme des Retinoblastoms und des bösartigen Melanomas der Aderhaut. Ophthalmologica. *151:* 231—259, 1966.

Vogel, M.: Angiogliomatosis der Papille. Klin. Monatsbl. Augenh. *147:* 44—50, 1965.

Tuberous Sclerosis
(Figures 158—159)

Tuberous sclerosis is a rare congenital, heredofamilial disease characterized by adenoma sebaceum, mental deficiency and epilepsy.

Adenoma sebaceum, which may be present from infancy, is characterized by highly vascularized skin papules usually arranged about the nose and cheeks. Mental retardation usually appears during childhood. The disease is usually fatal, the majority of patients dying before the age of 25 years as epileptic idiots, and multiple tuberous tumors may be present in the cerebrum as well as in other organs.

Involvement of the fundus is rare. The fundus lesions may occasionally give rise to visual disturbances and decreased vision.

OPHTHALMOSCOPICALLY, tuberous fundus lesions may appear in two different types. The first type is usually situated pre-papillary and is seen as a large nodular tumor about the size of the optic disc or even larger, and projecting forwards into the vitreous (Fig. 158). The surface of the tumor may be smooth or studded with nodules like a mulberry, and the color of the tumor is grayish-white or yellowish-white. Occasionally, buds may break off from this type of tumor and float freely into the vitreous or settle elsewhere in the retina. The second type of tuberous fundus lesion appears elsewhere in the fundus. It is seen as an oval or round, flat, white or grayish area in the retina, with an average diameter of about half that of the disc or less (Fig. 159).

Multiple tumors, especially of the second type, may be present in the same fundus. Both types of tuberous tumors appear to be relatively avascular, and the lesions are only slightly progressive.

Conditions that must be considered in the differential diagnosis are angiomatosis of the retina with papillary localization, and neurofibromatosis. The tuberous lesion is differentiated ophthalmoscopically from angiomatosis of the retina by the avascularity of the tuberous tumor and the lack of exudates. Furthermore the conditions are distinguished by differences in the general clinical appearance. In neurofibromatosis the fundus lesion may be very similar to that in tuberous sclerosis, and the conditions must therefore be separated by the general signs.

HISTOPATHOLOGICALLY, the tumors are composed of polymorphic fibrous astrocytes with an oval nucleus and indistinct cell boundaries. The tumors usually lie superficially and do not destroy the internal limiting membrane or infiltrate retinal structures other than the nerve fiber or the ganglion cell layers.

REFERENCES:
Garron, L. K. & W. H. Spencer: Retinal glioneuroma associated with tuberous sclerosis. Trans. Amer. Acad. Ophthal. Otolaryng. *68:* 1018—1021, 1964.
Reese, A. B.: Tumors of the eye. *2nd ed.* Hoeber, New York. 173, 1963.
Schwab, F.: Die Tumoren der Netzhaut und der Aderhaut mit Ausnahme des Retinoblastoms und des bösartigen Melanoms der Aderhaut. Ophthalmologica. *151:* 231—259, 1966.

Neurofibromatosis

Neurofibromatosis is a heredofamilial disease which is of congenital origin, presenting as tumors and pigmentation of the skin, tumors derived from the Schwann cells of the peripheral and sympathetic nerves, neurinomas in the central nervous system, and skeletal changes. The skin of the eyelids, the bony orbit, conjunctiva, uvea or retina may be affected.

The clinical picture may show extreme variation. The cutaneous lesions are present most frequently, and vary from café-aux-lait spots to true neurofibromas. Manifestations in the central nervous system include neurofibromas particularly affecting the acoustic and the optic nerves, giving rise to a varied picture of signs from the central nervous system. Skeletal changes may be present in the form of deformities and cystic changes in the bones.

Localized in the uveal tract, neurofibromas may give rise to buphthalmos.

Neurofibromas in the fundus may give rise to some reduction of the vision, depending on the localization of the tumor.

OPHTHALMOSCOPICALLY, neurofibromas in the fundus closely resemble those described in tuberous sclerosis (see Fig. 158).

In differential diagnosis tuberous sclerosis and angiomatosis of the retina must be considered.

HISTOPATHOLOGICALLY, the tumor is a neuroma consisting of bundles of neurocytes and neurofibrils, together with cystic spaces and areas of hyaline degeneration.

REFERENCES:

Bloch, F. J.: Retinal tumor associated with neurofibromatosis (von Recklinghausen's disease). Report of a case. A.M.A. Arch. Ophthal. *40:* 433—437, 1948.

Reese, A. B.: Tumors of the eye. *2nd ed.* Hoeber, New York. 190, 1963.

Schwab, F.: Die Tumoren der Netzhaut und der Aderhaut mit Ausnahme des Retinoblastoms und des bösartigen Melanoms der Aderhaut. Ophthalmologica. *151:* 231—259, 1966.

Sturge-Weber's Syndrome
(Figures 120 and 160—161)

Sturge-Weber's syndrome consists of a triad of symptoms: facial capillary angioma, intracranial angioma, and choroidal angioma with or without buphthalmos. All symptoms may not be present at the same time. Incomplete forms are more frequent than the complete syndrome.

The cutaneous capillary angioma, nevus flammeus, may be present at birth. It is usually unilateral and limited to the distribution of the first and second divisions of the trigeminal nerve.

Intracranial angiomas in the pia are usually situated on the same side as the nevus flammeus and are later associated with progressive calcification within the underlying cerebral cortex. Sooner or later a variable degree of cerebral atrophy develops, and this atrophy is followed by progressive mental deterioration and epileptiform attacks.

Choroidal angiomas may give rise to raised intraocular tension with or without buphthalmos. Visual disturbances and visual field defects may subsequently occur as a result of the raised intraocular tension.

OPHTHALMOSCOPICALLY, choroidal angiomas are seen as localized (Fig. 161) or more diffuse (Fig. 160) yellowish or yellowish-gray flat areas anywhere in the fundus. The retinal vessels may be tortuous and somewhat dilated (Fig. 120) and sometimes show a bizarre configuration (Fig. 160).

In cases with long-standing glaucoma, glaucomatous optic disc changes may occur in the form of atrophy and cupping of the optic nerve head (Figs. 120 and 161).

In the differential diagnosis, malignant choroidal melanoma must be considered. The two conditions can sometimes be distinguished by fluorescein angiography, as choroidal angiomas may show a fluorescein pattern, differing from that seen in malignant choroidal melanoma.

HISTOPATHOLOGICALLY, choroidal angiomas consist of endothelial-lined spaces of varying sizes, engorged with blood and separated by scanty connective tissue stroma. Over the tumor the retina may show degenerative changes in the form of microcyst formation. The optic disc may show glaucomatous cupping and atrophy, and there may be cavernous atrophy of the optic nerve.

REFERENCES:
Bölcs, S. & Gy. Bajnok: Über die meningo-okulo-faziale Angiomatose. Klin. Monatsbl. Augenh. *150:* 702—706, 1967.
Norton, E. W. D. & F. Gutman: Fluorescein angiography and hemangiomas of the choroid. A.M.A. Arch. Ophthal. *78:* 121—125, 1967.
Reese, A. B.: Tumors of the eye. *2nd ed.* Hoeber, New York. 396, 1963.
Schwab, F.: Die Tumoren der Netzhaut und der Aderhaut mit Ausnahme des Retinoblastoms und des bösartigen Melanoms des Aderhaut. Ophthalmologica. *151:* 231—259, 1966.
Wessing, A.: Fluoreszenzangiographie der Retina. Lehrbuch und Atlas. Thieme, Stuttgart. 143, 1968.

Sclerosis of the Retinal Vessels

(Figures 162—167, 180—181, 209, 218—220, 238—239 and 252—253)

As the retinal vessels are visible ophthalmoscopically, the development of retinal vascular sclerosis can readily be followed in the fundus.

Retinal vascular sclerosis is indicated by some of the following lesions: changes in the arterial light reflex, arteriovenous crossing phenomena, variations in caliber or course, or sheathing of the retinal vessels.

Involuntary sclerosis of the retinal vessels is an almost physiological process related to aging, normally found in healthy persons in the sixties and later. The condition is seldom present before the age of 50 years, and never in the young. The fundus changes consist of some narrowing and slight variations in caliber of the retinal arteries, broadening of the arterial light reflex (copper-wire arteries) and slight or moderate arteriovenous crossing phenomena.

More advanced retinal vascular sclerosis occurs in cases of involuntary sclerosis associated with hypertension, and in cases of long-standing hypertension and long-standing diabetes where the disease itself produces or accelerates the development of retinal vascular sclerosis. Advanced vascular sclerosis is characterized by moderate narrowing and some variation in caliber of the retinal arteries, copper- or silver-wire arteries, moderate or pronounced crossing phenomena and sometimes, atheromatous plaques or sheathing of the retinal vessels.

Involuntary retinal vascular sclerosis as a rule does not affect the visual acuity.

In advanced vascular sclerosis, however, degenerative retinal changes may induce visual disturbances.

OPHTHALMOSCOPICALLY, in involuntary or moderate sclerosis, the retinal arteries are slightly narrowed and the axial arterial light reflex is less bright, more diffuse and broader than normal (Figs. 162, 164—165), giving the artery the appearance of a copper-wire (copper-wire arteries). In advanced sclerosis, the arteries are narrow and the axial reflex is broad, very pale and whitish (Figs. 180—181), giving the artery the appearance of a silver-wire (silver-wire arteries).

Arteriovenous crossing phenomena may occur as Gunn's sign or Salus' sign. Gunn's sign is seen as a pale zone of the vein or a concealment of the vein on both sides of the crossing artery (Figs. 163—167). The width of this pale zone varies. In involuntary or moderate sclerosis, the pale zone of the vein is always small or only slightly indicated, while in advanced sclerosis the vein may show tapered ends or terminate abruptly at some distance from the artery, leaving a pale zone on each side of the artery (Figs. 180—181). At the arteriovenous crossing, the artery and the vein have a common adventitial coat and the apparent narrowing or concealment of the vein is due to a gradual loss of transparency in the arterial wall and the perivascular tissue.

At times, the vein shows some twisting and distension peripheral to the crossing, centrally it is straighter and narrower for a short distance and then resumes its normal appearance, a phenomenon known as "banking" (Figs. 163, 166). Salus' sign is seen as an S-formed bend or a U-formed displacement or deflection of the vein which crosses under the artery at right angles instead of obliquely, and associated with some pallor or concealment of the vein on both sides of the crossing artery (Fig. 167).

The sclerosed retinal arteries usually have a straighter course than normal (Fig. 164), branch more acutely, and show some variations in caliber. The retinal veins show slight irregular tortuosities and more or less irregular variations in caliber.

Sheathing of the retinal vessels is due to loss of transparency of the vessel wall. Slight sheathing is often not observed in ordinary ophthalmoscopy, but may readily be seen in red-free light ophthalmoscopy. Advanced sheathing is seen in ordinary ophthalmoscopy as pale, whitish parallel lines along the borders of the blood column (parallel sheathing) (Figs. 209, 220, 252). If sheathing progresses, the blood column may be completely hidden, so that a shorter or longer part of the vessel appears as a solid white strand (pipe-stem sheathing) (Figs. 219, 238—239, 253). Atheromatous plaques may also obscure an artery for a short distance (Fig. 218). Sheathing seems to be due to changes either in the perivascular adventitial sheaths or in the subendothelial tissue. The condition is not only related to the aging process, atheromatous dis-

ease or hypertension, but several factors may be concerned and therefore the etiology is still a matter of discussion.

In advanced vascular sclerosis, fundus changes may be present in the form of patchy retinal atrophies, small superficial and deep retinal hemorrhages and small glistening, well-defined white or yellowish-white exudates in the posterior part of the fundus.

Senile macular degeneration and vascular atrophy of the optic disc are discussed elsewhere.

HISTOPATHOLOGICALLY, the retinal vessels present varying degrees of arteriolosclerosis and phlebosclerosis. Fully developed, the sclerosed vessels show localized or generalized thickening, hyalinization and fibrosis of their walls and narrowing of their lumen. Occasionally, atheromatous lesions may be present in the larger retinal vessels. Hemorrhages are superficial and deep. The exudates are deeply situated and composed of albuminous and hyaline material.

REFERENCES:
Leishman, R.: The eye in general vascular disease, hypertension and arteriosclerosis. Brit. J. Ophthal. *41*: 641—701, 1957.
Prince, J. H.: Introduction to aging and pathology of the retina. Thomas, Springfield. 1965.
Seitz, R.: Klinik und Pathologie der Netzhautgefässe. Enke, Stuttgart. 1968.
Utermann, D. & E. J. Klempien: Über Beziehungen zwischen den Erscheinungsformen der Arteriosklerose am Augenhintergrund und degenerativen Erkrankungen am allgemeinen Gefässsystem. Docum. ophthal. *24*: 201—274, 1968.

Fundus Changes in Hypertension
(Figures 96 and 168—197)

The basic fundus lesion in hypertension is an angiospasm, seen as a generalized or localized narrowing of the retinal arteries. If, however, the hypertension is preceded by involuntary sclerosis of the retinal vessels, this angiospasm is more or less obscured by the sclerotic changes.

Hypertensive fundus changes may be classified into retinal angiopathy, retinopathy and neuroretinopathy, and in discussing these changes the various forms of hypertension must be distinguished, as the fundus changes and their course vary according to the different conditions.

Moderate chronic hypertension as observed in essential hypertension, some chronic renal, vascular and endocrine disorders etc., may be present for years without any visible fundus changes or may only present a slight narrowing of the retinal arteries. If hypertension persists, retinal angiopathy develops and this angiopathy is mainly seen as an accelerated sclerosis of the retinal vessels. In periods of exacerbation, however, the fundus picture may be altered by the occurrence of hypertensive retinopathy, while neuroretinopathy seldom develops.

Hypertensive fundus changes occurring in acute glumerulonephritis, eclampsia or pre-eclampsia of pregnancy, pheochromocytoma etc., are characterized in the early stages by retinal angiopathy, which is seen as generalized or localized narrowing of the retinal arteries. If blood pressure is not normalized within a short time, the fundus changes progress and retinopathy or even neuroretinopathy develops. The fundus picture, however, usually alters in accordance with remission and exacerbation of the hypertension. If hypertension has been present for a long time, secondary sclerosis invariably develops in the retinal vessels. However, if normal blood pressure is reestablished within a short time, the fundus changes may disappear entirely.

Keith, Wagener and Barker classified the hypertensive fundus changes into four grades according to the prognosis for life. Grade 1 was characterized by mild narrowing or sclerosis of the retinal arteries; grade 2 by generalized or localized irregular narrowing, moderate or marked sclerosis of the retinal arteries and arteriovenous crossing phenomena; grade 3 by the aforementioned vascular changes and retinal edema, cotton-wool exudates and retinal hemorrhages; grade 4 by papilledema in addition to the changes found in grade 3.

As the fundus picture usually alters in accordance with the hypertensive state, the ophthalmoscopic examination is of great value for the clinician. The retinal vascular changes, however, are not always in step with the vascular changes in kidney, heart and brain, so that an evaluation of the general prognosis must include evidence of changes in all vascular areas, severity and duration of hypertension, the age of the patient and the response to treatment.

Vision is not altered in hypertensive angiopathy. In hypertensive retinopathy central vision may be reduced if the macula is involved. In hypertensive neuroretinopathy, vision is usually decreased although the degree of visual reduction may vary considerably.

Ophthalmoscopically, hypertensive angiopathy without vascular sclerosis (Figs. 168—173) is characterized by generalized or localized narrowing of the retinal arteries. In long-standing hypertension or involuntary vascular sclerosis associated with hypertension, however, arteriovenous crossing phenomena and signs of vascular sclerosis are also present (Figs. 174—176). At times, the hypertensive angiopathy is associated with retinal edema (Figs. 172—173). This occurs most frequently in eclampsia or preeclampsia of pregnancy, and in cases with acute exacerbation of hypertension.

Hypertensive retinopathy (Figs. 177—184) is characterized by the addition of retinal hemorrhages and exudates and some retinal edema. The hemorrhages consist of superficial, flame-shaped and deep, rounded hemorrhages. The exudates consist of grayish-white or whitish cotton-wool patches, discrete or confluent yellowish-white exudates, and sometimes a macular star, composed of whitish exudates radiating in all directions from the fovea. Slight retinal edema is indicated by an increase in the fundal reflexes, while moderate edema gives the retina a more grayish color. In eclampsia, edema may even cause a reversible serous retinal detachment.

Retinal hemorrhages and cotton-wool exudates are often absorbed in the course of some weeks or a few months, leaving no ophthalmoscopic trace, but as new hemorrhages and exudates may develop simultaneously, the general ophthalmoscopic picture is often maintained.

Hypertensive neuroretinopathy (Figs. 96, 185—188, 192) is characterized by the addition of papilledema.

Hypertensive neuroretinopathy should not be confused with occlusion of the central retinal vein or papilledema.

If normal blood pressure is re-established within a short time, retinal edema subsides quickly, and papilledema, retinal hemorrhages and woolly exudates disappear in the course of some weeks or a few months, while hard yellowish-white exudates and a macular star subside very slowly over a period of months (Figs. 192—197), and discrete exudates may persist even for years (Fig. 190). The disappearance of a macular star is often followed by depigmentation and pigment clumping in the macular area (Figs. 196—197), and not infrequently by some persistent reduction of the visual acuity. Retinal hemorrhages and woolly exudates usually disappear leaving no ophthalmoscopic traces, but occasionally visible patchy retinal atrophy develops (Fig. 191). If hypertension has been present for a long time, retinal vascular sclerosis persists even if the blood pressure is normalized (Fig. 189).

Histopathologically, in early stages of hypertension, the ophthalmoscopically visible generalized and localized narrowing of the retinal arteries cannot be demonstrated. In long-standing hypertension, however, the retinal arteries show arteriolosclerosis with medial proliferation and hyalinization, localized adventitial proliferation and fibrosis, and narrowing of the lumen. Flame-shaped hemorrhages are formed in the superficial retinal layers and rounded hemorrhages in the deep layers. The retinal edema involves all layers. The discrete, yellowish-white exudates are found in spaces in the nuclear layers and consist of lipoid, albuminous and fibrinous material. Cotton-wool exudates are localized to the nerve fiber layer, which is swollen and includes the cytoid bodies. These are cell-like bodies possibly representing degenerative changes in the nerve fibers. The cotton-wool exudates probably represent minute ischemic infarcts. A macular star is situated in the outer plexiform layer and is formed by large, fat-filled microglia cells, interspersed by free masses of lipoid and by patches of hyalinized cellular debris.

REFERENCES:

Harry, J. & N. Ashton: The pathology of hypertensive retinopathy. Trans. ophthal. Soc. U.K. *83:* 71—90, 1963.

Heydenreich, A.: Die prognostische Bedeutung des Fundus hypertonicus. Klin. Monatsbl. Augenh. *151:* 312—319, 1967.

Leishman, R.: The eye in general vascular disease, hypertension and arteriosclerosis. Brit. J. Ophthal. *41:* 641—701, 1957.

Seitz, R.: Die Genese und Ätiologie des Kreuzungsphänomens und seine Bedeutung für die Diagnostik von Netzhautgefässerkrankungen. Klin. Monatsbl. Augenh. *139:* 491—512, 1961.

Seitz, R.: Klinik und Pathologie der Netzhautgefässe. Enke, Stuttgart. 1968.

Occlusion of the Central Retinal Artery and Its Branches

(Figures 198—221)

Occlusion of the central retinal artery or one of its branches may be the result of thrombotic closure of the lumen, blockage by an embolus or local vasomotor constriction of the vessels. Obstruction by thrombosis due to atheromatous disease with or without hypertension is by far the most common cause of obstruction of the retinal arterial blood flow. An occlusion by a proliferative endarteritis and terminal thrombosis may, however, occur in conditions such as giant-cell arteritis. Blockage of the arterial flow by an embolus is relatively rare. It may occur in conditions such as carotid insufficiency or carotid occlusion, rheumatic heart disease, in auricular fibrillation, and blood diseases such as polycythemia and paraproteinemia. Infective emboli may arise in subacute bacterial endocarditis and other infective illnesses. Fat emboli may occur after injury and air emboli have been recorded following carotid angiography. Blockage of the arterial blood flow by local vasomotor constrictions may also be of some importance.

Occlusion of the central retinal artery occurs most often in middle-aged or elderly persons. The occlusion is usually unilateral but may occur bilaterally.

In some cases, the occlusion is preceded by prodromal obscurations of vision for a variable period before the final attack. At the actual onset of the occlusion of the central retinal artery, the patient suddenly or within a few minutes experiences complete loss of vision in the affected eye, and the pupil becomes wide and does not react to direct light stimulation. If a branch of the central retinal artery is occluded, the visual defect is partial, corresponding to the area supplied by the involved branch. If the obstruction of the blood flow is total for more than one hour, the retina which was supplied by the occluded artery cannot survive and its function is lost. If the obstruction of the blood flow is incomplete or restored within an hour or so, recovery of vision may occur, but most frequently the improvement is incomplete and the eye often becomes blind.

Secondary glaucoma may follow an occlusion of the central retinal artery, usually one or two months after the vascular accident, but secondary glaucoma in this condition is rare compared to the frequency at which it occurs after central venous occlusion.

In rare cases, the clinical picture is altered by the presence of a cilioretinal artery, a branch from the short posterior ciliary arteries. In these cases the area supplied by the cilioretinal artery is normal and the corresponding visual field is spared.

In occlusion of a cilioretinal artery, however, the macular area is involved.

Central vision may be completely lost and a centrocoecal scotoma is present, while the rest of the visual field is spared.

OPHTHALMOSCOPICALLY, shortly after the occlusion of the central artery, the retinal arteries are seen as thin or even thread-like, more or less red lines of varying caliber. Sometimes the blood column is broken up into segments which may exhibit slight to-and-fro movements (Figs. 202—203). The arterial light reflexes are narrowed or absent, and arterial pulsation cannot be produced if the occlusion is complete. After a period of narrowing, the arteries may widen again (Figs. 198, 200, 204, 205), but pulsation still cannot be produced. Within a few hours after the occlusion, the retina becomes pale, opaque, grayish-white or milky, due to edema of the internal retinal layers, and particularly to a cloudy swelling of the ganglion cell layer (Figs. 198, 200, 202, 205). At the fovea, ganglion cells are lacking and the retina is thin. The fovea therefore retains its normal color and appears as a red-brown or cherry-red, rounded spot, contrasting markedly with the surrounding pale retina. The disc is pale and the disc margin indistinct. Retinal hemorrhages are usually absent, but if present they are few in number.

In cases which present a cilioretinal artery (Figs. 204, 210), the area supplied by this vessel is normal and contrasts markedly with the adjacent opaque retina.

In occlusion of a retinal arterial branch (Figs. 212, 214) or occlusion of a cilioretinal artery, the retinal pallor is confined to the area supplied by the occluded branch. In arterial branch occlusion, an embolus or an atheromatous plaque may be present and clearly visible at the site of the occlusion which is usually at a bifurcation of the artery (Figs. 214, 218).

After some time, a certain blood flow is usually re-established, and after some weeks or a few months the retinal edema gradually disappears (Figs. 198—201, 205—207, 212—215). Thereafter, the area involved may gradually assume a more or less granular, atrophic appearance (Fig. 211), often showing pigmentation and glistening, white exudates (Fig. 209). The retinal vessels become narrow and may show more or less pronounced sheathing (Figs. 208—209, 219—220), and in branch occlusion a certain collateral circulation may be established (Figs. 216—217, 221). In the late stage of central retinal artery occlusion, the optic disc becomes pale and atrophic (Figs. 199, 207—209).

The alterations in the retinal blood circulation can readily be followed by fluorescein angiography.

The ophthalmoscopic picture of central retinal artery occlusion is very characteristic and should not be confused with the ophthalmoscopic picture in Tay-Sachs' disease and Niemann-Pick's disease, which may appear very similar, although the pathogenesis is quite different. Furthermore, occlusion of the central retinal artery usually occurs in middle-aged or elderly persons, while the latter diseases occur only in infancy.

HISTOPATHOLOGICALLY, the central retinal artery may be occluded by a thrombus situated at or just behind the lamina cribrosa, but serial sections are often necessary to reveal the thrombus or its sequelae. The condition is often accompanied by phlebosclerosis of the central retinal vein.

In the early stages, there is marked swelling of the ganglion cells, marked edema and necrosis of the inner two thirds of the retina. Later, this part of

the retina becomes totally atrophic, while
the outer layers remain normal.

REFERENCES:

Ball, C. J.: Atheromatosis embolism to the
brain, retina and choroid. A.M.A. Arch. Ophthal. *76:* 690—695, 1966.

Bettelheim, H.: Beiträge zur Klinik und Diagnostik der Arteriitis cranialis. Klin. Monatsbl.
Augenh. *152:* 805—813, 1968.

Cullen, J. F.: Occult temporal arteritis. A common cause of blindness in old age. Brit. J.
Ophthal. *51:* 513—525, 1967.

David, N. J., E. W. D. Norton, J. D. Gass & J.
Beauchamp: Fluorescein angiography in cen-
tral retinal artery occlusion. A.M.A. Arch.
Ophthal. *77:* 619—629, 1967.

Dollery, C. T., D. W. Hill, J. W. Paterson, P. S.
Ramalho & E. M. Kohner: Collateral blood
flow after branch arteriolar occlusion in the
human retina. Brit. J. Ophthal. *51:* 249—255,
1967.

Duke-Elder, S. & J. H. Dobree: System of ophthalmology. *Vol. X.* Kimpton, London. 66,
1967.

Gass, J. D. M.: A fluorescein angiographic study
of macular dysfunction secondary to retinal
vascular disease. A.M.A. Arch. Ophthal. *80:*
535—617, 1968.

Meythaler, H.: Über die Verschlüsse von Blut-
gefässen der Netzhaut. Klin. Monatsbl. Augenh. *149:* 32—41, 1966.

Perraut, L. E. & L. E. Zimmerman: The occurrence of glaucoma following occlusion of the
central retinal artery. A clinicopathologic report of six new cases with a review of the
literature. A.M.A. Arch. Ophthal. *61:* 845—
865, 1959.

Snyder, W. B., L. Allen & O. Frazier: Fluorescence angiography. An aid in the diagnosis
of occluded vessels. A.M.A. Arch. Ophthal.
77: 168—175, 1967.

Vom Hofe, K. & E. Brossog: Über die Ergebnisse
vergleichender klinischer Untersuchungen
bei arteriellen und venösen Gefässverschlüssen der Netzhaut. Klin. Monatsbl. Augenh.
150: 16—26, 1967.

Zimmerman, L. E.: Embolism of central retinal
artery. A.M.A. Arch. Ophthal. *73:* 822—826,
1965.

Occlusion of the Central Retinal Vein and Its Branches

(Figures 222—239)

Obstruction of the central retinal vein or a branch of the central retinal vein is a result of a thrombus formation or occlusion of the lumen by proliferated endothelium and subendothelial connective tissue. Several factors may contribute to the obstruction. The most important factor is a sclerotic process involving the central vein as well as the central artery in the posterior part of the lamina cribrosa. A second important factor is stagnation of the circulation caused by the sclerotic process or by impairment of the arterial flow to the eye, or failure of the circulation, as seen in different conditions. Finally, degenerative and inflammatory processes in the veins, as well as primary simple glaucoma, may be factors in the pathogenesis.

In carotid insufficiency or carotid occlusion, cotton-wool exudates, small retinal hemorrhages and microaneurysms may occur without signs of true occlusion of the central retinal vein.

In occlusion of the central retinal vein and its branches, the retinal blood circulation is not completely blocked, but the blood flow is reduced. In the course of some months the circulation becomes more or less re-established by recanalization or the formation of a collateral circulation.

The condition occurs most frequently in elderly persons who exhibit signs of sclerosis of the retinal vessels and often hypertension, but it may also occur in long-standing diabetes, carotid insuffi-

ciency or carotid occlusion, polycythemia and other conditions with increased viscosity of the blood such as paraproteinemias, in simple chronic glaucoma, or it may complicate an acute orbitofacial inflammation. The occlusion is usually unilateral, but may also occur bilaterally.

Patients presenting obstruction of the central retinal vein often claim transient obscurations of vision lasting from a few minutes to some hours, some time before the actual onset of the venous blockage. When this occurs, vision becomes impaired within a few hours or characteristically the patients wake up in the morning with impaired vision. Although the vision is often reduced to counting of fingers or hand movements, light perception always remains.

Vision may improve in the course of some months, but as permanent macular damage is common, central vision may remain decreased or even be lost. In about 15 to 20 per cent of the cases, secondary (hemorrhagic) glaucoma develops about two or three months after the onset of the occlusion. In these cases the patient often presents a blind and painful eye, which may call for excision on account of the pain. At times, the fellow eye may also present glaucoma.

OPHTHALMOSCOPICALLY, incipient central venous occlusion is recognized by engorgement and tortuosity of the retinal veins, sometimes associated with a slight localized retinal edema, small retinal hemorrhages and some swelling of the optic disc. This ophthalmoscopic picture may precede the onset of central venous occlusion for a period varying from weeks to even months. The fully developed picture of occlusion of the central retinal vein (Figs. 222—225) is characterized by extensive flame-shaped, superficial retinal hemorrhages, and small, rounded, deep retinal hemorrhages, engorgement of the veins, swollen optic disc, fluffy exudates and edema throughout the fundus. The hemorrhages are larger near the disc than elsewhere. At times they break into the vitreous or form a preretinal hemorrhage. The veins are dark-red, dilated and tortuous. The arteries are usually narrow. The disc is red and swollen and the margin is blurred. Fluffy exudates may be present anywhere, but most frequently around the disc.

Recanalization of the vein is likely to occur in the course of some months, and hemorrhages and exudates tend to be absorbed. During that period, the retinal vessels usually become narrowed (Fig. 226), appear sclerotic and may sometimes be accompanied by pale sheaths, or be completely sheathed over a shorter or longer distance. Diffuse or patchy retinal atrophy is usually present. New-formed vascular channels sometimes develop a collateral circulation at or around the optic disc (Figs. 227, 236). In the late stage, bands or veils of connective tissue may also appear, preferentially around the disc area (Fig. 227). If glaucoma develops, glaucomatous atrophy of the disc may appear gradually.

The acute stage of central venous occlusion should not be confused with papilledema or hypertensive neuroretinopathy.

In branch vein occlusion, which is much more common than central vein occlusion, the visual symptoms depend on the site of the obstruction. If the macular area is involved, central vision is decreased or even lost. If a nasal branch is affected, however, there may be no symptoms at all. Secondary glaucoma is a rare complication in branch vein occlusion.

OPHTHALMOSCOPICALLY, an incipient branch vein occlusion is recognized by engorgement and tortuosity of a retinal vein (Fig. 230). In established occlusion of a branch of the central retinal vein (Figs. 231—233), the fundus changes, consisting of large superficial retinal hemorrhages and some cotton-wool exudates, are confined to a fan-shaped area drained by the obstructed vein. The occlusion is likely to develop at an arteriovenous crossing, and most commonly affects the upper temporal vein. Multiple branch vein occlusions may also occur (Figs. 228—229).

The retinal hemorrhages and the exudates tend to be absorbed in the course of some months, although numerous small round red dots, probably clusters of microaneurysms, may remain in the diseased area for a long period (Fig. 234). Ensheathing of retinal veins is often present in late stages of venous occlusion (Figs. 237—239). New-formed vascular channels sometimes develop a collateral circulation (Fig. 235). This collateral circulation starts as a fine network of dilated capillary vessels, gradually acquiring the form of a unipolar rete mirabile, which is subsequently transformed into a bipolar rete mirabile. Finally, it assumes the simple form of an anastomosis, consisting of a single large vascular communication.

The late stage of branch vein occlusion should not be confused with diabetic retinopathy.

In central retinal vein occlusion and branch vein occlusion, alterations in the retinal blood circulation can readily be followed by fluorescein angiography.

Histopathologically, the central retinal vein may be obstructed by a thrombus or occluded by endothelial or subendothelial proliferations at or just behind the lamina cribrosa, and the condition is often accompanied by an atheromatous process in the central retinal artery. When coming to histopathological examination, however, the central retinal vein has often become recanalized, and the condition may then be indicated only by a finely perforated septum in the lumen of the vein, which is detectable in serial sections only.

In the early stages, the retinal changes are dominated by hemorrhages and edema. In the late stages, there is pronounced atrophy and disorganization of the retinal layers, marked gliosis, and sometimes preretinal, new-formed vessels and connective tissue.

REFERENCES:

Ashton, N.: Studies of the retinal capillaries in relation to diabetic and other retinopathies. Brit. J. Ophthal. 47: 521—538, 1963.

Brændstrup, P.: Central retinal vein thrombosis and hemorrhagic glaucoma. Acta ophthal. (Kbh.). Suppl. 35, 1950.

David, N. J., E. W. C. Norton, J. D. Gass, R. Sexton & C. Gables: Fluorescein retinal angiography in carotid occlusion. A.M.A. Arch. Neurol. 14: 281—287, 1966.

Gass, J. D. M.: A fluorescein angiographic study of macular dysfunction secondary to retinal vascular disease. A.M.A. Arch. Ophthal. 80: 535—617, 1968.

Hill, D. W.: Fluorescein studies in retinal vascular occlusion. Brit. J. Ophthal. 52: 1—12, 1968.

Hollenhorst, R. W.: Ocular manifestations of insufficiency or thrombosis of the internal carotid artery. Amer. J. Ophthal. 47: 753—767, 1959.

Kearns, T. P. & R. W. Hollenhorst: Venous-stasis retinopathy of occlusive disease of the carotid artery. Proc. Mayo Clin. 38: 304—312, 1963.

Klien, B. A.: Sidelights on retinal venous occlusion. Amer. J. Ophthal. 61: 25—36, 1966.

Raitta, C.: Der Zentralvenen- und Netzhautvenenverschluss. Acta ophthal. (Kbh.). Suppl. 83, 1965.

Raitta, C.: Fluorescein Angiographie nach Zentralvenenverschluss. Acta ophthal. (Kbh.). 46: 207—210, 1968.

Vom Hofe, K. & E. Brossog: Über die Ergebnisse vergleichender klinischer Untersuchungen bei arteriellen und venösen Gefässverschlüssen der Netzhaut. Klin. Monatsbl. Augenh. 150: 16—26, 1967.

Fundus and Vitreous Hemorrhage

(Figures 186—188, 222—224, 240—245, 247, 255, 259, 278—279, 282—283, 287—291, 352—353, 366 and 368—370)

Fundus hemorrhage may appear as superficial or deep retinal hemorrhage, subretinal hemorrhage, preretinal hemorrhage or, if a hemorrhage bursts through the hyaloid membrane, as vitreous hemorrhage.

Fundus hemorrhage may occur in various conditions such as retinal vascular obstruction, retinal perivasculitis, papilledema, subarachnoidal hemorrhage, vascular disease such as arteriosclerosis, different retinopathies, particularly diabetic and hypertensive, diseases of the hematopoetic system or following trauma. Finally, fundus hemorrhage is not infrequent in the new-born due to trauma of the head and neck during normal labor or due to instrumental delivery.

Whether visual disturbances occur or not, and whether they are major or minor, depend on the size and the localization of the fundus hemorrhage. In vitreous hemorrhage, however, vision is always decreased to some extent.

OPHTHALMOSCOPICALLY, retinal hemorrhages vary according to the localization of the blood. If the retinal hemorrhage is superficial, lying in the nerve-fiber layer, it assumes a striated or flame-shaped appearance (Figs. 186—188, 222—224, 278—279, 282—283), while hemorrhages in the deeper part of the retina are rounded or irregularly shaped, and usually smaller than superficial hemorrhages (Figs. 247, 287—291).

Subretinal hemorrhages appear most frequently around the optic disc or in the macular area.

OPHTHALMOSCOPICALLY, they are seen as ill-defined, dark-red, slate-gray or even black hemorrhages of disc size or even larger, lying beneath the retinal vessels (Figs. 244—245, 352—353, 366, 368—370).

Ophthalmoscopically, the condition may sometimes be difficult to separate from a commencing malignant choroidal melanoma. The lesions, however, can be distinguished by fluorescein angiography as a subretinal hemorrhage shows no fluorescence, while a malignant choroidal melanoma shows a characteristic pattern of fluorescence.

OPHTHALMOSCOPICALLY, a preretinal hemorrhage is seen as a dark-red or nearly black mass in front of the retina (Figs. 240—243, 255). The upper border is usually horizontal or slightly concave, while the lower is as a rule convex.

At times, both retinal, preretinal and subretinal hemorrhages may all be present simultaneously, either originating in the retina or subretinally, and then penetrating into the other layers (Figs. 244—245).

Any retinal or preretinal hemorrhage which is sufficiently profuse may burst into the vitreous, producing diffuse haze of the vitreous, forming clots floating around in the vitreous (Fig. 259) or being so large that it fills the whole vitreous with blood, giving rise to a dark-red or nearly black reflex in the pupil.

In the differential diagnosis of vitreous hemorrhage, it is necessary to consider for example angiomatosis of the retina, Eales' disease, diabetic retinopathy, malignant choroidal melanoma and retinal detachment.

Fundal and vitreous hemorrhages may be absorbed very quickly, but sometimes they may persist for months or even years, giving rise to fundal degeneration or development of proliferative retinopathy.

HISTOPATHOLOGICALLY, superficial retinal hemorrhages lie in the nerve fiber layer while deep retinal hemorrhages lie in the outer and inner nuclear layers. Some degenerative changes are always present together with some glial proliferation. Subretinal hemorrhages lie between the choroid and the retinal pigment epithelium, often penetrating Bruch's membrane. Preretinal hemorrhages often lie behind the internal limiting membrane, which is detached from the nerve fiber layer, or penetrate the internal limiting membrane but remain behind the vitreous corpus.

REFERENCES:

Duke-Elder, S. & J. H. Dobree: System of ophthalmology. *Vol. X.* Kimpton, London. 137, 1967.

Fritz, A., G. Parent, A. Lambilliote & G. Beeckman: Physiopathologie des hémorragies rétiniennes obstétricales. Bull. Soc. Belge Ophtal. *142:* 475—489, 1966.

Krebs, W. & G. Jäger: Netzhautblutungen bei Neugeborenen und Geburtsverlauf. Klin. Monatsbl. Augenh. *148:* 483—490, 1966.

Pietruschka, G.: Zur Ätiologie und Therapie von Glaskörpereinblutungen. Klin. Monatsbl. Augenh. *144:* 641—670, 1964.

Reese, A. B. & I. S. Jones: Hematomas under the retinal pigment epithelium. Amer. J. Ophthal. *53:* 897—910, 1962.

Schenker, J. G. & G. M. Gombos: Retinal hemorrhage in the newborn. Obstet. and Gynec. *27:* 521—524, 1966.

Diabetic Retinopathy
(Figures 246—275)

Diabetes mellitus is probably that disease in which the most variegated picture of ocular complications or signs may be seen. These include retinopathy, cataract, changes in refraction, optic neuritis, lipemia retinalis, eye muscle palsies, rubeosis iridis and secondary glaucoma.

Diabetic retinopathy—which may be grouped into two main types, the simple and the proliferative retinopathy—is the ocular lesion which occurs most frequently. Like nephropathy, neuropathy, and cardiovascular changes, retinopathy is a late complication in diabetes and part of the diabetic angiopathy.

For many years, the incidence of diabetic retinopathy has been steadily increasing in all age-groups, particularly due to the increased longevity of diabetics since the introduction of insulin therapy.

In juveniles, diabetic retinopathy is never present when diabetes is demonstrated, and it occurs rarely before the age of 16 to 18 years, no matter how long the disease has lasted. In the older diabetics, however, retinopathy may be observed even before diabetes has been recognized clinically, although the diabetic state must have been present for years.

The incidence of retinopathy rises slowly during the first five years of diabetes, and more slowly in the younger age-groups than in the older age-groups. Then follows a sudden rise in incidence, and after about 10 years' duration, the incidence is nearly equal in all age-groups. After at least 15 years' duration, the incidence ranges from about 30 to 80 per cent, being lower in well controlled than in poorly controlled diabetics.

The incidence of diabetic retinopathy of the proliferative type has also shown a steady increase. In large series the incidence ranges from 2 to 8 per cent. Proliferative retinopathy is more frequent in the juvenile and middle-age groups than in the older age-groups. The average duration of diabetes before proliferative retinopathy develops, is 17 to 18 years in the younger age-groups and somewhat less in the older age-groups.

Various attempts have been made to classify diabetic retinopathy into different stages. It seems, however, more reasonable to consider diabetic retinopathy as two main types of retinopathy, the simple and the proliferative types, with a pre-proliferative stage interposed, and to consider the proliferative type not only as a progression of the simple type, but as a condition superimposed on the simple type.

In the proliferative type of diabetic retinopathy, emphasis should be paid to the site of the neovascularization, because new-formed vessels extending from the disc have a poorer prognosis than new-formed vessels occurring in the fundus periphery. Furthermore, attention should be drawn to vitreous detachment associated with neovascularization on the posterior surface of the hyaloid membrane, as such cases usually have a poor visual prognosis.

Of the two main types of diabetic retinopathy, the simple type presents fundus changes such as venous dilatation, retinal microaneurysms, retinal hemorrhages and exudates, sclerosis of the retinal vessels and sometimes sheathing of the vessels. The proliferative type presents formation of new-formed vessels and fibrous tissue in the fundus. The preproliferative stage, which is a warning of transition from the simple to the proliferative type of diabetic retinopathy, is characterized by marked venous changes, preretinal hemorrhages, degenerative changes in the hyaloid membrane, vitreous detachment and vitreous hemorrhage.

Although the retinopathy is still progressive, there is nevertheless a tendency for periodic remissions and exacerbations.

Visual disturbances may be present or not, depending on the size and the localization of the fundus lesions. If the retinal lesions are not localized in or around the macula, vision may remain unaltered for many years, but in cases dominated by confluent exudates in the macular area, vision is often reduced at an early stage. Generally, however, the visual prognosis in simple diabetic retinopathy is fairly good.

When retinopathy proceeds to the preproliferative or proliferative stage, reduction or loss of vision will follow.

In simple diabetic retinopathy, it may be difficult or impossible to evaluate ophthalmoscopically the visual prognosis in the individual cases, but generally the prognosis seems to be better in the older age-groups than in the other age-groups.

In these cases, a determination of the oscillatory potential in the b-wave of the electroretinogram may be of prognostic value. If the oscillatory potential is diminished or abolished, this is a warning

of transition from the simple to the proliferative type of diabetic retinopathy.

In many countries, however, diabetic retinopathy is now the major or one of the most important single causes of blindness.

OPHTHALMOSCOPICALLY, the earliest fundus changes in simple diabetic retinopathy (Figs. 246—249) are mostly situated in the posterior part of the fundus. They consist of scattered microaneurysms, punctate retinal hemorrhages and some venous dilatation. In older diabetics, sharply outlined exudates are also often present in the early stage of retinopathy. In juvenile diabetics, however, they are seldom present at this stage.

Retinal microaneurysms (Figs. 246, 247, 249) are seen ophthalmoscopically as small, round, distinctly outlined, darkred or nearly black spots, often with a central reflex. Their diameter is usually less than one half of the diameter of a large vein. Punctate retinal hemorrhages are seen as rounded red spots, often closely resembling microaneurysms.

In a single ophthalmoscopic examination, it is often difficult to distinguish microaneurysms from deep punctate hemorrhages, but repeated examinations show that microaneurysms remain unchanged for long periods, whereas hemorrhages tend to be absorbed quickly. However, the distinction is easily made by fluorescein angiography, since the aneurysms fluoresce while the hemorrhages do not fluoresce. As new retinal hemorrhages develop and disappear simultaneously, the general ophthalmoscopic picture, however, is often maintained.

Diabetic exudates (Figs. 248—249) consist of minute white or yellowish-white, well-defined flecks, of the same size as microaneurysms or punctate retinal hemorrhages, tending to coalesce into larger irregular patches. In long-standing diabetes, woolly exudates may occur in association with or without hypertension or nephropathy (Figs. 250—251).

As the diabetic retinopathy proceeds, the number of microaneurysms increases, the retinal hemorrhages enlarge in size and number, and superficial retinal hemorrhages sometimes develop. The exudates tend to be more numerous and to coalesce into larger, irregular, white or yellowish-white patches, or into large, glistening, waxy-looking masses, or tend to be arranged in a circinate manner.

In advanced retinopathy, the retinal vessels may show a varying degree of sclerosis and sheathing of the retinal vessels (Figs. 252—253), and the fundus picture is often altered by the presence of hypertensive fundus changes.

The development of proliferative retinopathy is preceded or followed by marked variations in caliber of the retinal veins, often giving the veins an appearance of a string of sausages (Fig. 254), by preretinal hemorrhages (Figs. 255, 258), degenerative changes in the hyaloid membrane (Fig. 257), vitreous detachment (Fig. 256) and vitreous hemorrhage (Fig. 259).

Proliferative diabetic retinopathy is characterized by the formation of new-formed vessels and fibrous tissue in the fundus or by one of these changes only.

The new-formed vessels and fibrous tissue may develop anywhere in the fundus.

OPHTHALMOSCOPICALLY, the new-formed vessels extending from the disc (Figs. 260—266) are seen as small tufts of vessels lying in a delicate stroma and protruding forwards, waving to-and-fro

when the eye is moved, or extending preretinally towards the periphery. When they occur in the fundal periphery (Figs. 267—268), the new-formed vessels lie preretinally in tufts or fan-shaped figures, closely apposed to the retina on the posterior side of the hyaloid membrane. In most instances they retain the position unaltered when the eye is moved, but in vitreous detachment they follow the detached membrane, so that when the eye is moved, they wave to-and-fro.

In the course of time the new-formed vessels may show some atrophy and the delicate supporting stroma of the neovascularization is converted into fibrous tissue. However, new vascular proliferations may often develop at the border of the lesion, and hemorrhages, especially vitreous hemorrhage, may accelerate this process.

Fibrous tissue (Figs. 269—272) is seen as preretinal white or grayish-white veils or membranes, fibrous bands or solid masses, covering smaller or larger areas of the fundus. Following vitreous hemorrhage, fibrous tissue may develop in the vitreous. When the fibrous tissue contracts in the course of time, the retina is detached (Figs. 273—275).

By means of fluorescein angiography it is possible to follow closely the vascular alterations throughout the various stages of diabetic retinopathy.

In the late stage of diabetic retinopathy, rubeosis iridis and hemorrhagic glaucoma may develop. In these cases, the patient often presents a blind and painful eye, calling for excision on account of the pain.

HISTOPATHOLOGICALLY, the characteristic changes in simple diabetic retinopathy consist of microaneurysms, retinal hemorrhages and exudates. The microaneurysms are found on the venous side of the capillary network and mainly in the inner nuclear layer. They are sharply outlined, mulberry-like globules measuring 30 to 90 microns. Their walls are often thickened and contain deposits of hyaline PAS-positive material. The hemorrhages are mainly found in the outer plexiform and nuclear layers. The exudates lie in the same layers as the hemorrhages, and consist of albuminous, hyaline and fatty material. The retinal vessels show a varying degree of arteriolosclerosis, phlebosclerosis, and capillary sclerosis, resulting from deposits of PAS-positive hyaline material in the vessel walls.

The histological picture in proliferative diabetic retinopathy is very complex, showing intraretinal new-formed channels and preretinal or prepapillary networks of new-formed vessels, sometimes piercing the internal limiting membrane and occupying a smaller or larger part of the vitreous. The new-formed vessels are supported in a delicate matrix of connective tissue, often transformed here and there into solid fibrous strands or masses, resulting in retinal detachment.

REFERENCES:

Amalric, P. & G. Coscas: Rétinopathie diabétique. I. Angiographie fluorescéinique dans la rétinopathie diabétique. Arch. Ophtal. (Paris). 27: 553—566, 1967.

Caird, F. I., A. Pirie & T. G. Ramsell: Diabetes and the eye. Blackwell, Oxford. 1969.

Davis, M. D.: Vitreous contraction in proliferative diabetic retinopathy. A.M.A. Arch. Ophthal. 74: 741—751, 1965.

Deckert, T., Sv. E. Simonsen & J. E. Poulsen: Prognosis of proliferative retinopathy in juvenile diabetics. Diabetes. 16: 728—733, 1967.

Dobree, J. H.: Proliferative diabetic retinopathy. Evolution of the retinal lesions. Brit. J. Ophthal. 48: 637—649, 1964.

Dolének, A. & A. Takáč: Atlas der Retinopathia diabetica. Fischer, Stuttgart. 1966.

Ferrer, O.: Two years fluorescein follow-up of diabetic microaneurysms. Ophthalmologica. 154: 6—20, 1967.

Gass, J. D. M.: A fluorescein angiographic study of macular dysfunction secondary to retinal vascular disease. A.M.A. Arch. Ophthal. 80: 535—617, 1968.

Larsen, H.-W.: Atlas of diabetic retinopathy. Acta ophthal. (Kbh.). Suppl. 55, 1959.

Larsen, H.-W.: Diabetic retinopathy. Acta ophthal. (Kbh.). Suppl. 60, 1960.

Lee, P. F.: Clinical and histologic findings in diabetic retinopathy. Amer. J. Ophthal. 65: 688—695, 1968.

Meyer-Schwickerath, G. R. E. & K. Schott: Diabetic retinopathy and photocoagulation. Amer. J. Ophthal. 66: 597—603, 1968.

Norton, E. W. D. & F. Gutman: Diabetic retinopathy studied by fluorescein angiography. Trans. Amer. ophthal. Soc. 63: 108—128, 1965.

Patz, A. & J. W. Berkow: Visual and systemic prognosis in diabetic retinopathy. Trans. Amer. Acad. Ophthal. Otolaryng. 72: 253—258, 1968.

Simonsen, Sv. E.: ERG in diabetics. In François, J. (Ed.): The clinical value of electroretinography. ISCERG symposium Ghent 1966. Karger, Basel. 403—412, 1968.

Tolentino, F. I., P. F. Lee & C. L. Schepens: Biomicroscopic study of vitreous cavity in diabetic retinopathy. A.M.A. Arch. Ophthal. 75: 238—246, 1966.

Unger, H.-H. & J. Unger: Retinale Angiolopathie juveniler Diabetiker. Klin. Monatsbl. Augenh. 150: 644—654, 1967.

Lipemia Retinalis
(Figures 276—277)

Lipemia retinalis is a rare condition due to a marked elevation of the serum lipids, either triglycerides or cholesterol or both. It occurs most often in xanthomatosis and in diabetic acidosis.

OPHTHALMOSCOPICALLY, the fundus (Figs. 276—277) appears slightly indistinct and lighter red than normal, due to a vitreous haze and accumulation of lipids in the retinal tissue. The color of the retinal vessels varies from salmon-pink to almost milky-white, and the vessels sometimes assume a ribbon-like appearance. The vascular light reflex is less brilliant than normal or may even disappear, and sometimes it may be difficult or impossible to distinguish the retinal vessels from the fundus background.

HISTOPATHOLOGICALLY, there is an accumulation of lipid in the retinal vessels and the perivascular tissue.

REFERENCES:

Appelmans, M., J. Michiels, N. de Vloo, L. Jamotton & J.-M. Massa: Lipémie rétinienne chez les diabétiques. Arch. Ophtal. (Paris). *21:* 5—13, 1961.

Ardouin, M., J. Lefranc, M. Simon, G. Le Bihan & J. Bernard: Lipémie rétinienne dans le cadre d'une hypertriglycéridémie dépendante des hydrates de carbone et révélée au cours d'un coma diabétique. Bull. Soc. Ophtal. Fr. *67:* 778—786, 1967.

Cullen, J. F. & W. D. H. Conacher: Idiopathic lipaemia retinalis. Brit. J. Ophthal. *49:* 11—17, 1965.

Laws, H. W. & E. R. Harpur: Lipemia retinalis. A.M.A. Arch. Ophthal. *59:* 521—526, 1958.

Fundus Changes in Anemia
(Figures 278—279)

Fundus changes may occur in all types of anemia, including macrocytic, microcytic and aplastic anemia, when the hemoglobin level falls to 6.0 g/100 ml or below. Evident fundus changes are therefore uncommon in anemia, and are most frequently observed in untreated cases of pernicious anemia.

Vision is not altered unless the macula is involved or optic atrophy develops.

OPHTHALMOSCOPICALLY, the fundus changes (Figs. 278—279) consist of superficial flame-shaped hemorrhages, often with a small fluffy whitish center, small rounded deep retinal hemorrhages, and some cotton-wool exudates. These lesions are mainly located around the disc. The retinal arteries are pale and the veins often dilated. The fundus may show a varying degree of pallor and not infrequently slight edema. The optic disc may be normal or show some pallor. In advanced cases papilledema may be present, and eventually optic atrophy may develop.

It is not possible from the ophthalmoscopic picture to differentiate the various forms of anemia.

REFERENCES:
Kearns, T. P.: Changes in the ocular fundus in blood diseases. Med. Clin. N. Amer. *40:* 1209—1216, 1956.
Marshall, R. A.: A review of lesions in the optic fundus in various diseases of the blood. Blood. *14:* 882—891, 1959.
Massa, J.-M., N. de Vloo & L. Jamotton: Les manifestations oculaires des hemopathies. Bull. Soc. Belge Ophtal. *142:* 1—413, 1966.
Merin, S. & M. Freund: Retinopathy in severe anemia. Amer. J. Ophthal. *66:* 1102—1106, 1968.

Polycythemia
(Figures 280—281)

Polycythemia is a condition characterized by a marked increase of red blood cells. The condition may be primary, as in polycythemia vera, or secondary as in congenital heart disease, severe pulmonary insufficiency or pulmonary vascular sclerosis. Both types, however, cause similar fundus changes.

Visual disturbances may occur as muscae volitantes and scotomas, and profound visual disturbances occur if the condition is complicated by retinal venous occlusion.

OPHTHALMOSCOPICALLY, the fundus in polycythemia (Figs. 280—281) has a deep-red color. The retinal vessels and especially the veins appear engorged and tortuous and the color is darker red than normal. The disc is hyperemic and may show a varying degree of edema. Retinal hemorrhages and exudates are usually absent or few in number, unless retinal venous thrombosis is present.

HISTOPATHOLOGICALLY, the retinal vessels are dilated, retinal hemorrhages may be present, and the optic disc may show a varying degree of edema.

REFERENCES:
Kearns, T. P.: Changes in the ocular fundus in blood diseases. Med. Clin. N. Amer. *40:* 1209—1216, 1956.
Massa, J.-M., N. de Vloo & L. Jamotton: Les manifestations oculaires des hemopathies. Bull. Soc. Belge Ophtal. *142:* 1—413, 1966.

Leukemia
(Figures 97 and 282—283)

All types of leukemia may present fundus lesions. The lesions are indistinguishable from one another and may occur at any stage of the disease, but are seen most frequently in acute leukemia, in late stages of chronic leukemia and in periods of severe anemia.

Visual disturbances occur only when the macula is involved, or when vitreous hemorrhage is present.

OPHTHALMOSCOPICALLY, the fundus lesions (Figs. 282—283) consist of retinal hemorrhages of varying size and shape, and frequently contain a fluffy whitish patch centrally. Whitish woolly exudates or infiltrates of varying size may be present in the posterior part of the fundus. Retinal microaneurysms may also occur. The retinal veins are frequently tortuous and dilated, and sometimes appear like a string of sausages or show pronounced sheathing. The fundus color often remains normal until the late stages, when fundus and retinal vessels become more orange-colored. At times the disc margin is slightly blurred and occasionally more pronounced papilledema is present, especially in children with intracranial leukemic infiltrations (Fig. 97).

The retinal hemorrhages with a pale center are characteristic of leukemia but not pathognomonic, and may also occur in conditions such as severe anemias, including pernicious anemia, and septicemias, including subacute bacterial endocarditis.

HISTOPATHOLOGICALLY, white blood cells may infiltrate the retina and accumulate in the perivascular areas. Hemorrhages and exudates may be present throughout the retina.

REFERENCES:

Allen, R. A. & B. R. Straatsma: Ocular involvement in leukemia and allied disorders. A.M.A. Arch. Ophthal. 66: 490—508, 1961.

Culler, A. M.: Fundus changes in leukemia. Trans. Amer. ophthal. Soc. 49: 445—473, 1951.

Duke, J. R., C. P. Wilkinson & S. Sigelman: Retinal microaneurysms in leukaemia. Brit. J. Ophthal. 52: 368—374, 1968.

Kearns, T. P.: Changes in the ocular fundus in blood diseases. Med. Clin. N. Amer. 40: 1209—1216, 1956.

Mahneke, A. & Å. Videbæk: On changes in the optic fundus in leukaemia. Aetiology, diagnostic and prognostic role. Acta ophthal. (Kbh.). 42: 201—210, 1964.

Marshall, R. A.: A review of lesions in the optic fundus in various diseases of the blood. Blood. 14: 882—891, 1959.

Massa, J.-M., N. de Vloo & L. Jamotton: Les manifestations oculaires des hemopathies. Bull. Soc. Belge Ophtal. 142: 1—413, 1966.

Myelomatosis or Multiple Myeloma
(Figures 99 and 284—287)

Myelomatosis or multiple myeloma is a rare, malignant disease of the reticulo-endothelial system characterized by widespread infiltration of the bone marrow throughout the body. The principal cell type in these infiltrates is the plasma cell.

Neurological symptoms, pain and a very high sedimentation rate are usually present. Hyperproteinemia occurs in many cases, with reversal of the normal albumin-globulin ratio, and paraproteins are often present as well as secondary anemia. In about 50 per cent of the cases, Bence-Jones protein is found in the urine. The skeletal lesions are seen radiologically mainly as round, well-defined bone defects.

Fundus lesions are uncommon. Unless the macula is involved, there are no visual disturbances.

OPHTHALMOSCOPICALLY, the most common lesions (Fig. 284) are superficial retinal hemorrhages and cotton-wool exudates located mainly around the optic disc.

In cases associated with paraproteinemia, the fundus changes may be much more pronounced (Figs. 285—287), showing a similarity with those changes found in macroglobulinemia. The veins are engorged and tortuous, and sometimes appear like a string of sausages. Small and large, rounded or streaky retinal hemorrhages are seen all over the fundus. In some areas the fundus is pale and yellowish due to retinal or subretinal exudation. Papilledema (Fig. 99) may also be present.

REFERENCES:

Danis, P., J. Braumann & P. Coppez: Les lesions du fond d'oeil au cours de certaines hyperproteinemies (Myélome à cryoglobuline, macroglobulinémie). Acta ophthal. (Kbh.). *33:* 33—52, 1955.

Clarke, E.: Ophthalmological complications of multiple myelomatosis. Brit. J. Ophthal. *39:* 233—236, 1955.

Massa, J.-M., N. de Vloo & L. Jamotton: Les manifestations oculaires des hemopathies. Bull. Soc. Belge Ophtal. *142:* 1—413, 1966.

Sanders, T. E., S. M. Podos & L. J. Rosenbaum: Intraocular manifestations of multipe myeloma. A.M.A. Arch. Ophthal. *77:* 789—794, 1967.

Macroglobulinemia (Waldenström)
(Figures 98 and 288—291)

Macroglobulinemia, which belongs to the dys- or paraproteinemias, is a rare, chronic condition characterized by purpura or bleeding from the mucous membranes of the nose and gums, some enlargement of the lymph nodes, and often enlargement of the liver and spleen. Neurological symptoms may sometimes be present.

There is a normochromic anemia and a markedly increased sedimentation rate. The serum is viscous, the total protein content high, the serum albumin lowered and the serum globulins dominated by a component of high-molecular weight, known as macroglobulin or the 20-S component. The platelet adhesivity is zero *in vivo*, but it is normal *in vitro*.

Characteristic fundus changes may occur in the course of the disease, and especially in cases with neurological symptoms.

Visual disturbances may be present or not, depending on the site and extension of the fundus lesions. When the lesions are extensive, secondary glaucoma may develop.

OPHTHALMOSCOPICALLY, the fundus lesions are characterized by venous changes, retinal hemorrhages, microaneurysms (Figs. 288—291), retinal or subretinal exudation, and sometimes by papilledema (Fig. 98).

The retinal veins are engorged and tortuous. Localized venous constrictions are often present, in some places giving the veins an appearance resembling a string of beads or sausages. Small or large, rounded and streaky retinal hemorrhages are seen all over the fundus but often most numerous in the fundus periphery. Clusters of small red dots, probably accumulations of microaneurysms, are often seen as red patches together with the hemorrhages. In some areas the fundus may be pale and yellowish due to retinal or subretinal exudation (Fig. 98). Fluffy exudates, however, are not characteristic. Papilledema often occurs in cases with involvement of the central nervous system.

Similar fundus changes may occur in cryoglobulinemia and other paraproteinemias.

The condition should not be confused with occlusion of the central retinal vein or diabetic retinopathy.

HISTOPATHOLOGICALLY, the veins are dilated and the retina presents hemorrhages and microaneurysms. Retinal and subretinal exudates may also be present, and the optic disc may show varying degrees of edema.

REFERENCES:

Ashton, N., D' A. Kok & W. S. Foulds: Ocular pathology in macroglobulinaemia. J. Path. Bact. *86:* 453—461, 1963.

Cagianut, B.: Le syndrome oculaire de la macroglobulinémie (Syndrome de Waldenström). Ann. Oculist (Paris). *191:* 579—591, 1958.

Carr, R. E. & P. Henkind: Retinal findings associated with serum hyperviscosity. Amer. J. Ophthal. *56:* 23—31, 1963.

Gates, R. F. & R. D. Richards: Macroglobulin-emia with unusual vascular changes. A.M.A. Arch. Ophthal. *64:* 77—80, 1960.

Massa, J.-M., N. de Vloo & L. Jamotton: Les manifestations oculaires des hemopathies. Bull. Soc. Belge Ophtal. *142:* 1—413, 1966.

Paufique, L. & J. Royer: Les signes oculaires des dysprotéinémies. Ann. Oculist (Paris). *192:* 721—735, 1959.

Rosen, E. S., A. V. Simmons & T. W. Warnes: Retinopathy of Waldenström's macroglobulinemia. Photographic assessment. Amer. J. Ophthal. *65:* 696—706, 1968.

Collagen Diseases

(Figures 292—293)

The collagen diseases are a group of diseases characterized by widespread alteration of the ground substance resulting in fibrinoid necrosis. These diseases are probably related to hypersensitivity or autoimmunity.

Cutaneous eruptions, joint pain, low-grade fever and hypertension are some of the characteristic clinical symptoms.

Among the collagen diseases, fundus changes are most often observed in polyarteritis nodosa, disseminated lupus erythematosus, dermatomyositis, scleroderma and anaphylactoid purpura, while fundus changes have not been observed in conditions such as rheumatic fever and rheumatoid arthritis.

Visual disturbances do not occur unless the macula is involved.

OPHTHALMOSCOPICALLY, the fundus changes are characterized (Figs. 292—293) by more or less numerous fluffy exudates of varying size and sometimes superficial retinal hemorrhages, both located around the disc and in the posterior pole. Hypertensive fundus changes and vascular occlusions may alter the ophthalmoscopic picture. Thus, the ophthalmoscopic appearance is not pathognomonic in any of these diseases.

HISTOPATHOLOGICALLY, the conditions are characterized by inflammatory changes in the vessel walls, cytoid bodies and superficial retinal hemorrhages.

REFERENCES:

Böke, W. & A. Bäumer: Klinische und histopathologische Augenbefunde beim akuten Lupus erythematodes disseminatus. Klin. Monatsbl. Augenh. *146:* 175—187, 1965.

Dubois, E. L. & D. L. Tuffanelli: Clinical manifestations of systemic lupus erythematosus. J.A.M.A. *190:* 104—111, 1964.

Goder, G.: Vaskuläre Augenveränderungen bei der generalisierten Sklerodermie. Klin. Monatsbl. Augenh. *144:* 370—383, 1964,

Hollenhorst, R. W. & J. W. Henderson: The ocular manifestations of the diffuse collagen diseases. Amer. J. med. Sci. *221:* 211—222, 1951.

Jütte, A.: Über Augenhintergrundsveränderungen beim akuten Lupus erythematodes visceralis. Klin. Monatsbl. Augenh. *137:* 765—772, 1960.

Munro, S.: Fundus appearances in a case of acute dermatomyositis. Brit. J. Ophthal. *43:* 548—558, 1959.

Pollack, I. P. & B. Becker: Cytoid bodies of the retina. In a patient with scleroderma. Amer. J. Ophthal. *54:* 655—660, 1962.

Vancea, P., Gh. Popa, V. Vaighel & L. Gavrilita: Périartérite noueuse a localisation oculaire. Ann. Oculist (Paris). *195:* 632—651, 1962.

Choroideremia
(Figures 294—295)

Choroideremia is a rare tapeto-choroidal dystrophy inherited in an intermediate sex-linked manner, presenting a progressive dystrophy in males and a non-progressive dystrophy in females.

In affected males the earliest and most prominent symptom is night blindness, which usually becomes evident during childhood and is later followed by a concentric contraction of the visual field. Central vision usually remains good until the age of about 40 years. After that time, central vision becomes gradually reduced. The electroretinographic response shows a gradual reduction and finally becomes extinguished.

Female carriers show no visual disturbances and visual fields and dark adaption remain normal.

OPHTHALMOSCOPICALLY, fundus changes in the affected males are seen in the earliest stage as a salt-and-pepper configuration. When this pigmentary atrophy progresses, the choroidal vessels become exposed in wide areas, but simultaneously the choroidal vessels show a progressive disappearance. When fully developed (Figs. 294—295), there is only a central patch of choroidal tissue left in the macular area while elsewhere the atrophic choroid is exposed, and small pigment deposits are scattered throughout the fundus. The optic disc remains normal, while the retinal vessels show some narrowing.

The condition should not be confused with primary choroidal atrophy.

In female carriers the ophthalmoscopic changes are limited to the peripheral salt-and-pepper configuration seen in the early stages of the affected males.

HISTOPATHOLOGICALLY, in the late stage the choroid, pigment epithelium and rods and cones are completely absent except in the macular area.

REFERENCES:

Franceschetti, A., J. François & J. Babel: Les hérédo-dégénérescences chorio-rétiniennes. Masson, Paris. 729, 1963.

François, J., J. de Brabandere & L. Stockmans: Choroïdérémie (dégénérescence chorio-rétinienne progressive). Bull. Soc. Belge Ophtal. *146:* 384—400, 1967.

Harris, G. S. & J. R. Miller: Choroideremia. Visual defects in a heterozygote. A.M.A. Arch. Ophthal. *80:* 423—429, 1968.

McCulloch, J. C.: The pathologic findings in two cases of choroideremia. Trans. Amer. Acad. Ophthal. Otolaryng. *54:* 565—572, 1950.

Rubin, M. L., R. S. Fishman & R. A. McKay: Choroideremia. Study of a family and literature review. A.M.A. Arch. Ophthal. *76:* 563—574, 1966.

Sorsby, A., A. Franceschetti, R. Joseph & J. B. Davey: Choroideremia. Clinical and genetic aspects. Brit. J. Ophthal. *36:* 547—581, 1952.

Straub, W.: Das Elektroretinogramm. Klin. Monatsbl. Augenh. *Suppl. 36:* 126, 1961.

Gyrate Atrophy of the Choroid and Retina
(Figures 296—297)

Gyrate atrophy is a rare, slowly progressive, heredodegenerative chorioretinal disease affecting both sexes equally.

The symptoms may commence during childhood or early adult life. The first symptom is usually the observation of night blindness, which is later followed by a progressive contraction of the visual field and a progressive reduction of vision. A progressive myopia is frequently present in these cases.

In early stages, the electroretinographic response is normal, later it becomes subnormal and finally extinguished.

OPHTHALMOSCOPICALLY, the condition usually commences in the fundal periphery with irregular or rounded, well-defined, more or less confluent areas of chorioretinal atrophy. As the condition progresses, wide areas of the fundus may be involved (Figs. 296—297), but the macula is usually spared. In the atrophic areas the exposed sclera has a whitish or yellowish-white color, the choroidal vessels are practically absent, and scattered clumps of retinal pigment are seen plainly. The retinal vessels appear normal or slightly contracted.

In the final stage the ophthalmoscopic appearance resembles to some extent that in choroideremia. Gyrate atrophy of the choroid must not be confused with primary choroidal atrophy.

REFERENCES:

Collier, M.: L'atrophie gyrée de la chorio-rétine et ses relations syndromiques. Bull. Soc. Ophtal. Fr. *62:* 163—167, 1962.

Franceschetti, A., J. François & J. Babel: Les hérédo-dégénérescences chorio-rétiniennes. Masson, Paris. 647, 1963.

François, J., F. Barbier & A. de Rouck: Les conducteurs du gène de l'Atrophia Gyrata Chorioideae et Retinae de Fuchs. (Anomalie d'Alder). Bull. Soc. Belge Ophtal. *122:* 367—382, 1959.

Gillespie, F. D.: Gyrate atrophy of choroid and retina. Amer. J. Ophthal. *57:* 317—320, 1964.

Straub, W.: Das Elektroretinogramm. Klin. Monatsbl. Augenh. *Suppl. 36:* 126, 1961.

Sæbø, J.: Atrophia gyrata chorioideae et retinae. Brit. J. Ophthal. *32:* 824—847, 1948.

Retinitis Pigmentosa
(Figures 298—301)

Retinitis pigmentosa or pigmentary retinal dystrophy is a degenerative disease of the retina, commencing in the retinal neuroepithelium, particularly in the rods.

The condition is characterized by widespread pigmentary changes in the retina, narrowing of the retinal vessels, optic atrophy, and is associated with night blindness and constriction of the visual fields. The electroretinographic response is markedly subnormal or completely extinguished at an early stage, while central vision becomes reduced in the late stage.

The disease is progressive and bilateral. A hereditary tendency is observed in about two-thirds of the cases, and in the majority of these the inheritance is recessive. The two sexes are affected almost equally. However, the condition may occur rarely in a sex-linked form. The incidence of retinitis pigmentosa is estimated at about five per 1,000 individuals.

The first symptom is night blindness, commonly noticed in childhood. As the disease progresses, a ring scotoma is produced, which increases gradually in a central and peripheral direction until it involves the whole peripheral field. Finally, the visual field shows a marked constriction, so that only tubular vision remains. When the visual field is reduced to about 10°, central vision also becomes markedly diminished.

The disease runs a variable course, but considerable disturbance of vision usually occurs in the thirties, leading to practical blindness in the forties and fifties.

The condition is often associated with myopia, and cataract frequently develops in the course of the disease.

Ophthalmoscopically, there are no visible fundus changes in the early stages, but the electroretinographic response is markedly subnormal or completely extinguished. The earliest retinal changes are seen as scattered accumulations of dark-brown or black pigment, assuming a bone corpuscle configuration (Figs. 298—301). The initial pigment changes occur at the equator and progress towards the periphery and the macular area. The amount of pigment gradually increases, and in advanced cases pigment deposits are also arranged around the retinal vessels, the pigment sheathing of which becomes a characteristic feature of the disease. Depigmented areas are left in which the choroidal vessels are seen plainly. The retinal vessels show a marked narrowing (Fig. 301), and this may appear even before obvious pigmentary changes are present. The optic disc shows a progressive pallor and assumes a grayish or yellowish-gray color (Fig. 301). In the advanced stage, the macula may assume a moth-eaten appearance (Fig. 301).

In the typical case the diagnosis is not difficult. Atypical cases may occur, however, with little or no pigment, abnormal pigment distribution or sectorial pigment accumulation. Even unilateral cases may occur. In all those cases the diagnosis is confirmed by the abnormal electroretinographic response. The condition must be distinguished from other degenerative fundus diseases, and also from disseminated choroiditis.

HISTOPATHOLOGICALLY, the condition is characterized by a disappearance of the retinal neuroepithelial cells, at first the rods and later the cones. Glial cells and pigment epithelium proliferate, and cellular strands of pigment epithelium migrate into the retinal tissue and frequently accumulate around the retinal vessels. The vessels show thickening of their walls and a diminished lumen. In the optic nerve the nerve fibers are often replaced by glial tissue, and a glial membrane is sometimes formed in front of the optic disc. The inner retinal layers rarely show severe changes until a late stage of the disease.

REFERENCES:

Duke-Elder, S. & J. H. Dobree: System of ophthalmology. *Vol. X.* Kimpton, London. 577, 1967.

Franceschetti, A., J. François & J. Babel: Les hérédo-dégénérescences chorio-rétiniennes. Masson, Paris. 212, 1963.

Hogan, M. J. & L. E. Zimmerman (Ed.): Ophthalmic pathology. *2nd ed.* Saunders, Philadelphia. 543, 1962.

Straub, W.: Das Elektroretinogramm. Klin. Monatsbl. Augenh. *Suppl. 36:* 109, 1961.

Sunga, R. N. & L. L. Sloan: Pigmentary degeneration of the retina: Early diagnosis and natural history. Invest. Ophthal. *6:* 309—325, 1967.

Retinitis Punctata Albescens
(Figures 302—305)

Retinitis punctata albescens or albipunctate dystrophy is a rare heredofamilial disease characterized by innumerable small white dots scattered over the fundus and associated with night blindness.

The condition occurs in a stationary and a progressive form.

The stationary form commences in childhood with night blindness, but vision, visual fields, color sense and usually also electroretinographic response remain normal.

OPHTHALMOSCOPICALLY, the fundus shows a multitude of minute white dots diffusely scattered in the fundus, leaving the macular area free. The disc and retinal vessels appear normal.

In the progressive form, night blindness is present from childhood. The visual fields show a progressive contraction and central vision gradually deteriorates.

The electroretinographic response is subnormal or extinguished.

OPHTHALMOSCOPICALLY, the progressive form, like the stationary form, shows a multitude of minute white dots scattered in the fundus (Figs. 302—303, 305), but small pigment deposits (Fig. 303) often showing a bone corpuscle configuration may also be present. The retinal vessels show some narrowing and the optic disc some pallor (Fig. 304). At times the macular area is involved (Fig. 304), showing depigmentation and pigment accumulation.

REFERENCES:

Franceschetti, A., J. François & J. Babel: Les hérédo-dégénérescences chorio-rétiniennes. Masson, Paris. 283, 1963.

Krill, A. E. & B. A. Klien: Flecked retina syndrome. A.M.A. Arch. Ophthal. 74: 496—508, 1965.

Tamai, A., T. Setogawa & F. Kandori: Electroretinographic studies on retinitis punctata albescens. Amer. J. Ophthal. 62: 125—131, 1966.

Fundus Flavimaculatus
(Figures 306—307)

Fundus flavimaculatus is a rare, possibly congenital condition characterized by white or yellowish-white, irregular patches in the fundus, confined to the posterior pole and often associated with degenerative changes at the macula.

Vision may be normal, but if the macula is involved central vision decreases. The visual fields are usually normal and the condition is seldom associated with night blindness. The electroretinographic response is usualy normal or subnormal.

OPHTHALMOSCOPICALLY, the condition is characterized (Figs. 306—307) by small or large, irregular, yellow or yellowish-white patches or lines mainly confined to the posterior pole. The macula may show degenerative changes, but the retinal vessels and the optic disc are normal.

In juvenile heredomacular degeneration (Figs. 324—325), fundus changes may occasionally occur similar to those seen in fundus flavimaculatus.

REFERENCES:
Amalric, P., H. Kment & H. Remky: Fundus flavimaculatus. Klin. Monatsbl. Augenh. *150:* 625—636, 1967.
Brown, N. & D. W. Hill: Fundus flavimaculatus. Two familial cases with macular degeneration. Brit. J. Ophthal. *52:* 849—852, 1968.
Franceschetti, A., J. François & J. Babel: Les hérédo-dégénérescences chorio-rétiniennes. Masson, Paris. 426, 1963.
Klien, B. A. & A. E. Krill: Fundus flavimaculatus. Clinical, functional and histopathologic observations. Amer. J. Ophthal. *64:* 2—23, 1967.

Amaurotic Family Idiocy
(Figures 308—313)

Amaurotic family idiocy is a rare, recessive, familial disease belonging to the lipoidoses. It is characterized by degenerative changes in the retina and the central nervous system and accumulation of gangliosides in the ganglion cells in the central nervous system as well as in the retina.

It occurs in two types, the infantile, known as Tay-Sachs' disease and the juvenile, known as Spielmeyer-Vogt, Spielmeyer-Stock or Batten-Mayou's disease.

THE INFANTILE TYPE, which is predominant among Jews, commences during the first year of life. It is rapidly progressive and death occurs usually within one or two years. It is characterized by the lack of mental development, progressive muscular weakness, paralyses, convulsions and rapidly developing blindness. The electroretinogram, however, is normal.

OPHTHALMOSCOPICALLY, both foveae are surrounded in the early stage by an opaque, whitish zone, not unlike that seen in central retinal artery occlusion, and the foveae are seen as cherry-red spots (Fig. 308). The disc and the retinal vessels appear normal. Later, however, the opacification clears somewhat, the cherry-red spots become less distinct, the discs atrophic and the retinal vessels narrow.

The condition should not be confused with occlusion of the central retinal artery, and it is distinguished from Niemann-Pick's disease and Gaucher's disease by the general clinical symptoms.

HISTOPATHOLOGICALLY, there is diffuse lipoidal degeneration of the cytoplasm of the ganglion cells of the retina and the central nervous system, and the ganglion cells are PAS-positive and contain gangliosides.

In Niemann-Pick's disease, which is a rare congenital condition belonging to the lipoidoses and characterized by widespread deposits of sphingomyelin and possibly cerebrosides in the retina, the central nervous system and the viscera, particularly the liver and spleen, fundus changes may occur (Fig. 309) similar to those described in Tay-Sachs' disease, although not as frequently as in the latter disease.

A similar ophthalmoscopic picture has been described in Gaucher's disease, which also belongs to the lipoidoses and is characterized by the accumulation of cerebrosides, mainly in the reticulo-endothelial system.

THE JUVENILE TYPE of amaurotic family idiocy, also belonging to the lipoidoses and usually showing a recessive, familial character, often commences before or at puberty. It is more slowly progressive than the infantile type. Symptoms usually start with a progressive loss of vision, later followed by mental deterioration and neurological symptoms in the form of progressive dementia and apathy, epileptiform attacks, ataxy, rigidity, and tremor. The electroretinographic response is extinguished already in the early stage. Death usually occurs about the age of 18 years.

OPHTHALMOSCOPICALLY, the fundus lesion is seen in the early stage as a small white spot in the fovea, while the optic disc and the retinal vessels are normal. The white spot is subsequently transformed into a larger pigmented spot, which is usually surrounded by a red halo (Fig. 310). As the disease progresses, the disc becomes pale and atrophic (Fig. 311), the retinal vessels narrow (Fig. 312), and the macular lesions increase in size. Depigmentation and fine pigmentations are seen in both maculae (Fig. 312) and in the periphery (Fig. 313) of the fundi. At times, a number of fine whitish branching streaks radiate from the macula, but cherry-red spots or whitish zones in the maculae, as seen in the infantile type, do not occur.

The condition is easily distinguished from heredomacular degeneration and central choroiditis by the electroretinographic response, which is subnormal or extinguished in the juvenile form of amaurotic idiocy.

HISTOPATHOLOGICALLY, the retinal lesions are characterized by degeneration of the rods and cones and the pigment epithelium, simultaneous lipoidal degeneration of the ganglion cells, and glial proliferation.

In the central nervous system the changes are of the same type as in the infantile form, but in the juvenile type the affection is milder and unevenly distributed.

In the juvenile type of amaurotic family idiocy, vacuolated lymphocytes may occur as in Niemann-Pick's disease and in different acute infective conditions. Vacuolated lymphocytes, however, are not present in the infantile form of amaurotic family idiocy.

REFERENCES:

Anderson, B., G. Margolis & W. S. Lynn: Ocular lesions related to disturbances in fat metabolism. Amer. J. Ophthal. 45 (April—Part II): 23—41, 1958.

Bergaust, B.: Juvenile amaurotic idiocy. Acta ophthal. (Kbh.). 40: 202—205, 1962.

Cogan, D. G. & T. Kuwabara: The sphingolipidoses and the eye. A.M.A. Arch. Ophthal. 79: 437—452, 1968.

Copenhaver, R. M. & G. Goodman: The electroretinogram in infantile, late infantile, and juvenile amaurotic family idiocy. A.M.A. Arch. Ophthal. 63: 559—566, 1960.

Danis, P., C. Bégaux & G. Decock: Bases ophtalmologiques d'une classification des idioties amaurotiques. J. Génét. hum. 6: 91—155, 1957.

Franceschetti, A., J. François & J. Babel: Les hérédo-dégénérescences chorio-rétiniennes. Masson, Paris. 907, 1963.

Gartner, S. & M. Bronstein: Infantile cerebroretinal lipidosis (Tay-Sachs disease). A.M.A. Arch. Ophthal. 59: 584—589, 1958.

Larsen, H.-W. & N. Ehlers: Ocular manifestations in Tay-Sachs' and Niemann-Pick's diseases. Acta ophthal. (Kbh.). 43: 285—293, 1965.

Manschot, W. A.: Retinal histology in amaurotic idiocies and tapeto-retinal degenerations. Ophthalmologica. 156: 28—37, 1968.

Heredomacular Degeneration

(Figures 314—325)

Heredomacular degeneration is a slowly progressive, often bilateral, degenerative condition affecting the macula. Although cases may occur without any family history, there is usually a strong family incidence, and the inheritance is most frequently recessive.

Heredomacular degeneration may start at any age. According to the age of onset, the condition can be grouped into the following types: infantile (Best's type), juvenile (Stargardt's type), adult (Behr's type), presenile and senile. Most frequently, however, the condition appears in childhood or at puberty.

The principle complaint is a gradual, usually bilateral diminution of central vision. There is a relative or absolute central scotoma, the extent of which depends on the size of the macular lesion. The peripheral visual field is intact and the electroretinogram is normal. There are, however, no general symptoms.

OPHTHALMOSCOPICALLY, the infantile type commences as a vitelliform disc or cyst which is indistinguishable from a congenital vitelline macular cyst (Figs. 28—29). The evolution of the lesion is exceedingly slow. Finally, the lesion is converted into an atrophic scar with or without pigmentation.

OPHTHALMOSCOPICALLY, in the juvenile and adult type, the macular changes commence with a slight irregularity in pigmentation and are followed by some depigmentation and fine clumping of pigment.

At the early stage, a small whitish spot is frequently present in the fovea (Figs. 316—317), surrounded by a red halo, and fine whitish branching lines may radiate from the fovea (Figs. 314—315). This small whitish spot later disappears. Fully developed (Figs. 318—325), the macular degeneration is seen as a sharply demarcated, round or oval, reddish-brown or deep-red, often worm-eaten area measuring from one half to two disc diameters. Varying amounts of fine and coarse pigment deposits and depigmentations are situated in the macular lesion. Finally, the lesion may sometimes be surrounded by whitish patches resembling those seen in fundus flavimaculatus (Figs. 324—325).

The foveal reflex is absent from the onset, and the macular reflex disappears later. Occasionally, fine pigment accumulations are seen in the fundus periphery, but elsewhere the fundi appear normal. The optic discs and retinal vessels are normal.

The condition is in the early stage distinguished from the juvenile form of amaurotic family idiocy by the lack of electroretinographic changes, and later by differences in the ophthalmoscopic picture and a lack of general symptoms.

The condition must not be confused with central choroiditis.

In the presenile and senile type, the macular lesions closely resemble those seen in senile macular degeneration.

HISTOPATHOLOGICALLY, there is degeneration of the neuroepithelium in the affected area, and degeneration and some proliferation of the retinal pigment epithelium.

REFERENCES:

Biró, I.: Die Umbildung der zentralen Netzhautdegenerationen und die "Cysta vitelliformis". Klin. Monatsbl. Augenh. *153:* 363—370, 1968.

Blodi, F. C.: The pathology of central tapetoretinal dystrophy (hereditary macular degenerations). Trans. Amer. Acad. Ophthal. Otolaryng. *70:* 1047—1053, 1966.

Braley, A. E.: Dystrophy of the macula. Amer. J. Ophthal. *61:* 1—24, 1966.

Falls, H. F.: A classification and clinical description of hereditary macular lesions. Trans. Amer. Acad. Ophthal. Otolaryng. *70:* 1034—1046, 1966.

Franceschetti, A., J. François & J. Babel: Les hérédo-dégénérescences chorio-rétiniennes. Masson, Paris. 436, 464, 477, 1963.

François, J.: Vitelliform degeneration of the macula. Bull. N.Y. Acad. Med. *44:* 18—27, 1968.

François, J., G. Verriest & A. de Rouck: Hérédodégénérescence maculaire juvénile avec atteinte prédominante de la vision photopique. Ann. Oculist (Paris). *195:* 1137—1191, 1962.

Krill, A. E., P. A. Morse, A. M. Potts & B. A. Klien: Hereditary vitelliruptive macular degeneration. Amer. J. Ophthal. *61:* 1405—1415, 1966.

Remky, H., J. Rix & K. F. Klier: Dominantautosomale Maculadegeneration (Best, Sorsby) mit zystischen und vitelliformen Stadien (Huysmans, Zanen). Klin. Monatsbl. Augenh. *146:* 473—497, 1965.

Straub, W.: Das Elektroretinogramm. Klin. Monatsbl. Augenh. *Suppl. 36:* 153, 1961.

Toxic Macular Degeneration

(Figures 326—331)

Toxic macular degeneration with pigmentary changes may be the result of various toxic substances or drugs, particularly tranquilizers such as chlorpromazine and thioridazine, and antimalarials such as chloroquine and its derivatives.

Visual disturbances may occur together with central, pericentral or paracentral scotomas, and the visual field may show concentric contraction.

Ophthalmoscopically, the macular area shows in the early stage a fine diffuse mottling, pigment clumping, depigmentation (Figs. 328—329) or a small hemorrhage. The condition is sometimes associated with slight edema in the adjacent area (Figs. 330—331). Later, a pale ring may surround the fovea to form a ring-shaped lesion (Figs. 326—327) called "bull's eye", or the lesion shows some pigment clumping. Pigmentary changes may also develop in the periphery. The retinal vessels may show a varying degree of contraction, and finally the optic disc may become atrophic.

References:

Alkemade, P. P. H.: Phenothiazine-retinopathy. Ophthalmologica. *155:* 70—76, 1968.

Burns, C. A.: Indomethacin, reduced retinal sensitivity, and corneal deposits. Amer. J. Ophthal. *66:* 824—835, 1968.

Böke, W., A. Bäumer, W. Müller-Limmroth & M. Mludek: Zur Frage der Chloroquinschädigungen des Auges. Klin. Monatsbl. Augenh. *151:* 617—633, 1967.

Carlberg, O.: Three cases of choroquine retinopathy. A follow-up investigation. Acta ophthal. (Kbh.). *44:* 367—374, 1966.

Carr, R. E., P. Henkind, N. Rothfield & I. M. Siegel: Ocular toxicity of antimalarial drugs. Long-term follow-up. Amer. J. Ophthal. *66:* 738—744, 1968.

Henkind, P., R. E. Carr & I. M. Siegel: Early chloroquine retinopathy: Clinical and functional findings. A.M.A. Arch. Ophthal. *71:* 157—165, 1964.

Kearns, T. P. & R. W. Hollenhorst: Chloroquine retinopathy. Evaluation by fluorescein fundus angiography. A.M.A. Arch. Ophthal. *76:* 378—384, 1966.

Lawwill, T., B. Appleton & L. Altstatt: Chloroquine accumulation in human eyes. Amer. J. Ophthal. *65:* 530—532, 1968.

Meier-Ruge, W.: Medikamentöse Retinopathie. Thieme, Stuttgart. 1967.

Nylander, U.: Ocular damage in chloroquine therapy. Acta ophthal. (Kbh.). *Suppl. 92,* 1967.

Shearer, R. V. & E. L. Dubois: Ocular changes induced by long-term hydroxychloroquine (Plaquenil) therapy. Amer. J. Ophthal. *64:* 245—252, 1967.

Senile Macular Degeneration
(Figures 332—341)

Senile macular degeneration is a condition resulting from vascular sclerosis, and it may often be closely related to senile disciform macular degeneration. At times, the process starts as senile macular degeneration and ends as disciform degeneration. Sometimes the former is seen in one eye and the latter in the other eye. Bilateral occurrence is frequent, although the degree of involvement may differ in the two eyes.

Senile macular degeneration occurs most frequently in the sixties and later.

Frequently, there is no correlation between the apparent extent of the fundus lesions and the degree of the visual disturbances. Central vision may either be normal or severely reduced, and reduction of vision may commence slowly or develop within a few days. Once developed, the visual disturbances are permanent.

OPHTHALMOSCOPICALLY, senile macular degeneration is seen at the early stage as fine pigment accumulation and depigmentation in the macular area (Figs. 332—333). In the course of months or years, the depigmented atrophic spots become enlarged and there may be a varying amount of pigment accumulation (Figs. 334—336). Frequently, the condition is accompanied by few or numerous, small or large colloid bodies (Figs. 337—341) in and around the macular area. In the latter case, the condition closely resembles the fundus lesion described as Doyne's honeycomb choroiditis or dystrophy.

The retinal vessels show a varying degree of sclerosis. The optic disc is normal and retinal hemorrhages are not characteristic.

HISTOPATHOLOGICALLY, the macular changes are characterized by depigmentation and atrophy of the retinal pigment cells, isolated pigment cell proliferation and degenerative changes in the layers of rods and cones. There are degenerative changes in Bruch's membrane, often associated with colloid bodies, and sclerosis and some atrophy of the choroidal vessels in the macular area.

REFERENCES:
Braley, A. E.: Dystrophy of the macula. Amer. J. Ophthal. *61:* 1—24, 1966.
Franceschetti, A., J. François & J. Babel: Les hérédo-dégénérescences chorio-rétiniennes. Masson, Paris. 518, 1963.
Klien, B. A.: Some aspects of classification and differential diagnosis of senile macular degeneration. Amer. J. Ophthal. *58:* 927—939, 1964.
Pearce, W. G.: Doyne's honeycomb retinal degeneration. Brit. J. Ophthal. *52:* 73—78, 1968.

Cystoid Degeneration of the Macula
(Figures 342—343)

Cystoid degeneration of the macula, just as cystoid degeneration in the fundal periphery, is due to a degenerative process with formation of small cystic cavities in the internuclear layer of the retina.

The condition occurs most often in old people, and visual disturbances may vary widely, from practically no complaints to the occurrence of a central scotoma.

OPHTHALMOSCOPICALLY, the lesion may be difficult to recognize in the early stage where small irregular reflexes may be the only sign of the condition. Later, however, the degeneration gives the macula a honeycombed appearance. Finally, a larger cystic cavity (Fig. 342) may be formed in the macula by coalescence of the small cystic spaces. If the anterior wall of this cystic cavity ruptures, it gives rise to a lamellar macular hole (Fig. 343). The distinction between a cystic cavity and a hole may be difficult in ordinary ophthalmoscopy, but is easily distinguished by using a slit-lamp together with a Hruby lens. The retinal vessels show a varying degree of sclerosis, and the optic disc is normal.

In cystoid macular degeneration, a lamellar macular hole very seldom gives rise to retinal detachment.

HISTOPATHOLOGICALLY, the condition is seen as cystoid spaces especially in the internuclear retinal layer, and is associated with some retinal degeneration. At times, the fovea presents a large cystic cavity or even a lamellar retinal hole. The underlying choroid usually shows sclerotic changes.

REFERENCES:

Busacca, A., H. Goldmann & S. Schiff-Wertheimer: Biomicroscopie du corps vitré et du fond de l'oeil. Masson, Paris. 196, 1957.

Favre, M.: Trou dans la macula et décollement de la rétine. Ophthalmologica. *140:* 94—98, 1960.

Franceschetti, A., J. François & J. Babel: Les hérédo-dégénérescences chorio-rétiniennes. Masson, Paris. 787, 1963.

Hruby, K. & A. Posner: Slitlamp examination of vitreous and retina. Williams & Wilkins, Baltimore. 98, 1967.

Marsol, C. & J. Bouchat: Le trou maculaire. Arch. Ophtal. (Paris). 27: 387—396, 1967.

Slezak, H.: Über loch- und cystenähnliche Befunde des hinteren Augenspols. Graefes Arch. Ophth. *173:* 168—174, 1967.

Primary Choroidal Atrophy
(Figures 344—349)

Primary choroidal atrophy is a degenerative condition showing a heredofamilial tendency and characterized by choroidal atrophy and degenerative changes in the retina. The condition can be divided into three separate entities, central areolar choroidal atrophy, peripapillary choroidal atrophy and diffuse choroidal atrophy.

Central areolar choroidal atrophy
(Figs. 344—347).

Central areolar choroidal atrophy, which is usually bilateral, occurs most frequently in middle-aged or older persons, but may already become evident at ages between 20 and 40 years.

Central vision may be severely reduced in early stages. However, central vision is often only slightly impaired in the early stage, but shows progressive diminution. When central vision is decreased, there is a central scotoma of varying extension but the peripheral field is intact.

OPHTHALMOSCOPICALLY, the early lesion is seen in the macular area as an ill-defined, sometimes irregular patch with retinal pigment atrophy and exposure of the choroidal vessels (Figs. 344—345). Sometimes slight edema and small hemorrhages may also be present. The fully developed macular lesion (Figs. 346—347) is well-defined, oval or round, measuring from one to four disc diameters. The affected area is whitish or yellowish-white due to choroidal atrophy. The choroidal vessels are diminished in number and the remaining vessels are sclerosed. Retinal pigment is nearly absent in the affected area.

Peripapillary choroidal atrophy
(Fig. 348).

Peripapillary choroidal atrophy usually occurs in middle-aged or older persons.

The fundal lesion produces a visual field defect, and if the macula is also involved there is a central scotoma, but the peripheral field remains intact.

OPHTHALMOSCOPICALLY, the lesion (Fig. 348) is seen as an ill-defined area with exposure of the atrophic choroid and sclerosed choroidal vessels, together with some pigment clumping. At first, the lesion is located around the optic disc, but later it may also involve the macular area.

Diffuse choroidal atrophy
(Fig. 349).

Diffuse choroidal atrophy usually occurs in middle-aged persons, but is not infrequently seen already in the thirties.

Visual symptoms may be absent in the early stages, while later the visual fields usually show a progressive contraction. If the macular area is involved, central vision is markedly reduced. Night blindness is often present and the electroretinographic response is subnormal or even extinguished.

OPHTHALMOSCOPICALLY, there is a more or less diffuse exposure of the choroidal vessels (Fig. 349), seen as a network of grayish or grayish-white lines, and between these lines the fundus has assumed a grayish or grayish-brown color. Small or large irregular masses of pigment clumping are often present in the equatorial region. The optic disc and the retinal vessels usually appear normal.

Primary choroidal atrophy should not be confused with choroideremia or gyrate choroidal atrophy.

REFERENCES:

Brooser, G. & G. Uzonyi: Verwendung der Fluoreszein-Angiographie bei der Diagnose der primären Chorioideasklerose. Klin. Monatsbl. Augenh. *152:* 219—225, 1968.

Carr, R. E.: Central areolar choroidal dystrophy. A.M.A. Arch. Ophthal. *73:* 32—35, 1965.

Franceschetti, A., J. François & J. Babel: Les hérédo-dégénérescences chorio-rétiniennes. Masson, Paris. 627, 1963.

Howard, G. M. & E. Wolf: Central choroidal sclerosis. A clinical and pathological study. Trans. Amer. Acad. Ophthal. Otolaryng. *68:* 647—660, 1964.

McKay, R. A. & B. E. Spivey: Generalized choroidal angiosclerosis. A.M.A. Arch. Ophthal. *67:* 727—735, 1962.

Sandvig, K.: Central, areolar choroidal atrophy. A report on four cases. Acta ophthal. (Kbh.). *37:* 325—329, 1959.

Sorsby, A. & J. B. Davey: Generalized choroidal sclerosis. Course and mode of inheritance. Brit. J. Ophthal. *39:* 257—275, 1955.

Juvenile Disciform Degeneration
of the Macula
(Figures 350—361)

Juvenile disciform macular degeneration most frequently affects individuals in the twenties. The ophthalmoscopic appearance is very much like the senile form of disciform macular degeneration, but in the juvenile group there is no evidence of vascular disease. The condition becomes bilateral in about 50 per cent of the cases.

The visual complaints vary considerably depending on the localization and extension of the fundal lesion. In the early stage, the patients most often complain of metamorphopsia and blurring of vision. In some cases a permanent central scotoma may develop, in others a paracentral scotoma develops and central vision remains normal or becomes slightly reduced. The peripheral visual field remains intact.

OPHTHALMOSCOPICALLY, the fundus lesion may start in one of two ways. In the one, it starts as a small indistinct edematous, grayish or yellowish-white fleck in the central part of the macula (Figs. 359—360) or perifoveally in the macular area (Figs. 356—357). The fleck, which soon enlarges, seldom becomes larger than two disc diameters. Small subretinal hemorrhages may often border the lesion. In the other process, fundus changes start with a rounded, dark-red or slate-gray subretinal hemorrhage of about disc size (Figs. 350—353). The hemorrhage is gradually absorbed, leaving a grayish or yellowish-white area.

In nearly all cases, a final fibrotic stage is reached, which is the same in both processes described. At this stage (Figs. 354—355, 358), the lesion is seen as a rounded, whitish or yellowish-white, slightly elevated mass, measuring from one to two disc diameters. The fibrotic mass may be surrounded by small glistening white exudates (Fig. 354). Occasionally, the final stage shows a more diffuse chorioretinal scarring (Fig. 361). The retinal vessels and the optic disc appear normal.

In the early stage, the condition may be confused with a commencing malignant choroidal melanoma and an acute choroiditis, but the conditions may be distinguished by fluorescein angiography, as they usually show different patterns of fluorescence. Clinically they are soon distinguished, as their course differs.

HISTOPATHOLOGICALLY, the changes resemble those of the senile type of disciform macular degeneration, but the choroid shows no evidence of vascular disease.

REFERENCES:

Braley, A. E.: Dystrophy of the macula. Amer. J. Ophthal. 61: 1—24, 1966.

Gass, J. D. M.: Pathogenesis of disciform detachment of the neuroepithelium. Amer. J. Ophthal. 63: 573—711, 1967.

Pau, H.: Chorioretinitis exsudativa centralis (haemorrhagica). Klin. Monatsbl. Augenh. 152: 348—357, 1968.

Thomann, H.: Die disziformen Maculopathien. Klin. Monatsbl. Augenh. 152: 625—639, 1968.

Senile Disciform Degeneration of the Macula

(Figures 362—371)

Senile disciform macular degeneration most frequently affects individuals over the age of 60 years. The condition is closely related to vascular sclerosis and often to senile macular degeneration. At times, senile macular degeneration is found in one eye and disciform degeneration in the other. The condition becomes bilateral in about 50 per cent of the cases.

The patients complain of suddenly occurring metamorphopsia and blurred vision, which is soon followed by a permanent central scotoma. The peripheral visual field, however, remains intact.

OPHTHALMOSCOPICALLY, the fundus lesion may start in one of two different ways. In the one, it starts as a small, slightly elevated, grayish-red or yellowish, often edematous indistinct fleck in the macula (Figs. 362, 364, 368—369). The fleck soon enlarges, and gradually involves the whole macular area. During progression, subretinal hemorrhages often border the lesion (Fig. 368). In the other process, fundus changes (Figs. 366, 370) start with a rounded, irregular, dark-red, grayish-green or greenish subretinal hemorrhage, which is gradually absorbed, leaving a grayish or yellowish-white area.

Finally, a fibrotic stage is reached, which is the same in both processes described (Figs. 363, 365, 367, 371). In this stage, there is a rounded, grayish or yellowish-white mass in the macular area, measuring from a few to several disc diameters, and often projecting forward for several diopters. Not infrequently, the central mass is surrounded by glistening white exudates arranged in a circinate manner (Fig. 365). The retinal vessels may show a varying degree of sclerosis. The disc, however, is normal.

In the early stage, senile disciform macular degeneration may be confused with a commencing malignant choroidal melanoma and an acute choroiditis, but the conditions may be distinguished by fluorescein angiography, as they usually show different patterns of fluorescence. Clinically they are soon distinguished, as their course differs.

HISTOPATHOLOGICALLY, the lesions are largely confined to the macular area. In the early stage, fresh blood or albuminous exudate is accumulated beneath the retinal pigment epithelium, between the pigment epithelium and the neuroepithelium, and in the subretinal area. Ruptures are found in Bruch's membrane and the retinal layers are pushed forward by the blood or exudate. Later, the process becomes organized, the retinal pigment epithelium proliferates, and new-formed vessels and connective tissue cells extend from the choroid into the exudate or blood. Finally, the retina is elevated by a dense layer of relatively avascular connective tissue. The outer retinal elements show complete degeneration, leaving cystic spaces, and the inner layers show marked atrophy. In the macular area there is also marked sclerosis and atrophy of the choroidal vessels.

REFERENCES:

Braley, A. E.: Dystrophy of the macula. Amer. J. Ophthal. *61:* 1—24, 1966.

Frayer, W. C.: Elevated lesions of the macular area. A.M.A. Arch. Ophthal. *53:* 82—92, 1955.

Gass, J. D. M.: Pathogenesis of disciform detachment of the neuroepithelium. Amer. J. Ophthal. *63:* 573—711, 1967.

Sautter, H. & D. Utermann: Der Pseudotumor der Macula. Klin. Monatsbl. Augenh. *145:* 1—18, 1964.

Slezak, H.: Zur Differentialdiagnose tumorähnlicher Veränderungen des Augenhintergrundes. Klin. Monatsbl. Augenh. *153:* 465—475, 1968.

Thomann, H.: Die disziformen Maculopathien. Klin. Monatsbl. Augenh. *152:* 625—639, 1968.

Circinate Retinopathy
(Figures 372—373)

Circinate retinopathy or retinitis circinata is a relatively uncommon condition characterized by a girdle of exudates surrounding the macular area. In the majority of cases, the condition is seen in elderly persons showing evidence of senile vascular disease, and is often associated with conditions such as senile macular degeneration or senile disciform macular degeneration. Circinate retinopathy, however, may also occur in other conditions with disturbances of the fundal circulation, especially diabetic retinopathy, venous occlusion and sometimes in Coats' syndrome or angiomatosis of the retina.

Visual disturbances depend on the degree of macular involvement, but central vision usually becomes gradually diminished and a central scotoma develops. The peripheral visual field, however, is left intact.

In senile cases the condition is frequently bilateral, although the eyes may be unequally affected or the development in the second eye may be delayed for some years.

OPHTHALMOSCOPICALLY, circinate retinopathy (Figs. 372—373) is seen as a complete or incomplete girdle of sharply defined, deep, discrete or confluent, glistening white or yellowish-white exudates surrounding the macular area. The lesion is usually bound by the upper and lower temporal retinal vessels. The macular area frequently shows degenerative changes (Fig. 373) resembling those seen in senile macular degeneration or senile disciform macular degeneration. In advanced cases, the exudates may also involve the macula, and small retinal hemorrhages may occur among the exudates. The condition usually shows a steady progression, but in some cases the exudates may be absorbed again, leaving only small pigmentary changes while the macular lesion remains. The retinal vessels show some sclerosis and the optic disc is usually normal.

HISTOPATHOLOGICALLY, the condition is characterized by an accumulation of fat-filled phagocytes in the middle and outer retinal layers, interspersed by free masses of lipid material. The adjacent retinal elements show a varying degree of degeneration. The area enclosed by the exudates shows varying degrees of cystoid, senile or disciform degeneration.

REFERENCES:

Houston, W. R. & G. N. Wise: Circinate retinopathy. A.M.A. Arch. Ophthal. 58: 777—782, and 783—796, 1957.

Larsen, H.-W.: Atlas of diabetic retinopathy. Acta ophthal. (Kbh.). Suppl. 55, 1959.

Larsen, H.-W.: Diabetic retinopathy. Acta ophthal. (Kbh.). Suppl. 60: 32, 1960.

Raitta, C.: Der Zentralvenen- und Netzhautvenenverschluss. Acta ophthal. (Kbh.). Suppl. 83: 61, 1965.

Colloid Bodies (Drusen)
(Figures 333, 337—341 and 374—376)

Colloid bodies, also known as hyaline bodies or drusen, are mound-like excrescences in Bruch's membrane. Their nature is not quite clear. Colloid bodies may occur in otherwise normally appearing fundi (Figs. 374, 376), they may be present as a senile phenomenon (Figs. 333, 337—341, 375) or as a degenerative phenomenon in vascular, inflammatory or neoplastic fundal conditions.

A certain condition presenting an accumulation of colloid bodies in the macular area, and occurring as a heredo-familial disease, initially without visual symptoms but eventually showing some degree of macular degeneration is known as Doyne's honeycomb choroiditis or dystrophy.

Colloid bodies may be seen at all ages, but occur most frequently in individuals over 60 years. In themselves, they do not cause any visual disturbances.

OPHTHALMOSCOPICALLY, they are seen as yellowish or yellowish-white pinpoint dots or larger rounded spots situated beneath the retinal vessels (Figs. 374—376). They may be few in number or numerous, scattered anywhere in the fundus, and often form large aggregates, especially in the macular area and around the disc. When large, they may be slightly elevated. At times, the single lesion is bordered by slight pigmentation.

HISTOPATHOLOGICALLY, the membrane of Bruch is thickened and shows flat, round or mound-like PAS-positive projections. In early stages, the projections are covered by retinal pigment epithelium, but when the excrescences enlarge the pigment epithelium becomes flattened, depigmented or disappears entirely at the site of the excrescences.

REFERENCES:
Braley, A. E.: Dystrophy of the macula. Amer. J. Ophthal. *61:* 1—24, 1966.
Ernest, J. T. & A. E. Krill: Fluorescein studies in fundus flavimaculatus and drusen. Amer. J. Ophthal. *62:* 1—6, 1966.
Forni, S. & J. Babel: Etude clinique et histologique de la malattia leventinese. Ophthalmologica. *143:* 313—322, 1962.
Franceschetti, A., J. François & J. Babel: Les hérédo-dégénérescences chorio-rétiniennes. Masson, Paris. 490, 1963.
Krill, A. E. & B. A. Klien: Flecked retina syndrome. A.M.A. Arch. Ophthal. *74:* 496—508, 1965.
Pearce, W. G.: Doyne's honeycomb retinal degeneration. Brit. J. Ophthal. *52:* 73—78, 1968.

Central Serous Retinopathy
(Figures 377—378)

The etiology of central serous retinopathy is unknown, but several theories have been advanced, including vasomotor instability and allergy. The term central serous retinopathy is applied to different conditions, all presenting a well-defined edema in the macular area and clinically behaving in the same way, even if in some cases the edema is located in the retina and in others is located preretinally or subretinally.

The condition is usually unilateral and affects most often young or middle-aged males.

The patient complains of hazy vision, metamorphopsia, micropsia, positive central or paracentral scotoma, and objects may appear as if seen through sun-glasses. In most cases, there is complete recovery of vision in the course of weeks or some months. However, recurrences are common and may occasionally lead to permanent impairment of vision.

OPHTHALMOSCOPICALLY, central serous retinopathy is seen as a slightly elevated zone of indistinctness in the macular area, measuring from one to two disc diameters (Figs. 377—378). The involved area resembles a flat vesicle and is sharply outlined by a circular or oval light reflex. The color is grayish-red or deeper red than normal, and the retinal vessels in the affected area are slightly tortuous and contracted. Small white dots are frequently present within the affected area (Fig. 378). The condition may subside, leaving a normal macular area or one with some atrophy and pigment disturbances, or even cystoid degeneration, eventually followed by a lamellar macular hole.

Central serous retinopathy is relatively often associated with an optic pit or hole in the temporal part of the optic disc (Fig. 377).

In ordinary ophthalmoscopy it is usually impossible to determine whether the edema is preretinal, retinal or subretinal. Using a slit-lamp together with a Hruby lens, however, it is easy to determine the position of the serous fluid.

HISTOPATHOLOGICALLY, there is a preretinal, retinal or subretinal accumulation of serous fluid together with some degenerative changes in the retina in the foveal region.

REFERENCES:

Farpour, H. & J. Babel: Les fossettes papillaires; Diagnostic différentiel, anomalies vasculaires et cas limites. Ann. Oculist (Paris). *201:* 1—17, 1968.

Gass, J. D. M.: Pathogenesis of disciform detachment of the neuroepithelium. Amer. J. Ophthal. *63:* 573—711, 1967.

Hruby, K. & A. Posner: Slitlamp examination of vitreous and retina. Williams & Wilkins, Baltimore. 100, 1967.

Klien, B. A.: Central serous retinopathy and chorioretinopathy. Trans. Amer. Acad. Ophthal. Otolaryng. *69:* 614—620, 1965.

Kranenburg, E. W.: Crater-like holes in the optic disc and central serous retinopathy. A.M.A. Arch. Ophthal. *64:* 912—924, 1960.

Maumenee, A. E.: Further advances in the study of the macula. A.M.A. Arch. Ophthal. *78:* 151—165, 1967.

Peabody, R. R., H. C. Zweng & H. L. Little: Treatment of persistent central serous retino-

pathy. A.M.A. Arch. Ophthal. *79:* 166—169,
1968.
Spalter, H. F.: Photocoagulation of central serous retinopathy. A.M.A. Arch. Ophthal. *79:*
247—253, 1968.

Sugar, H. S.: Congenital pits in the optic disc.
Amer. J. Ophthal. *63:* 298—307, 1967.
Wessing, A.: Zur Pathogenese und Therapie der
sogenannten Retinitis centralis serosa. Ophthalmologica. *153:* 259—276, 1967.

Coats' Syndrome
(Figures 379—384)

Coats' syndrome may be divided into two groups. The first is characterized from the very beginning by massive retinal and subretinal exudate, with or without gross vascular disease. The second, also called Leber's multiple miliary aneurysms, commences with retinal arterial aneurysms and only slight exudative changes. The exudates, however, usually progress, so that the late stages may be indistinguishable. The condition is probably always due to a vascular malformation, primarily affecting the retinal vessels in the diseased area of the fundus.

The syndrome occurs most frequently in apparently healthy young persons, especially males, and usually affects one eye only. In most cases the disease is slowly and steadily progressive, but may remain stationary for long periods.

In early stages there are no or only slight visual complaints. Later, vision may be reduced to a varying degree, depending on the localization and extension of the pathological process.

OPHTHALMOSCOPICALLY, the fundus changes in the first group are characterized (Figs. 379—383) by well-defined or soft-edged, yellowish or whitish, flat or prominent, single or confluent exudates situated beneath the retinal vessels. The exudates are usually localized near the optic disc (Fig. 379) or the macula (Fig. 382), but may also occur in the periphery (Fig. 381). Small retinal hemorrhages may be diffusely scattered in the fundus. Fusiform or spherical dilatations (Figs. 380—382) and tortuosities preferentially of the retinal arteries frequently occur at several sites. Occasionally, angioma-like lesions (Fig. 383) may also be present. Sheathing of the retinal vessels is common (Fig. 380). In the early stage, some vitreous haze may be present. In the late stages, the exudates may cover the whole fundus and finally retinitis proliferans and retinal detachment may develop.

In the second group the fundus changes (Fig. 384) commence with fusiform or spherical dilatations, arterial and sometimes also venous aneurysms, and tortuosities of the retinal vessels in different areas of the fundus. At first, there may be no exudates, only some sheathing of the diseased vessels or slight exudation around the diseased vessels. In the course of time, however, the exudates usually enlarge so that the late stages and final appearance may be indistinguishable from that described in the first group.

In the differential diagnosis, it is necessary to consider retinoblastoma, angiomatosis of the retina and posterior uveitis.

HISTOPATHOLOGICALLY, the early stages are characterized by a serofibrinous exudate involving all retinal layers. Necroses are often present in the outer retinal layers, and widely dilated and thin-walled capillary vessels are frequently found in the inner layers. An extensive exudate, invaded by characteristic large, pale-staining histiocytes, is formed between the retinal pigment epithelium and the main retina, which then becomes detached. Finally, the exudate is replaced by fibrous tissue deep in the retina or between the retina and the choroid.

REFERENCES:

Gass, J. D. M.: A fluorescein angiographic study of macular dysfunction secondary to retinal vascular disease. A.M.A. Arch. Ophthal. *80:* 535—617, 1968.

Imre, G.: Coats' disease. Amer. J. Ophthal. *54:* 175—191, 1962.

Manschot, W. A. & W. C. de Bruijn: Coats's disease: Definition and pathogenesis. Brit. J. Ophthal. *51:* 145—157, 1967.

Morales, A. G.: Coats' disease. Natural history and results of treatment. Amer. J. Ophthal. *60:* 855—865, 1965.

Reese, A. B.: Telangiectasis of the retina and Coats' disease. Amer. J. Ophthal. *42:* 1—8, 1956.

Woods, A. C. & J. R. Duke: Coats's disease. Review of the literature, diagnostic criteria, clinical findings and plasma lipid studies. Brit. J. Ophthal. *47:* 385—412, 1963.

Angioid Streaks
(Figures 385—395)

Angioid streaks are a rare, slowly progressive degenerative condition characterized by ruptures in Bruch's membrane and frequently associated with macular degeneration.

Angioid streaks may occur with or without evidence of systemic disease. Most frequently the condition is found in association with pseudoxanthoma elasticum, which is an uncommon systemic disease, having a familial character and showing a heredity of the recessive type. It is characterized by a generalized degeneration of the elastic tissue of the body, mainly affecting the skin, ocular fundus and cardiovascular system. The complex of angioid streaks and pseudoxanthoma elasticum is known as the Grönblad-Strandberg syndrome. Occasionally, angioid streaks have been observed in Ehlers-Danlos' syndrome, Paget's disease and sickle-cell anemia.

Angioid streaks may occur at all ages. The condition is always bilateral, but the eyes are usually unequally affected.

In early stages, there are usually no visual complaints. In long-standing cases, however, the macula is usually involved and this may seriously affect the visual acuity. Finally, vision may be further impaired by visual field defects occurring in association with an extensive choroidal atrophy.

Angioid streaks are often associated with systemic diseases and especially with pseudoxanthoma elasticum, with wide-spread degeneration of the elastic tissue. In these cases the vascular changes may lead to serious disturbances of function in other systems, and the general prognosis is determined by the systemic disease.

OPHTHALMOSCOPICALLY, the angioid streaks are seen as fine or broad, brown, red or grayish wavy bands with tapering ends, situated beneath the retinal vessels (Figs. 385—387). They may resemble blood vessels and are often bordered by some pigment or a whitish line (Fig. 388). The angioid streaks frequently anastomose near the optic disc, forming an irregular ring around it, and then radiating towards the equatorial region. In the macular and perimacular area and sometimes also in the fundus periphery, coarse granulation may be present, giving rise to the so-called peau d'orange configuration (Figs. 387—388). In the fundus periphery, scattered, yellowish-white or whitish spots, known as salmon spots (Fig. 389), often associated with some pigment deposits resembling small chorioretinal scars or colloid bodies, are often present in long-standing cases. Small or large retinal or preretinal hemorrhages may also occur. Macular changes usually develop about the age of 50 years. The lesions resemble disciform macular degeneration (Figs. 390—394). Finally, patchy areas of choroidal sclerosis appear and become confluent. They form large, sharply defined lobulated zones of atrophy, with exposure of the choroidal vessels and pigment deposits (Fig. 395), and the angioid streaks disappear entirely in these atrophic areas.

HISTOPATHOLOGICALLY, irregular defects
and ruptures in Bruch's membrane are
found at the site of the angioid streaks,
and the breaks show jagged edges and
vary in breadth. Connective tissue from
the choroid may fill the defects and the
pigment epithelium may show both
hypertrophy and atrophy in association
with the defects. In the advanced stage,
disciform degeneration is found in the
macula. The choriocapillaris may be atrophic and replaced by collagenous connective tissue.

REFERENCES:

Britten, M. J. A.: Unusual traumatic retinal
  haemorrhages associated with angioid
  streaks. Brit. J. Ophthal. *50:* 540—542, 1966.
Carlborg, U., B. Ejrup, E. Grönblad & F. Lund:
  Vascular studies in pseudoxanthoma elas-
ticum and angioid streaks. Acta med. scan-
  dinav. *Suppl. 350,* 1960.
Domke, H. & M. Tost: Zur Histologie der "Angioid streaks". Klin. Monatsbl. Augenh. *145:*
  18—29, 1964.
Franceschetti, A., J. François & J. Babel: Les
  hérédo-dégénérescences   chorio-rétiniennes.
  Masson, Paris. 546, 1963.
Gills, J. P. & D. Paton: Mottled fundus oculi
  in pseudoxanthoma elasticum. A.M.A. Arch.
  Ophthal. *73:* 792—795, 1965.
Goodman, R. M., E. W. Smith, D. Paton, R. A.
  Bergman, C. L. Siegel, O. E. Ottesen, W. M.
  Shelley, A. L. Pusch & V. A. McKusick: Pseudoxanthoma elasticum: A clinical and histopathological study. Medicine (Balt.). *42:*
  297—334, 1963.
Green, W. R., A. Friedman-Kien & W. G. Ban-
  field: Angioid streaks in Ehlers-Danlos syndrome. A.M.A. Arch. Ophthal. *76:* 197—204,
  1966.
Percival, S. P. B.: Angioid streaks and elastor-
  rhexis. Brit. J. Ophthal. *52:* 297—309, 1968.
Rosen, E.: Fundus in pseudoxanthoma elasticum. Amer. J. Ophthal. *66:* 236—244, 1968.

Retinal Perivasculitis
(Figures 396—397, 399—401, 403, 408, 410 and 412—413)

Retinal perivasculitis is an inflammatory condition including both periphlebitis and periarteritis. Most frequently the retinal veins are involved, more rarely the retinal arteries. Sometimes, however, both arteries and veins are affected.

Retinal perivasculitis may occur in conditions as for example Eales' disease, multiple sclerosis, uveitis and acute retinochoroiditis or in diseases such as tuberculosis and syphilis.

Eales' Disease
(Figures 396—399)

Eales' disease is a condition of unknown etiology characterized by retinal periphlebitis and a tendency to recurrent vitreous hemorrhages.

As a rule, both eyes are affected, and in the early stages one more than the other.

The disease occurs most frequently in healthy young individuals, especially males. Occasionally there is a history of tuberculosis.

In the periphlebitic stage, there are no or only slight visual disturbances. The occurrence of vitreous hemorrhage, however, causes a blurring or loss of vision. Following the first few attacks the vitreous may clear again in the course of some weeks or months, but recurrent vitreous hemorrhages may develop after varying intervals, causing permanent damage with reduction of vision.

OPHTHALMOSCOPICALLY, the early stage is characterized by perivasculitic and mainly periphlebitic changes in different areas, especially towards the periphery (Figs. 396—397). Small retinal hemorrhages and chorioretinal foci are often present and small fan-shaped preretinal neovascularizations (Figs. 397—398) may occur in the periphery. The first vitreous hemorrhages may be absorbed and leave only some vitreous opacities. Recurrent hemorrhages, however, may be absorbed very slowly, often leading to retinitis proliferans (Figs. 398—399) with formation of new-formed vessels and connective tissue, preretinally and in the vitreous. The proliferative retinopathy may sooner or later cause traction on the retina, resulting in retinal detachment.

In the periphlebitic stage, the condition must be distinguished from periphlebitis in multiple sclerosis and in uveitis.

In the proliferative stage, it must be distinguished from proliferative diabetic retinopathy.

In the differential diagnosis of vitreous hemorrhage it is necessary to consider for example Eales' disease, angiomatosis of the retina, diabetic retinopathy, malignant choroidal melanoma and retinal detachment.

HISTOPATHOLOGICALLY, the retinal vessels and especially the veins show vasculitis and perivasculitis. The vessel walls are inflamed, their lumina sometimes occluded and they are often surrounded by lymphocytes. The late stages show retinitis proliferans and retinal detachment.

REFERENCES:

Brandt, H. P.: Katamnestische Untersuchungen bei Periphlebitis retinae. Klin. Monatsbl. Augenh. *149:* 41—49, 1966.

Doden, W. & A. Adams: Ergebnisse neurologischer Untersuchungen von Kranken mit Periphlebitis retinae. Klin. Monatsbl. Augenh. *129:* 305—317, 1956.

Donders, P. C.: Eales' disease. Docum. ophthal. *12:* 1—105, 1958.

Elliot, A. J.: Recurrent intraocular hemorrhage in young adults (Eales's disease). Trans. Amer. ophthal. Soc. *52:* 811—875, 1954.

Jütte, A. & L. Lemke: Kapillardefekte im Netzhautkreislauf bei Periphlebitis retinae. Klin. Monatsbl. Augenh. *149:* 334—340, 1966.

Multiple Sclerosis
(Figures 400—401)

Transient retinal periphlebitis is a frequent occurrence in the course of multiple sclerosis, in addition to retrobulbar neuritis, optic atrophy and eye muscle palsies. The periphlebitis, however, does not cause any visual disturbances.

OPHTHALMOSCOPICALLY, the periphlebitic changes are mainly found in the periphery of the fundus (Figs. 400—401). The veins are more or less obscured by whitish fluffy exudates which ensheath a single or several veins for a shorter or longer distance, and whitish plaques sometimes lie in front of the veins. The periphlebitic changes persist for some time and then disappear, but frequently new ones appear elsewhere. Occasionally, the retinal periphlebitis is associated with uveitis, but retinal hemorrhages and retinitis proliferans do not occur.

The condition must be distinguished from periphlebitis in Eales' disease and in uveitis.

HISTOPATHOLOGICALLY, the fundal lesions present a picture of retinal periphlebitis.

REFERENCES:

Breger, B. C. & I. H. Leopold: The incidence of uveitis in multiple sclerosis. Amer. J. Ophthal. *62:* 540—545, 1966.

Collier, M.: Uvéite et sclérose en plaques. Bull. Soc. franç. Ophtal. *76:* 624—635, 1963.

Haarr, M.: Uveitis with neurological symptoms. Acta ophthal. (Kbh.). *39:* 60—70, 1961.

Møller, P. M. & P. E. Hammerberg: Retinal periphlebitis in multiple sclerosis. Acta neurol. scandinav. *Suppl. 4:* 263—269, 1963.

Paufique, L. & R. Etienne: Un signe peu connu de la sclérose en plaques: La périphlébite des veines rétiniennes. Ann. Oculist (Paris). *188:* 701—707, 1955.

Fundus Changes in Uveitis

(Figures 402—406 and 472)

Fundus changes in uveitis consist mainly of retinal edema and periphlebitis.

OPHTHALMOSCOPICALLY, the retinal edema in this condition may be localized to the macular area or widespread (Fig. 402), giving the retina a dull appearance with abnormal light reflexes. Occasionally, an exudative retinal detachment develops (Fig. 472). When the edema subsides, hard exudates may develop in the macular area (Figs. 404—405).

Retinal periphlebitis (Fig. 403) may occur with sheathing of the veins for a variable distance, and in sarcoidosis this sheathing is often associated with dense preretinal vitreous opacities (Fig. 406), which may remain unchanged after the uveitis and periphlebitis have subsided.

In the differential diagnosis, periphlebitic changes in Eales' disease and in multiple sclerosis have to be considered.

REFERENCES:
Crick, R. P.: Ocular sarcoidosis. Trans. ophthal. Soc. U.K. *75:* 189—206, 1955.
Duke-Elder, S. & J. H. Dobree: System of ophthalmology. *Vol. X.* Kimpton, London. 213, 218, 1967.
Ortlepp, J., A. Heydenreich & E. Hauschild: Maculaschäden bei Uveitis anterior. Klin. Monatsbl. Augenh. *150:* 221—225, 1967.
Paul, W. & J. Dabels: Beitrag zur Periphlebitis retinae. Klin. Monatsbl. Augenh. *152:* 145—158, 1968.

Scintillatio Albescens and Synchysis Scintillans
(Figure 407)

Scintillatio albescens is a rare condition of unknown etiology. It usually affects individuals about the age of 60 years and is bilateral in about 75 per cent of the cases. Visual acuity is slightly reduced or normal.

OPHTHALMOSCOPICALLY, scintillatio albescens is seen as numerous small, round or disc-shaped, white, snowball-like vitreous opacities showing only slight movements when the eye is moved, and typically occurring in a vitreous which is otherwise of normal appearance.

HISTOPATHOLOGICAL AND HISTOCHEMICAL studies support the view that these vitreous opacities consist chiefly of calcium soaps.

Synchysis scintillans occurs most often in young adults and is frequently bilateral. The condition is often the consequence of other ocular diseases such as chronic degeneration, trauma, hemorrhage or inflammation.

OPHTHALMOSCOPICALLY, synchysis scintillans (Fig. 407) is seen as innumerable freely movable, glistening flakes in a fluid vitreous, often reflecting the ophthalmoscopic light with a golden sheen.

HISTOPATHOLOGICALLY AND HISTOCHEMICALLY, the opacities consist chiefly of crystalline deposits of cholesterol.

REFERENCES:
Rodman, H. I., F. B. Johnson & L. E. Zimmerman: New histopathological and histochemical observations concerning asteroid hyalitis. A.M.A. Arch. Ophthal. *66:* 552—563, 1961.
Wichser, J.: Kristalline Einlagerungen im Glaskörper. Docum. ophthal. *24:* 3—40, 1968.

Retinal Arteritis and Periarteritis
(Figures 408—413)

Retinal arteritis and periarteritis may occur as the only manifestation of retinal vasculitis. More frequently, however, the condition is seen in association with retinal periphlebitis.

OPHTHALMOSCOPICALLY, numerous whitish patches border and partially cover the retinal arteries from the disc and a variable distance into the fundus (Fig. 408). The arteritis may subside leaving no trace, or giving rise to some constriction of the retinal arteries (Fig. 409) or even the formation of an arterial occlusion.

Sometimes, retinal arteritis is observed in association with acute chorioretinitis (Figs. 410—413).

In uveitis and Eales' disease, periarteritic changes may be present together with periphlebitic changes in the fundus periphery.

REFERENCES:
Duke-Elder, S. & J. H. Dobree: System of ophthalmology. *Vol. X.* Kimpton, London. 218, 1967.

Choroiditis
(Figures 414—436)

Choroiditis or posterior uveitis is an inflammatory condition usually starting in the choroid and subsequently involving the retina. Sometimes, however, it may be secondary to retinitis and anterior uveitis.

Choroiditis is most frequently a nonsuppurative inflammation of endogenous origin, caused by bacterial, viral, mycotic or parasitic agents, or very often a reaction due to toxic or allergic insults.

Choroiditis may occur in conditions such as tuberculosis, congenital syphilis, the secondary and tertiary stages of acquired syphilis, congenital or acquired toxoplasmosis, brucellosis, prenatal rubella infection, sarcoidosis, etc. In the vast majority of cases, however, the etiology is difficult or impossible to determine clinically in spite of extensive examination, including serological tests.

Choroiditis may occur at any age and is frequently bilateral. It may start insidiously, with no or only slight visual disturbances, or may be acute with hazy vision, metamorphopsia, macropsia, micropsia, and positive or negative scotomas, depending on the site and extension of the focal process. Pain is not present unless the condition is associated with iridocyclitis or scleritis. The inflammation may run a self-limited course, but frequently it is chronic and progressive, showing recurrent attacks. Not infrequently, however, symptomless chorioretinal scars are found on routine ophthalmoscopy.

Ophthalmoscopically, the choroidal lesions appear as small or large, solitary or multiple, central, peripheral or diffusely spread lesions in the fundus, all resembling each other and giving no basis for an etiological diagnosis.

In the acute exudative stage (Figs. 414, 416, 418), there is diffuse subretinal and retinal edema which is soon followed by lesions appearing as ill-defined, slightly elevated, fluffy, pale, yellowish-white patches in the fundus. In front of the patches there is usually some vitreous haze. The retinal vessels may show some perivasculitis, and the disc may be edematous.

When healing starts after some time, the fluffy patches subside and are converted into chorioretinal scars, usually seen as sharply outlined, whitish, atrophic areas with or without pigment accumulation or bordered by irregular pigment deposits (Figs. 415, 417, 419—425). The atrophic area may be avascular or crossed by fragments of the choroidal vessels.

In disseminated choroiditis the chorioretinal scars are indistinct and more or less confluent, and the pigment clumping is irregular and often widespread (Figs. 426—430).

In diffuse choroiditis the fundus may assume a nearly salt-and-pepper appearance, as seen for example in intrauterine rubella infection (Figs. 431—432). The fundus may also be dotted with minute chorioretinal scars (Fig. 433) or show a more diffuse chorioretinal degeneration (Figs. 434—435) and a varying amount of pigment accumulation (Figs. 434, 436).

Occasionally, a small lesion of acute choroiditis may be confused ophthalmoscopically with a commencing malignant choroidal melanoma or a commencing disciform macular degeneration, but using fluorescein angiography it is often possible to distinguish these conditions by their different patterns of fluorescence.

In the scar stage, choroiditis should not be confused with colobomas, angioid streaks, old choroidal ruptures, fundus changes in excessive myopia or conditions associated with pigmentary degeneration in the fundus.

HISTOPATHOLOGICALLY, acute choroiditis is characterized by a granulomatous or non-granulomatous inflammation.

The granulomatous type is usually related to bacterial, viral, mycotic or parasitic inflammation, and to conditions such as tuberculosis, syphilis, toxoplasmosis, brucellosis and sarcoidosis. It consists of focal or diffuse infiltration of the choroid by epitheloid cells, lymphocytes and plasma cells. Infective agents are sometimes found in the lesion. The overlying retina usually shows considerable degeneration, and perivasculitis is found in the adjacent areas. The scar stage is characterized by fibrosis of the choroid, destruction of retinal pigment epithelium and rods and cones, together with a varying degree of disorganization of the other retinal layers.

The non-granulomatous type is usually related to toxic or allergic insults or bacterial or viral inflammation of low virulence. It consists mainly of diffuse choroidal and retinal exudate, together with some infiltration of the choroid by lymphocytes and subsequently plasma cells. The condition subsides, leaving no or only slight degenerative changes in the choroid and the retinal pigment epithelium.

REFERENCES:

Duke-Elder, S. & E. S. Perkins: System of ophthalmology. *Vol. IX.* Kimpton, London. 148, 1966.

Krill, A. E.: The retinal disease of rubella. A.M.A. Arch. Ophthal. 77: 445—449, 1967.

Lemke, L. & A. Jütte: Das Fluoreszenz-Angiogramm der Chorioiditis. Klin. Monatsbl. Augenh. *149:* 19—31, 1966.

Wessing, A.: Fluoreszenzangiographie der Retina. Lehrbuch und Atlas. Thieme, Stuttgart. 98, 1968.

Woods, A. C.: Endogenous inflammations of the uveal tract. Williams & Wilkins, Baltimore. 1961.

Retinochoroiditis Juxtapapillaris (Jensen)
(Figures 437—442)

Retinochoroiditis juxtapapillaris is an inflammatory condition of unknown etiology. It is characterized by circumscribed fundal lesions, adjacent to or involving the optic disc, together with a sector-shaped scotoma, often spreading fan-wise from the blind spot, and due to a lesion of the nerve fibers. Recurrences are frequent *in loco,* but the inflammation runs a self-limited course and the visual prognosis is frequently good.

Retinochoroiditis juxtapapillaris may occur at any age, but predominantly in young adults, and is usually unilateral.

In the acute stage, there is hazy vision. Visual acuity is moderately or severely reduced and a sector-formed field defect can be demonstrated. The hazy vision disappears in the course of some weeks or a few months, and vision often becomes normal or nearly normal again unless the papillomacular bundle is damaged, but the field defect remains stationary. Recurrences are frequent *in loco* and the field defect usually remains unchanged.

OPHTHALMOSCOPICALLY, the acute stage (Figs. 437, 439, 441) is characterized by vitreous haze and diffuse edema adjacent to or surrounding the optic disc, and frequently some edema of the disc. In the edematous area there is a circumscribed exudate of disc size or larger, often accompanied by a few retinal hemorrhages. The retinal vessels are more or less obscured by the exudate, the veins engorged and the arteries normal or slightly narrowed.

When the inflammation subsides, the exudative patch is converted into a chorioretinal scar (Figs. 438, 440—442), just as in choroiditis. In subsequent attacks (Fig. 441), new exudates appear adjacent to the chorioretinal scar.

HISTOPATHOLOGICALLY, there are too few microscopic reports to give a definitive description of the condition, but both retina, choroid and optic nerve head may be involved.

REFERENCES:

Graeber, W.: Ist die Retinochorioiditis juxtapapillaris (Jensen) eine Neurofibrillitis? Klin. Monatsbl. Augenh. *142:* 1030—1038, 1963.

Klien, B. A.: Jensen's juxtapapillary retinopathy. Amer. J. Ophthal. *42:* 9—14, 1956.

Théodoridis, A.: Sur la rétinite de Jensen. Ann. Oculist (Paris). *199:* 615—618, 1966.

Retinoschisis and Retinal Cysts

(Figures 443—450)

Retinoschisis can be divided into two forms.

The juvenile or idiopathic form, which shows a hereditary tendency and often is sex-linked, affecting young males, is probably congenital in origin and due to degenerative changes both in the vitreous and the retina, resulting in splitting of the retina into two layers and the formation of cyst-like spaces which may sometimes be converted into giant cysts in the fundal periphery.

The senile form, which occurs most frequently between the ages of 50 and 70 years, is closely related to cystoid degeneration of the retina. In this condition the retina becomes split into two layers by coalescence of the cystic spaces.

Both forms are frequently bilateral and slowly progressive. The lesion starts in the fundus periphery and in the juvenile form it is often confined to the lower temporal quadrants, producing an absolute scotoma corresponding to the site of the lesion. The condition is often not noticed by the patient, and is thus first discovered on routine examination, unless the macular area is involved and central vision decreased.

Retinoschisis and a retinal cyst may be present in the same eye. The major complication in both conditions is the development of retinal detachment by the formation of holes in the outer retinal layers.

OPHTHALMOSCOPICALLY, retinoschisis is seen (Figs. 444—448) as a flat or slightly elevated area with fairly well-defined, branching whitish lines or bands lying beneath or in front of the retinal vessels, or lying as a thin opaque web (Figs. 446—447), partly obscuring the retinal vessels and protruding slightly into the vitreous. At times, the whitish lines are bordered by some pigment. In the affected area, small oval or round intraretinal cavities may be seen plainly (Fig. 443). The lesion always starts in the fundal periphery and gradually progresses towards the optic disc. In the senile form, cystoid degeneration is present in the fundal periphery.

Retinal cysts, which often occur together with retinoschisis, are most often located in the lower temporal quadrants. They appear as grayish-pink, yellowish-pink or grayish (Figs. 448—450), well-defined globules, projecting forward for a variable distance and containing stretched retinal vessels in the projecting wall. At times, a tear develops in the wall of the cyst, leading to retinal detachment (Fig. 449).

In typical cases the diagnosis is not difficult. In less advanced cases, however, the diagnosis may be difficult to establish using ordinary ophthalmoscopy and is only confirmed by using the slit-lamp with a Hruby lens or the Goldmann three-mirror contact lens. In cases where retinoschisis is complicated by retinal detachment, it may be difficult to distinguish it from "primary" retinal detachment. In cases associated with retinal cysts, the condition has to be distinguished from cysts of other origin, including traumatic cysts and parasitic cysts.

HISTOPATHOLOGICALLY, juvenile retinoschisis is seen as a splitting of the retinal layers immediately under the ganglion cell layer, or even more superficially, while senile retinoschisis is seen as a splitting of the retinal layers by coalescence of numerous small cysts in the external plexiform layer, producing more or less atrophy of the other retinal layers. A retinal cyst is lined internally by a very delicate glial membrane containing the retinal vessels and externally by relatively intact neuroepithelium and pigment epithelium.

REFERENCES:

Bengtsson, B. & B. Linder: Sex-linked hereditary juvenile retinoschisis. Presentation of two affected families. Acta ophthal. (Kbh.). 45: 411—423, 1967.

Byer, N. E.: Clinical study of senile retinoschisis. A.M.A. Arch. Ophthal. 79: 36—44, 1968.

Cibis, P. A.: Retinoschisis—retinal cysts. Trans. Amer. ophthal. Soc. 63: 417—453, 1965.

Franceschetti, A., J. François & J. Babel: Les hérédo-dégénérescences chorio-rétiniennes. Masson, Paris. 828, 1963.

Hagler, W. S. & A. W. North: Intraretinal macrocysts and retinal detachment. Trans. Amer. Acad. Ophthal. Otolaryng. 71: 442—454, 1967.

Keith, C. G.: Retinal cysts and retinoschisis. Brit. J. Ophthal. 50: 617—628, 1966.

Ricci, A.: Clinique et transmission héréditaire des dégénérescences vitréo-rétiniennes. Bull. Soc. Ophtal. Fr. 61: 618—662, 1961.

Sabates, F. N.: Juvenile retinoschisis. Amer. J. Ophthal. 62: 683—688, 1966.

Shea, M., C. L. Schepens & S. R. von Pirquet: Retinoschisis I. Senile type: A clinical report of one hundred seven cases. A.M.A. Arch. Ophthal. 63: 1—9, 1960.

Yanoff, M., E. K. Rahn & L. E. Zimmerman: Histopathology of juvenile retinoschisis. A.M.A. Arch. Ophthal. 79: 49—53, 1968.

Choroidal Detachment
(Figures 451—453)

Choroidal detachment is a condition in which the choroid has been separated from the sclera by an effusion of fluid. It may occur spontaneously without any apparent cause, follow intraocular surgery or be related to inflammation or trauma.

Spontaneous choroidal detachment is a rare condition, most often affecting males between the ages of 30 and 60 years. The condition is frequently bilateral, and often progressive over a period of some years. Reattachment may, however, occur spontaneously after a varying number of years.

In the early stage vision is not affected, but visual field defects are present corresponding to the extension of the detachment. Later, however, central vision may be reduced or even lost.

Choroidal detachment following intraocular surgery may occur just after the operation or appear some days later, and the condition is considered among other things to be due to insufficient wound closure. The early occurrence is very common, but usually the choroid is reattached spontaneously within a few days. The choroidal detachment appearing some days after surgery occurs in about 10 to 15 per cent of the cases. The detachment usually disappears within 2 to 3 weeks.

Postoperative choroidal detachment is usually associated with diminution or abolition of the anterior chamber, lowering of the intraocular tension and visual field defects. If the anterior chamber remains flat for a longer period, it may result in the development of closed-angle glaucoma.

The choroidal detachment associated with inflammatory conditions or trauma is principally determined by the primary disease.

OPHTHALMOSCOPICALLY, choroidal detachment is seen as a dark grayish-brown smooth elevation in the fundus periphery or an elevation containing fine whitish parallel lines (Figs. 451—452). The lesion often shows well-defined bounderies, the convexity of which is towards the optic disc. The detachment may be confined to a single quadrant, usually the lower temporal, or may involve the whole periphery. If the detachment is extensive, the detached areas may bulge forwards like balloons separated by ridges caused by the anchorage of the vortex veins. On transillumination, the detached area usually appears lighter than the non-detached areas. The retinal vessels appear normal when passing over the detached area. On moving the eye, the lesion shows no wave-like motions as may be seen in retinal detachment. In long-standing cases clumping of pigment may occur in the affected area (Fig. 453), giving it a moth-eaten appearance.

In the differential diagnosis, retinal detachment as well as malignant choroidal melanoma have to be considered.

HISTOPATHOLOGICALLY, the choroid is detached from the sclera by an albuminous fluid and there is marked congestion and dilation of the choroidal vessels.

REFERENCES:
Bernard, P.: Le décollement de la choroïde. Bull. Soc. Ophtal. Fr. *Suppl.:* I—CCXXV, 1963.

Hawkins, W. R. & C. L. Schepens: Choroidal detachment and retinal surgery. A clinical and experimental study. Amer. J. Ophthal. *62:* 812—819, 1966.
Hilsdorf, C., J. Marxer & H. Schönenberger: Beitrag zur Behandlung der postoperativen Chorioidalabhebung. Ophthalmologica. *152:* 294—302, 1966.
Rosen, E. & A. Lyne: Uveal effusion. Amer. J. Ophthal. *65:* 509—518, 1968.

Vitreous Detachment

(Figure 454)

Vitreous detachment is a common condition frequently associated with the aging process, and therefore frequently found after the age of 50 years. Vitreous detachment may, however, also occur in conditions such as myopia, and vitreous retraction may follow inflammatory or degenerative conditions.

Vitreous detachment is not infrequently associated with retinal tears, and may in some cases eventually be followed by retinal detachment.

The condition is often unnoticed by the patient, but sometimes the detaching vitreous may cause photopsia due to traction in the retina. If vitreous detachment is complicated by retinal detachment, symptoms of the latter condition will supervene.

OPHTHALMOSCOPICALLY, the condition may give rise to abnormal reflexes in the fundus, and occasionally the posterior hyaloid membrane may show some condensation (Fig. 454), seen as a slightly opaque membranous veil around the disc and the macular area, where the vitreous is firmly attached. The condition is easily recognized by using the slit-lamp together with a Hruby lens or a Goldmann three-mirror contact lens.

REFERENCES:
Busacca, A., H. Goldmann & S. Schiff-Wertheimer: Biomicroscopie de corps vitré et du fond de l'oeil. Masson, Paris. 115, 1957.
Goldmann, H.: Senescenz des Glaskörpers. Ophthalmologica. *143:* 253—279, 1962.
Hruby, K. & A. Posner: Slitlamp examination of vitreous and retina. Williams & Wilkins, Baltimore. 48, 1967.
Jaffe, N. S.: Complications of acute posterior vitreous detachment. A.M.A. Arch. Ophthal. *79:* 568—571, 1968.
Linder, B.: Acute posterior vitreous detachment and its retinal complications. A clinical biomicroscopic study. Acta ophthal. (Kbh.). *Suppl. 87,* 1966.
Tasman, W. S.: Posterior vitreous detachment and peripheral retinal breaks. Trans. Amer. Acad. Ophthal. Otolaryng. *72:* 217—224, 1968.

Detachment of the Retina
(Figures 37—39, 148—149, 455—472 and 488)

The condition known as retinal detachment is a separation of the main retina from the retinal pigment epithelium. The separation occurs between the pigment epithelium and the layer of the rods and cones, as these layers are only loosely attached to each other except at the optic disc and the ora serrata, while the pigment epithelium is firmly attached to the choroid. The loose attachment between the pigment epithelium and the rods and cones represents a potential space, the original cavity in the embryonic optic vesicle.

Retinal detachment is probably always secondary to some local ocular disease.

In the majority of cases, detachment is due to some primary, often obscure retinal or vitreal degeneration, producing a tear or hole in the retina, through which fluid can escape into the potential space between the pigment epithelium and the neuroepithelium. This condition, often named "primary" retinal detachment, occurs most frequently in the age group between 40 and 70 years and is more common in males (60 to 70 per cent of the cases) than in females. It becomes bilateral in about 15 to 30 per cent of the cases, and is more common in myopic eyes (about two-thirds of the cases) than in emmetropic or hypermetropic eyes. Some cases show a hereditary tendency, but in most cases the hereditary element is considered to be a disposition to retinal or retino-vitreal degeneration rather than a disposition to retinal detachment itself.

In the minority of cases, in which there is usually no tear or hole in the retina, the detachment is secondary to neoplastic conditions such as retinal or choroidal tumors (Fig. 488), circulatory conditions such as angiomatosis of the retina (Figs. 148—149), toxemia of pregnancy, Eales' disease, Coats' syndrome, inflammatory conditions such as severe uveitis (Fig. 472) and sympathetic ophthalmitis. In proliferative diabetic retinopathy, Eales' disease and retrolental fibroplasia (Figs. 37—39), or following perforating traumas of the eye, retinal detachment may occur due to traction in the retina by the organized tissue. In such cases detachment is seen primarily without a retinal hole, but the continuous pull in the retina may give rise to a secondary retinal tear (Fig. 471).

Retinal detachment may also occur after ocular surgery, particularly cataract extraction. It occurs in about 2 per cent of all cataract extractions and especially in cases with loss of vitreous fluid.

A retinal detachment may appear with or without prodromal symptoms. In the former case, which is rather frequent, the patient notices some muscae volitantes, metamorphopsia and flashes or flickers of light in part of the visual field, some days or even weeks before the detachment becomes evident. The symptoms of retinal detachment may vary considerably according to the site and extension of the detachment. When detachment is large and involves the macular area, central vision becomes suddenly reduced. When detachment starts in the periphery, a cloudy shadow suddenly appears in the visual field, and as the detachment spreads towards the macula the shadow enlarges and vision becomes increasingly impaired. If, however, the detachment is flat and localized in the lower part of the fundus it may escape the notice of the patient until it is discovered on routine examination. The detachment is usually progressive, and therefore if untreated it usually becomes total and vision is lost.

OPHTHALMOSCOPICALLY, retinal detachment shows wide variations depending on the site, extension, projection and duration of the detachment, and on the site and form of the retinal tears or holes.

When a detachment has been present for some time, the detached retina loses its normal transparency and becomes visible as an opaque, grayish-white membrane. The detached area is either sharply limited, or passes without sharp limits into the attached, normal-looking retina.

In shallow or flat detachment (Figs. 455—460), the detached retina assumes a rippled surface which is recognized by discrete, wavy, whitish lines, and the retinal vessels in this area show slight bending. In deep or far projecting detachment (Figs. 461—462, 465), the retina is seen as a grayish-white, uneven membrane resembling hills and valleys, or as a large balloon sometimes obscuring the optic disc. The detached retina projects forward for a varying distance and usually shows wave-like motions when the eye is moved. In the detached area the retinal vessels appear more tortuous and darker than normal.

In the early stage, the retinal detachment is usually limited to a segment of the fundus and is often situated in the upper quadrants. As the subretinal fluid

tends to gravitate to the lower part of the eye, detachment gradually becomes total. The upper part of the retinal detachment, however, often becomes flat when the subretinal fluid has settled below.

In "primary" retinal detachment, retinal tears or holes are almost invariably present (Figs. 465—470). The tears are mainly located in the equatorial region or at the ora serrata and most often they appear in the upper temporal quadrant. Frequently, more than one hole is present in the fundus.

According to size and form, the holes are classified as horseshoe-shaped tears with operculum, linear tears with serrated margins, small rounded holes occurring mainly in areas of cystoid degeneration, and arcuate holes due to disinsertion or dialysis of the retina at the ora serrata.

When the retinal tear or hole is situated in an area of far projecting detachment, it is seen plainly as a sharply outlined area through which the red color of the choroid becomes apparent, contrasting sharply with the surrounding retina. When the hole is situated in a shallow detachment or non-detached area, however, it may be difficult to detect because of the small contrast in color (Figs. 463—464).

In detachment in the macular area, a distinctly outlined red patch, usually a macular pseudo-hole (Fig. 457), may be difficult to distinguish from a true macular hole.

In the diagnosis of retinal detachment, direct and indirect ophthalmoscopy and examination with the Goldmann three-mirror goniolens should always be performed to trace and localize the retinal holes very accurately as this is of greatest importance for a successful operative treatment.

In the differential diagnosis, ultrasonography is of particular value because this method allows the distinction between "primary", spontaneous retinal detachment and detachment due to a solid process, usually a malignant choroidal melanoma. Transillumination as well as fluorescein angiography may also provide valuable information in such cases.

Retinoschisis and retinal cysts are discussed elsewhere.

HISTOPATHOLOGICALLY, retinal detachment is seen as a separation of the main retina from the pigment epithelium. The retinal changes are characterized by cystoid degeneration, areas of atrophy and tears. The choroid and the vitreous show various degrees of degeneration.

REFERENCES:

Byer, N. E.: Clinical study of retinal breaks. Trans. Amer. Acad. Ophthal. Otolaryng. *71:* 461—473, 1967.

Cibis, P. A.: Vitreoretinal pathology and surgery in retinal detachment. Mosby, St. Louis. 1965.

Edmund, J.: The clinical picture and prognosis of retinal detachment. Acta ophthal. (Kbh.). *42:* 980—1014, 1964.

Havener, W. H. & S. Gloeckner: Atlas of diagnostic techniques and treatment of retinal detachment. Mosby, St. Louis. 1967.

Hruby, K.: Die juvenile Netzhautablösung. Klin. Monatsbl. Augenh. *152:* 305—312, 1968.

Klöti, R.: Netzhautablösung. Klinisch-therapeutische und experimentelle Aspekte. Ophthalmologica. *Suppl. 67,* 1965.

Liesenhoff, H.: Ursachen der Netzhautablösung im Kindesalter und ihre Behandlungsmöglichkeiten. Klin. Monatsbl. Augenh. *152:* 60—69, 1968.

Schepens, C. L. & D. Marden: Data on the natural history of retinal detachment. Amer. J. Ophthal. *61:* 213—226, 1966.

Tassman, W.: Retinal detachment in children. Trans. Amer. Acad. Ophthal. Otolaryng. *71:* 455—460, 1967.

Tulloh, C. G.: Trauma in retinal detachment. Brit. J. Ophthal. *52:* 317—321, 1968.

Urrets-Zavalia, A.: Le décollement de la rétine. Masson, Paris. 1968.

Grouped Pigmentation of the Retina

(Figures 473—474)

Grouped pigmentation of the retina is a rare congenital anomaly characterized by non-progressive patchy aggregations of the pigment in the retina. The basis of this anomaly is hyperplasia of the pigment cells of the retinal epithelium. The condition is nearly always unilateral.

The pigmentation does not cause any visual or other functional disturbances.

Ophthalmoscopically, the pigmentations are seen (Figs. 473—474) as sharply defined, rounded or angular, grayish-brown, dark-brown or nearly black patches, frequently grouped in a manner resembling the footprints of an animal or arranged in quite irregular masses. The size varies from small dots to disc size. The pigmentations are frequently confined to a single sector of the fundus, becoming larger as they approach the periphery. The posterior pole and the macula are usually not involved. The retinal vessels pass in front of the pigmentations.

The ophthalmoscopic picture of grouped pigmentation of the retina is very characteristic, and should not be confused with choroidal nevi or malignant choroidal melanoma.

Histopathologically, the condition is characterized by areas of varying size, showing proliferation and aggregation of deeply pigmented retinal pigment epithelium cells, some of which may have migrated into the retina. The overlying neuroepithelium shows failure of development of rods and cones.

References:

Franceschetti, A., J. François & J. Babel: Les hérédo-dégénérescences chorio-rétiniennes. Masson, Paris. 607, 1963.

Lindsay, A.: Retinal pigmentation due to choroidal melano-sarcoma with observations on congenital grouped pigmentation of the retina. Brit. J. Ophthal. 39: 114—118, 1955.

Meunier, A. & P. Boursin: La pigmentation groupée de la rétine. Bull. Soc. Belge Ophtal. 99: 470—478, 1951.

Choroidal Nevus
(Figures 475—478)

Choroidal nevus or benign choroidal melanoma is a relatively common neoplasm consisting of melanocytes.

Choroidal nevi have a congenital basis although they do not become evident ophthalmoscopically until about puberty or during pregnancy, when all melanocytic cells of the body become active.

Choroidal nevi are usually stationary and benign, but a nevus may sometimes be transformed into a malignant choroidal melanoma.

Choroidal nevi do not cause visual disturbances. A small scotoma may, however, be present in the visual field.

OPHTHALMOSCOPICALLY, a nevus is seen (Figs. 475—478) as a flat, circular or oval, slate-gray, grayish-green or bluish patch of nearly uniform density, with ill-defined, often somewhat feathered margins and usually about the size of the optic disc. It is most frequently situated near the disc, but it may occur in the macular area or elsewhere in the fundus. The overlying retina is flat or slightly elevated, and the retinal vessels lying in front of the nevus appear darker than normal. At times, small drusen-like light dots are present on the surface of the nevus.

In the differential diagnosis of choroidal nevus, grouped pigmentation of the retina and malignant choroidal melanoma have to be considered. Ophthalmoscopically, the distinction between a choroidal nevus and a malignant choroidal melanoma is usually not difficult. In some cases, however, it may be rather difficult. In these cases fluorescein angiography may be of some help. If the choroidal lesion shows no staining it is a choroidal nevus, but if the lesion shows fluorescence the conditions cannot be distinguished by fluorescein angiography, and the patient must be kept under further control.

HISTOPATHOLOGICALLY, choroidal nevi are highly cellular tumors composed of oval or spindle-shaped, well-differentiated, mature pigment-bearing cells showing no or only few mitotic figures, and the cells do not infiltrate the surrounding tissues.

REFERENCES:

Naumann, G., M. Yanoff & L. E. Zimmerman: Histogenesis of malignant melanomas of the uvea. I. Histopathologic characteristics of nevi of the choroid and ciliary body. A.M.A. Arch. Ophthal. 76: 784—796, 1966.

Tamler, E. & A. E. Maumenee: A clinical study of choroidal nevi. A.M.A. Arch. Ophthal. 62: 196—202, 1959.

Wessing, A.: Fluoreszenzangiographie der Retina. Lehrbuch und Atlas. Thieme, Stuttgart. 149, 165, 1968.

Malignant Melanoma of the Choroid
(Figures 479—490)

Malignant choroidal melanoma is the most common malignant intraocular neoplasm. It may arise anywhere in the uveal tract, but most often in the choroid. Bilateral occurrence is extremely rare.

The malignancy depends on the cell type. The prognosis is best in cases where the tumor is composed of spindle cells and tumors containing heavy deposits of reticulin, and poorest in mixed and epithelioid tumors, and those containing sparse or no reticulin. The average ten-year mortality rate of malignant choroidal melanoma, including all cell types, is about 50 per cent.

Malignant melanoma occurs most frequently in middle life, and is exceedingly rare in children.

The symptoms depend on the site and extension of the tumor. Tumors localized at or near the macula early give rise to metamorphopsia, blurred vision and central scotoma. Tumors localized elsewhere in the fundus may be unnoticed for a long time, but sooner or later give rise to defects in the visual field. Secondary glaucoma may sometimes develop as a result of intraocular extension of the tumor. Occasionally, the tumor causes an intraocular hemorrhage with a sudden loss of vision.

Extraocular extension of the tumor and metastases may occur early, and may occasionally be the first sign of a malignant choroidal melanoma. The tumor extends along the ciliary nerves and vessels, or infiltrates the sclera directly. Invasion through the substance of the optic nerve into the meninges is unusual. The metastases are hematogenous. They may involve almost any organ of the body, but most frequently the liver.

OPHTHALMOSCOPICALLY, malignant melanoma is seen in the early stage as an indistinctly outlined, often mottled, yellowish-red, grayish or brownish, flat or slightly elevated patch in the fundus, and the retinal vessels overlying the tumor appear darker than normal (Figs. 479—480). As the tumor grows, extension takes place in the plane of the choroid (Figs. 481—484) and towards the retina (Figs. 486—487). When the tumor has penetrated Bruch's membrane, the retina is pushed forwards (Figs. 488—489) and detached to a variable extent, but retinal tears or holes are usually not present. The color of the tumor varies with the degree of pigmentation, from yellow or yellowish-pink to grayish-red or even dark brown, but the color is usually not uniform, as the pigment is irregularly distributed.

In malignant choroidal melanomas penetrating into the vitreous, pigmented tumor cell aggregations may occasionally be dispersed into the vitreous or diffusely spread on the retinal surface (Fig. 485).

A benign medulloepithelioma, which is a rare condition, may ophthalmoscopically be indistinguishable from a malignant choroidal melanoma (Fig. 490).

Malignant choroidal melanoma can be both easy and difficult to diagnose. In early stages, it may be confused with a choroidal nevus, commencing disciform degeneration of the macula, subretinal hemorrhage, metastatic carcinoma of the choroid, angioma of the choroid, acute choroiditis or tuberculoma of the choroid. In the late stages, it may be confused with simple retinal detachment, detachment of the choroid or cysts of the retina. Complicating secondary glaucoma, intraocular hemorrhage, uveitis or panophthalmitis may also make the diagnosis difficult. A blind and phthisic eye should always arouse suspicion of malignant choroidal melanoma.

In the diagnosis of malignant choroidal melanoma, direct as well as indirect ophthalmoscopy should be performed together with transillumination of the eye and slit-lamp examination aided by a Hruby lens or a Goldmann three-mirror goniolens.

Fluorescein angiography may be of value in the diagnosis and differential diagnosis, as some of the conditions to be considered often show characteristic patterns of fluorescence different from those in malignant choroidal melanoma (commencing disciform macular degeneration, acute choroiditis, and, sometimes, choroidal angioma), or show no fluorescence (subretinal hemorrhage and, frequently, choroidal nevus).

Using ultrasonography it is possible to distinguish between a solid process and simple retinal detachment.

Finally, the color and growth of the patological process is of great value in differentiating the conditions.

Melanin in the urine is probably only present when extensive metastases are present.

HISTOPATHOLOGICALLY, malignant melanomas are classified according to the cell type as spindle A and B, fascicular, mixed and epithelioid tumors. The tumors are usually highly cellular, containing varying amounts of reticulin and often showing areas of necrosis.

REFERENCES:

Benthien, H.: Klinischer Verlauf, Prognose und Therapie des malignen Melanoms der Uvea. Klin. Monatsbl. Augenh. *153:* 4—16, 1968.

François, J.: Diagnostic des mélanomes malins de la choroïde. Ophthalmologica. *151:* 114—134, 1966.

François, J. & M. Hanssens: Histopathologie des mélanomes malins de la choroïde. Ophthalmologica. *151:* 135—160, 1966.

Gitter, K. A., D. Meyer, L. K. Sarin, A. H. Keeney & J. Justice: Fluorescein and ultrasound in diagnosis of intraocular tumors. Amer. J. Ophthal. *66:* 719—731, 1968.

Hogan, M. J. & L. E. Zimmerman (Ed.): Ophthalmic pathology. *2nd ed.* Saunders, Philadelphia. 419, 1962.

Jensen, O. A.: Malignant melanomas of the uvea in Denmark 1943—1952. Acta ophthal. (Kbh.). *Suppl. 75,* 1963.

Lemke, L., A. Jütte & A. Scheibe: Differential-diagnose des Melanocytoblastoms der Aderhaut mit Fluorescein-Natrium. Graefes Arch. Ophth. *175:* 58—67, 1968.

Oosterhuis, J. A. & Ch. W. van Waveren: Fluorescein photography in malignant melanoma. Ophthalmologica. *156:* 101—116, 1968.

Reese, A. B.: Tumors of the eye. *2nd ed.* Hoeber, New York. 232, 1963.

Snyder, W. B., L. Allen & O. Frazier: Fluorescence angiography of ocular tumors. Trans. Amer. Acad. Ophthal. Otolaryng. *71:* 820—832, 1967.

Wessing, A.: Fluoreszenzangiographie der Retina. Lehrbuch und Atlas. Thieme, Stuttgart. 151, 1968.

Metastatic Carcinoma of the Choroid
(Figures 491—492)

Metastatic tumors in the choroid may arise from carcinoma, hypernephroma, malignant melanoma or chorionepithelioma. Although rare, metastatic carcinoma is the most common secondary tumor in the choroid.

Metastatic carcinomas of the choroid are the results of emboli of malignant cells reaching the eye through the posterior ciliary vessels. Lodged in the choriocapillaris, the cells multiply and infiltrate the choroid, forming a secondary tumor.

The most frequent site of the primary carcinoma is the breast and the lung. However, the primary tumor may also be a carcinoma of the gastro-intestinal tract, kidney, prostate, ovary, parotid gland, liver, testicle, pancreas or thyroid.

The occurrence of visual disturbances depends exclusively on the site and extension of the choroidal metastases. There may be no ocular symptoms, or a history of failing vision in one eye. Bilateral occurrence, however, is not infrequent. Symptoms of secondary glaucoma and pain sometimes become evident in the late stages, but these symptoms may occur earlier if the ciliary body and iris are affected.

OPHTHALMOSCOPICALLY, metastatic choroidal tumors are seen (Figs. 491—492) as well- or ill-defined, rounded, slightly raised, opaque, often mottled, grayish, yellowish or yellowish-white areas of varying extension. They are either single or multiple, and typically they appear on the temporal side near the optic disc.

Small hemorrhages may occur but they are not a prominent feature. The metastases extend chiefly in the plane of the choroid with relatively little increase in thickness. Sometimes, a shallow, more or less wide-spread retinal detachment may develop.

In typical cases presenting a history of carcinoma elsewhere, the diagnosis is not difficult. In cases with no apparent primary tumor, however, the condition has to be differentiated from malignant choroidal melanoma, acute choroiditis and the acute stage of retinal arterial occlusion.

HISTOPATHOLOGICALLY, the cells of a metastatic carcinoma of the choroid are often less differentiated than those of the primary tumor. It may be difficult or impossible, therefore, to determine the site of the primary carcinoma by examining the metastatic tumor.

REFERENCES:
Albert, D. M., R. A. Rubenstein & H. G. Scheie: Tumor metastasis to the eye. Amer. J. Ophthal. 63: 723—726, 1967.
Greear, J. N.: Metastatic carcinoma of the eye. Amer. J. Ophthal. 33: 1015—1025, 1950.
Greer, C. H.: Choroidal carcinoma metastatic from the male breast. Brit. J. Ophthal. 38: 312—315, 1954.
Reese, A. B.: Tumors of the eye. 2nd ed. Hoeber, New York. 514, 1963.
Seddik, N., C. Gailloud & R. Faggioni: Les métastases oculaires, orbitaires et palpébrales. Ophthalmologica. 156: 273—284, 1968.
Snyder, W. B., L. Allen & O. Frazier: Fluorescence angiography of ocular tumors. Trans. Amer. Acad. Ophthal. Otolaryng. 71: 820—832, 1967.

Fundus Changes in Retrobulbar Tumor
(Figures 493—494)

Any orbital tumor of sufficient size may cause indentation of the eye and give rise to retinal folding or ridging.

Ophthalmoscopically, the indentation is seen in the fundus as horizontal or slightly oblique, parallel retinal folds or ripples (Figs. 493—494), most often situated in the macular area. When the tumor is removed the folds usually disappear, unless permanent shrinkage has developed.

References:

Hedges, Th. R. & I. H. Leopold: Parallel retinal folds. Their significance in orbital space-taking lesions. A.M.A. Arch. Ophthal. *62:* 353—355, 1959.

Wolter, J. R.: Parallel horizontal retinal folding. Amer. J. Ophthal. *53:* 26—29, 1962.

Retinoblastoma
(Figures 495—499)

Retinoblastoma is a retinal tumor composed of undifferentiated neuroblastic cells, and occurring most frequently in childhood. The tumor is probably always congenital in origin, and bilateral in about 20 to 25 per cent of the cases. In bilateral cases, the extension of the tumor is often different in the two eyes when noticed, or the tumor may be unilateral at first observation, and not appear in the second eye until months or even years after the tumor is noticed in the first eye. Although most cases are sporadic, familial cases occur. The offspring of survivors of the disease show a high incidence of retinoblastoma.

Most frequently, retinoblastoma is observed clinically during the first four years of life. After that age, the incidence declines abruptly, and it is extremely rare in adults.

As retinoblastoma occurs predominantly in small children, the first evidence of disease is frequently observed by the parents as lack of fixation, development of strabismus and most frequently as an anomalous whitish pupillary reflex, known as "amaurotic cat's eye" (Fig. 495).

The tumor may spread within the eye by local extension producing an enlargement of the globe, an endophthalmitic reaction in the eye or even painful secondary glaucoma. Most frequently, the tumor spreads by direct extension along the optic nerve, reaching the intracranial cavity. Less frequently, it penetrates the walls of the bulb into the orbit and the surrounding structures. In these cases lymphatic spread may occur along the orbital lymphatics, at first to the preauricular and cervical lymph nodes and later showing a more diffuse involvement of the lymph nodes. Hematogenous metastases are common and involve primarily the bones and the viscera, especially the liver.

The prognosis after careful treatment of the tumor in the early stage is fairly good, but in advanced cases with extension into the orbit, into the central nervous system, or where metastases have appeared, the condition is invariably fatal in spite of any treatment.

In successfully treated cases of retinoblastoma, the patient should be examined at short intervals for a period of at least two to four years, as new tumor growth may occur in the treated eye or in the previously unaffected eye.

OPHTHALMOSCOPICALLY, a retinoblastoma is seen in the early stage as a sharply defined, rounded, yellowish-white, grayish-white or pinkish-white tumor of varying size, situated anywhere in the fundus. The irregularly projecting surface of the tumor shows fine tortuous vessels (Fig. 498), often also pearly-white, calcareous deposits and, occasionally, small hemorrhages. The tumor may be single (Figs. 497—498) or present a number of lesions of similar size, or consist of a larger lesion surrounded by several small ones (Fig. 496).

The tumor growth may be either endophytic or exophytic.

In the former case, tumor growth takes place on the anterior surface of the retina, proliferates into the vitreous, and tumor implants may be seeded anywhere in the unaffected parts of the retina. Occasionally, a vitreous haze due to an endophthalmitic tumor reaction may partly obscure the fundus.

In the latter case, tumor growth takes place on the posterior surface of the retina and is therefore not as easily detected as the endophytic type of extension. In the early stages, exophytic extension appears as an elevated grayish zone in the fundus. In the later stages it is accompanied by a progressive detachment of the retina.

When the tumor has grown sufficiently large it becomes visible to the naked eye as a whitish pupillary reflex, the well-known condition of "amaurotic cat's eye" (Fig. 495).

After successful treatment, the retinoblastoma subsides, leaving an atrophic zone and often some calcareous deposits (Fig. 499).

In the diagnosis, scleral transillumination, ultrasonography and sometimes fluorescein angiography may be of value.

The early diagnosis of retinoblastoma is of great importance. The diagnosis may sometimes, however, be difficult and the condition may be confused with nonmalignant conditions such as Coats' syndrome, angiomatosis of the retina, choroidal tuberculoma, persistence of the primary vitreous, retrolental fibroplasia, falciform retinal detachment and endophthalmitis.

HISTOPATHOLOGICALLY, a retinoblastoma is composed principally of undifferentiated neuroblastic cells which exhibit large hyperchromatic nuclei and scanty cytoplasm. The tumor cells show a varying degree of differentiation and have a tendency to form retinoblastoma-rosettes. There are usually numerous mitotic figures, and areas of necrosis are often present, except in the perivascular area.

REFERENCES:
Holland, G. & H. Thiers: Beitrag zum Glioma retinae. Ophthalmologica. *146:* 377—394, 1963.
Howard, G. M. & R. M. Ellsworth: Differential diagnosis of retinoblastoma. A statistic survey of 500 children. I. Relative frequency of the lesions which simulate retinoblastoma. Amer. J. Ophthal. *60:* 610—618, 1965.
Jensen, O. A.: Retinoblastoma in Denmark 1943—1958. Acta ophthal. (Kbh.). *43:* 821—840, 1965.
Morgan, S. S. & H. L. Bair: Hereditary retinoblastoma. Amer. J. Ophthal. *65:* 43—47, 1968.
Nielsen, M. & E. Goldschmidt: Retinoblastoma among offspring of adult survivors in Denmark. Acta ophthal. (Kbh.). *46:* 736—741, 1968.
Reese, A. B.: Tumors of the eye. *2nd ed.* Hoeber, New York. 84, 1963.
Sezer, N. & R. Barishak: The diagnosis of retinoblastomas. Ophthalmologica. *151:* 184—195, 1966.
Stallard, H. B.: Multiple islands of retinoblastoma. Incidence rate and time span of appearance. Brit. J. Ophthal. *39:* 241—243, 1955.
Wessing, A.: Fluoreszenzangiographie der Retina. Lehrbuch und Atlas. Thieme, Stuttgart. 140, 1968.
Wetzig, P. C. & C. N. Jepson: Fluorescein photography. In the differential diagnosis of retinoblastoma. Amer. J. Ophthal. *61:* 341—343, 1966.

Mechanical Injuries to the Eye
(Figures 500—519)

Mechanical injuries to the eye are common. They may involve every structure in the eye and be the result of contusion and concussion or due to perforating or penetrating lesions.

In the anterior part of the eye, the most common lesion due to contusion is anterior chamber hemorrhage (hyphema), rupture of the root of the iris (iridodialysis), rupture of the sphincter of the iris and luxation of the lens. Perforating wounds most often result in prolapse of the iris and in cataract.

In the posterior part of the eye, contusions may result in retinal edema, macular cyst- or hole-formation, retinal or choroidal hemorrhages, and choroidal ruptures. Perforating lesions following accidents or foreign bodies cause hemorrhage and varying degrees of tissue damage. Retinal detachment may be a late complication.

Traumatic retinal edema, also known as commotio retinae or Berlin's edema, is the most frequent retinal lesion resulting from blunt injury. Usually it develops within 24 hours after the injury and disappears in the course of some days or weeks. While the edema persists, visual acuity is reduced and field defects are present. When the edema subsides, normal vision is often restored.

OPHTHALMOSCOPICALLY, traumatic retinal edema is seen (Figs. 500—501) as a grayish-white or grayish, opaque, ill-defined, slightly elevated area most often situated in the posterior part of the fundus. The fovea is likely to appear as a cherry-red spot and the macular area is often surrounded by linear light reflexes (Figs. 500—501). The edema usually disappears leaving no trace, but sometimes the edema may result in permanent degenerative changes, including pigmentary abnormalities (Fig. 502) or macular cyst- or hole-formation (Fig. 505), with permanent impairment of central vision.

Retinal or preretinal hemorrhages (Fig. 503) may also be the result of a blunt injury. These hemorrhages often subside leaving no trace, but pigmentary changes (Fig. 504) may occasionally follow the hemorrhage.

Traumatic choroidal ruptures are frequently obscured in the acute stage by intraocular hemorrhage. The ruptures are first discovered when the vitreous clears in the course of some days or weeks.

OPHTHALMOSCOPICALLY, traumatic choroidal ruptures are seen (Figs. 506—507, 510—511) as crescentic or irregular white patches or lines of exposed sclera, commonly situated within 3 or 4 mm from the disc. Usually there is only a single choroidal rupture (Fig. 510), but several ruptures may be present in the same fundus (Figs. 507, 511). The ruptures are most frequently seen at the temporal side of the disc and not infrequently they may involve the macular area (Fig. 511). In the early stage, the rupture is surrounded and partly obscured by retinal and subretinal hemorrhages and by retinal edema (Figs. 508—509). In the scarring stage, the lesion is seen as an elongated, usually crescentic, whitish or grayish-white atrophic zone with a varying amount of pigment deposits (Figs. 510—511).

Intraocular foreign bodies (Figs. 512—513) may cause more or less extensive damage to the structures of the eye. Pigmentary changes and scar formation may occur after the foreign body has been removed (Figs. 514—515).

Retained intraocular foreign bodies of iron often cause siderosis, while retained foreign bodies of copper may cause diffuse intraocular degeneration (chalcosis) or a violent uveitis with subsequent phthisis. In early stages of siderosis, the electroretinogram is of the negative plus type. Later, it changes to the negative minus type, and finally the electroretinographic response becomes extinguished. If the foreign body is removed in the first stage, the electroretinogram may be normalized.

Perforating lesions (Figs. 517—518) may result in gross intraocular hemorrhage and more or less extensive damage to the structures of the eye, followed by scar formation (Fig. 519), and later in some cases by retinal detachment.

In rare instances, the perforating lesion may give rise to the occurrence of papilledema ex vacuo (Fig. 516).

REFERENCES:

Duke-Elder, S.: Text-book of ophthalmology. *Vol. VI.* Injuries. Kimpton, London. 1954.

Kutschera, E. & B. Kosmath: Augenverletzungen bei Jagdunfällen. Klin. Monatsbl. Augenh. *153:* 808—813, 1968.

Müller-Jensen, K. & W. Allmaras: Zur Prognose der Augenverletzungen bei Verkehersunfällen. Klin. Monatsbl. Augenh. *153:* 803—807, 1968.

Purtscher's Retinopathy
(Figure 520)

Purtscher's retinopathy, angiopathia retinae traumatica or retinopathy due to distant injury, is a condition occurring in association with injury to the skull or thoracic compression. The nature of the condition is not quite clear and, therefore, still a matter of discussion.

The condition appears within a few days after the injury and usually subsides within a few weeks.

In the acute stage, visual disturbances may occur if the macula is involved, but these disturbances usually disappear when the retinopathy subsides.

OPHTHALMOSCOPICALLY, the condition (Fig. 520) is characterized by woolly exudates and streaky hemorrhages, usually within the area bordered by the superior and inferior temporal vessels. The hemorrhages and exudates gradually become absorbed, usually leaving no trace.

REFERENCES:

Calmettes, L., F. Deodati & G. Bechac: L'embolie graisseuse de la rétine. Arch. Ophtal. (Paris). 27: 209—220, 1967.

Rask, J. A.: Post-traumatic fat embolism located in the retina. Acta ophthal. (Kbh.). 46: 218—222, 1968.

Schmidt, J. G. H.: Angiopathia retinae traumatica (Purtscher) und Fettembolie. Klin. Monatsbl. Augenh. 152: 672—679, 1968.

Verin, P. & M.-J. le Rebeller: Les embolies graisseuses. Incidences ophtalmologiques. Revue générale à propos de 9 cas. Arch. Ophtal. (Paris). 27: 123—144, 1967.

Fundus Changes after Strangulation
(Figure 521)

Fundus changes after strangulation are seldom observed, but may occur in the form of small or large retinal, preretinal or subretinal hemorrhages (Fig. 521).

Sun Eclipse Injury of the Retina
(Figures 522—523)

Every sun eclipse is watched by many people. In spite of warnings, some people do not wear dark, protecting lenses and some may afterwards show retinal lesions following the thermal effect of the sun.

Visual disturbances due to this thermal effect may occur as central scotomas or scotomas elsewhere in the visual field.

OPHTHALMOSCOPICALLY, the condition is seen in the scarring stage (Figs. 522—523) as a chorioretinal lesion with atrophy and pigment accumulations, preferentially in the macular area.

REFERENCES:

Penner, R. & J. N. McNair: Eclipse blindness. Report of an epidemic in the military population of Hawaii. Amer. J. Ophthal. *61:* 1452—1457, 1966.

COLOR ATLAS
OF THE
OCULAR FUNDUS

Figure 1. Composite picture. Right eye. Normal appearance of a medium pigmented fundus. The fundus has a uniform, warm red color. The macular area is slightly deeper red in color. The optic disc and the retinal vessels are normal.

CLINICAL NOTE: Figure 1 is from a female, aged 39. No general or ocular complaints.
Eye examination: Visual acuity, both eyes: 6/6, emmetropia. Anterior segments and fundi are normal.
General examination showed nothing abnormal.

Figure 2. Right eye. Normal fundus in a young person. The macular and foveal light reflexes are seen clearly. Fundus pigmentation is uniform. The optic disc and the retinal vessels are normal.

CLINICAL NOTE: Figure 2 is from the same patient as figures 54 and 64, a male, aged 21. No general or ocular complaints.

Eye examination: Visual acuity, both eyes: 6/6 with + 1.5 D sph. Anterior segments are normal. Right fundus is normal. Left fundus shows large optic disc with conus and pigmentation temporally. Left blind spot slightly enlarged.
General examination showed nothing abnormal.

Figure 3. Right eye. Normal appearance of a lightly pigmented fundus. The fundus has an orange-red color. Choroidal vessels are seen faintly. Disc and retinal vessels are normal.

CLINICAL NOTE: Figure 3 is from a female, aged 49. During the last few weeks gradually reduced vision in the left eye. No complaints from the right eye. No general symptoms.
Eye examination: Visual acuity, right eye: 6/6 with + 1.0 D sph.; left eye: 6/18 with + 1.0 D sph. Visual field, right eye: normal; left eye: small central scotoma. Intraocular tension and anterior segments are normal. Right fundus is normal. Left fundus shows presenile macular degeneration.
General examination showed nothing abnormal. Blood pressure: 130/80 mm Hg.

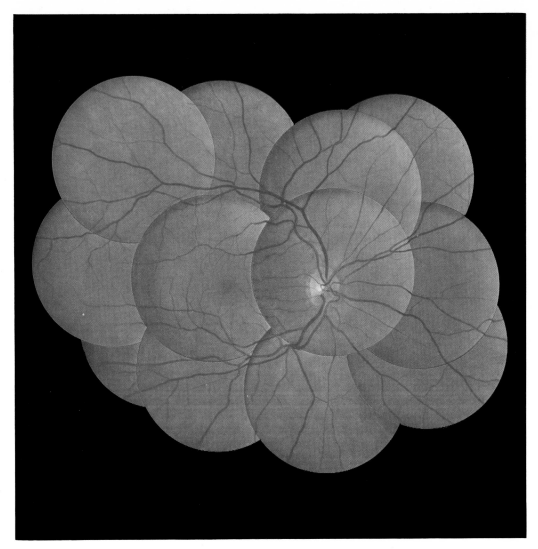

1

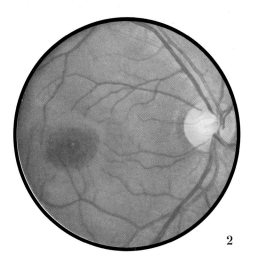

2

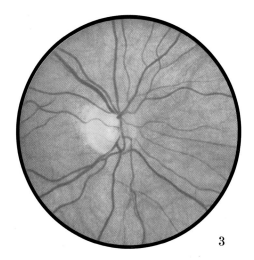

3

Figure 4. Right eye. Normal fundus in a Negro. The fundus is red-brown. Disc and retinal vessels are normal.

CLINICAL NOTE: Figure 4 is from the same patient as figure 57, a male, aged 30. No general or ocular complaints.
Eye examination: Visual acuity, both eyes: 6/6, emmetropia. Anterior segments and fundi are normal.
General examination showed nothing abnormal.

Figure 5. Right eye. Normal fundus in an Indian. The fundus has a light brown color with a tint of green. Disc and retinal vessels are normal.

CLINICAL NOTE: Figure 5 is from a male, aged 30. No general or ocular complaints.
Eye examination: Visual acuity, both eyes: 6/6, emmetropia. Anterior segments and fundi are normal.
General examination showed nothing abnormal.

Figure 6. Right eye. Normal fundus in a Chinese. The fundus is tessellated and shows slate-gray areas. Disc and retinal vessels are normal.

CLINICAL NOTE: Figure 6 is from a male, aged 49. No general or ocular complaints.
Eye examination: Visual acuity, both eyes: 6/6 with + 1.0 D sph. Anterior segments and fundi are normal.
General examination showed nothing abnormal.

Figure 7. Left eye. Normal fundus in a young Greenlander. The fundus has a red-brown color with a tint of green. The macular reflex is seen clearly. Disc and retinal vessels are normal.

CLINICAL NOTE: Figure 7 is from the same patient as figure 509, a female, aged 13. A fortnight ago she received a blunt injury to the right eye from a single shot fired from a shotgun. Since then central vision in the right eye has been severely reduced.
Eye examination: Visual acuity, right eye: 3/36, unimproved by lenses; left eye: 6/6, emmetropia. Anterior segments are normal. In the right fundus, there are fresh choroidal ruptures surrounded by retinal edema, and by retinal and subretinal hemorrhages. Visual field defect corresponds to the fundal lesion. The left fundus is normal.
General examination showed nothing abnormal.

Figures 8 and 9. Right eye. Temporal and nasal part of the same fundus. The fundus shows marked tessellation. The fundus color corresponds to a dark-haired person. The macula, optic disc and retinal vessels are normal.

CLINICAL NOTE: Figures 8 and 9 are from a female, aged 21. No general or ocular complaints.
Eye examination: Visual acuity, both eyes: 6/6 with − 4.0 D sph. Anterior segments and fundi are normal.
General examination showed nothing abnormal.

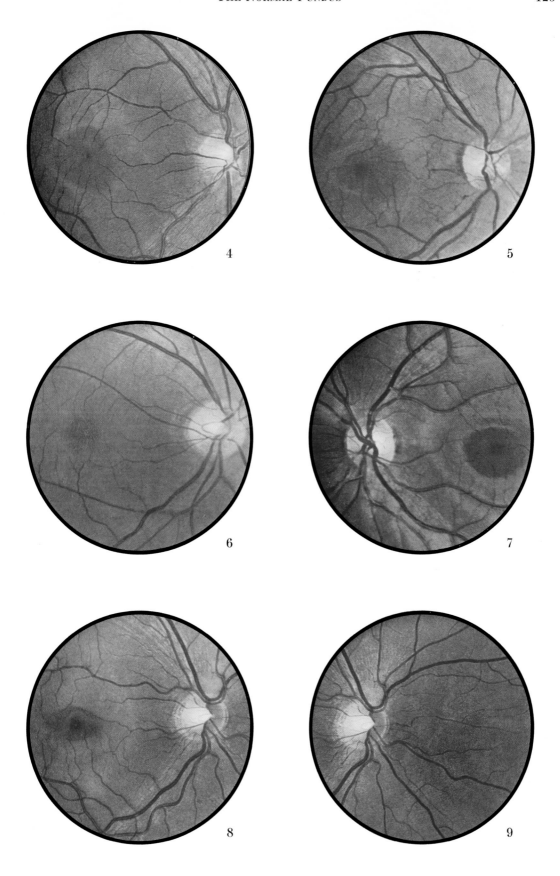

Figures 10 and 11. Right eye. Temporal and nasal part of the same pseudoalbinotic fundus. The fundus has an orange-red color and the choroidal vessels are seen plainly. The macular area has a normal appearance. Disc and retinal vessels are normal.

Clinical note: Figures 10 and 11 are from a male, aged 11. No general or ocular complaints. *Eye examination:* Visual acuity, both eyes: 6/6 with + 1.0 D sph. − 0.5 D cyl. axis 90°. Anterior segments are normal. Fundi are pseudo-albinotic.
General examination showed nothing abnormal.

Figures 12 and 13. Right eye. Temporal and nasal part of the same albinotic fundus. The macular area has a pink color and the fovea is absent. In the rest of the depigmented fundus the scleral color is dominating. Choroidal vessels are seen plainly. Disc and retinal vessels are normal.

Clinical note: Figures 12 and 13 are from a female, aged 20. Her mother's brother shows complete albinism. Since infancy she has had complete albinism with photophobia, nystagmus and poor vision.
Eye examination: Visual acuity, both eyes: 6/60 with − 2.0 D sph. − 3.0 D cyl. axis 0°. The iris is pink-gray and translucent in both eyes. The fundi are albinotic.
General examination showed complete albinism.

Figure 14. Right eye. Carrier of albinism. Nasal fundus periphery shows extensive coarse and irregular pigmentation and some depigmentation. Retinal vessels are normal.

Clinical note: Figure 14 is from a female, aged 18. Her father and a male cousin have ocular albinism and nystagmus. She has no sisters. A brother and all women in the family have no visual disturbances or known albinism.
Eye examination: Visual acuity, both eyes: 6/6, emmetropia. Anterior segments including the irides are normal. Both fundi present extensive coarse and irregular pigmentation and some depigmentation in the fundal periphery. Discs and retinal vessels are normal.
General examination showed nothing abnormal.

Figure 15. Right eye. Carrier of albinism. Nasal fundus periphery shows extensive coarse and irregular depigmentation. Retinal vessels are normal.

Clinical note: Figure 15 is from a female, aged 32. Her son has ocular albinism. Otherwise no visual disturbances or known albinism in the family.
Eye examination: Visual acuity, both eyes: 6/6, emmetropia. Anterior segments including the irides are normal. Both fundi present extensive coarse and irregular pigmentation and depigmentation in the fundal periphery. Disc and retinal vessels are normal.
General examination showed nothing abnormal.

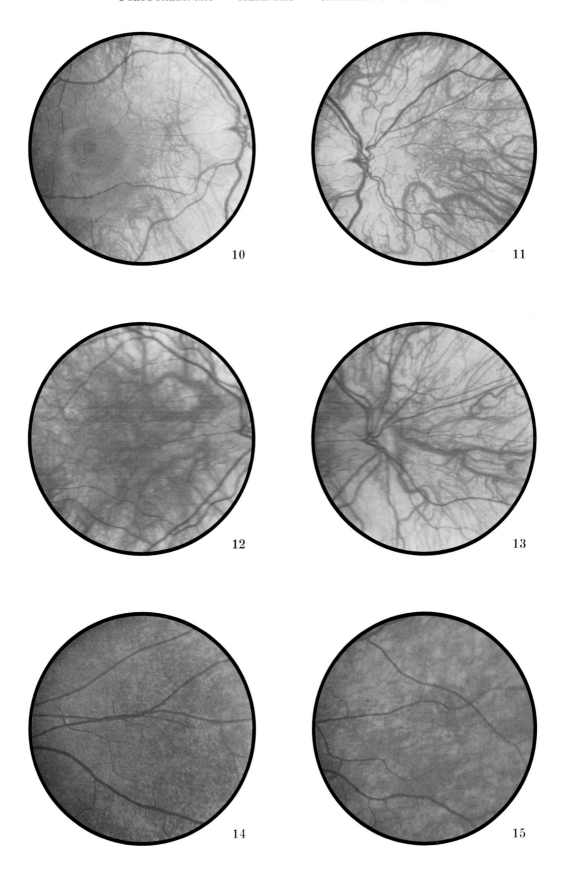

Figure 16. Left eye. A white, silky patch of medullated nerve fibers is situated just above the optic disc. The opaque fibers partly obscure some of the retinal vessels. Disc and retinal vessels are normal.

CLINICAL NOTE: Figure 16 is from a female, aged 41. She has no visual or general complaints.
Eye examination: Visual acuity, right eye: 6/6 with − 0.5 D cyl. axis 25°; left eye: 6/6 with + 1.0 D sph. + 0.75 D cyl. axis 75°. Anterior segments are normal. Both fundi present medullated nerve fibers at the disc. Visual field defect corresponds to the fundal changes.
General examination showed nothing abnormal.

Figure 17. Right eye. Isolated whitish, silky patch of medullated nerve fibers in the fundus periphery. The patch has a finely striated surface and a feathered margin.

CLINICAL NOTE: Figure 17 is from a male, aged 48. Acute monocytic leukemia demonstrated two months ago. No ocular complaints.
Eye examination: Visual acuity, both eyes: 6/6, emmetropia. Anterior segments are normal. Some flame-shaped retinal hemorrhages are seen in both fundi. In the right eye, there is an isolated patch of medullated nerve fibers in the upper temporal quadrant. Small visual field defect corresponds to the medullated nerve fibers. Optic discs and retinal vessels are normal.
General examination showed an anemic patient without enlargement of the spleen or lymph nodes. Hemoglobin: 7.2 g/100 ml. Sedimentation rate: 125 mm/hour. White blood cells: 6,700 per cu mm, with 30 per cent monoblasts, 15 per cent leucocytes, and 55 per cent lymphocytes.

Figure 18. Right eye. A large white patch of medullated nerve fibers surrounds and partly obscures the optic disc and the large retinal vessels. The patch has a feathered margin.

Figure 19. Left eye. From the same patient as figure 18. A large white patch of medullated nerve fibers obscures the optic disc and its surroundings but leaves the macular area free.

CLINICAL NOTE: Figures 18 and 19 are from a female, aged 19. No general or ocular complaints.
Eye examination: Visual acuity, both eyes: 6/6, emmetropia. Anterior segments are normal. Except for large patches of medullated nerve fibers in both eyes, the fundi are normal. Visual field defects correspond to the extension of medullated nerve fibers.
General examination showed nothing abnormal.

Figures 20 and 21. Left eye. Disc and macular area of the same fundus. Extensive area of medullated nerve fibers in the posterior pole, obscures the optic disc, macular area and many of the retinal vessels.

CLINICAL NOTE: Figures 20 and 21 are from a male, aged 7. Since infancy vision has been defective in his left eye. No complaints from the right eye.
Eye examination: Visual acuity, right eye: 6/6, emmetropia; left eye: 6/60, unimproved by lenses. No squint. Anterior segments are normal. The right fundus is normal. In the left fundus, the whole posterior pole is covered by medullated nerve fibers. Visual field defect corresponds to the fundus changes.
General examination showed nothing abnormal.

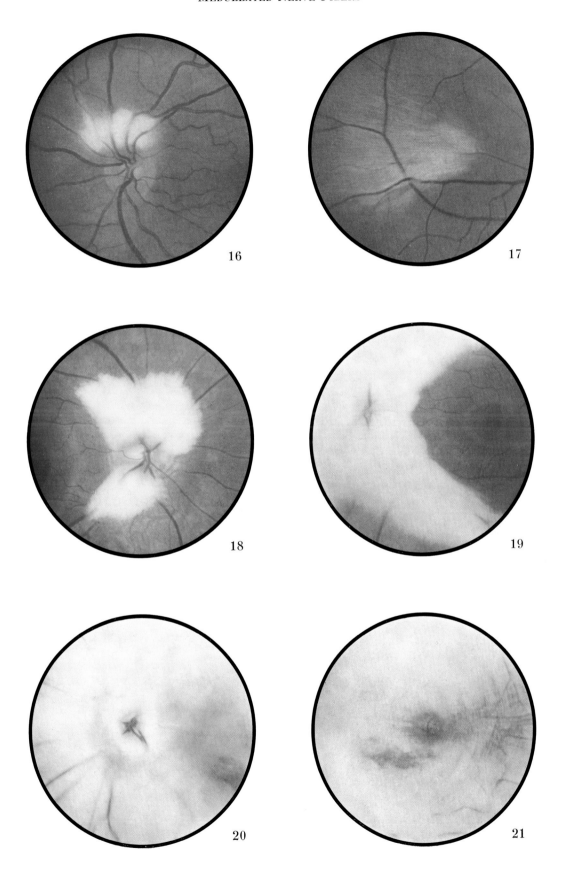

16

17

18

19

20

21

Figure 22. Right eye. Small crater-like hole in the temporal part of the optic disc. Otherwise disc and retinal vessels are normal.

CLINICAL NOTE: Figure 22 is from a male, aged 23. No general or ocular complaints.
Eye examination: Visual acuity, both eyes: 6/6, emmetropia. Anterior segments are normal. Except for crater-like hole in the right optic disc, the fundi are normal. No visual field defect.
General examination showed nothing abnormal.

Figure 23. Left eye. Small pigmented crater-like hole in the temporal part of the optic disc. Otherwise disc and retinal vessels are normal.

CLINICAL NOTE: Figure 23 is from a female, aged 22. No general or ocular complaints.
Eye examination: Visual acuity, both eyes: 6/6 with + 0.5 D sph. Anterior segments are normal. Except for crater-like hole in the left optic disc, the fundi are normal. No visual field defect.
General examination showed nothing abnormal.

Figure 24. Right eye. Incomplete coloboma of the optic disc and the choroid. Centrally, the optic disc coloboma, filled with whitish glial tissue, separates the upper and lower retinal vessels. Below, the choroidal coloboma is seen as a whitish crescent.

CLINICAL NOTE: Figure 24 is from a female, aged 30. Vision of her right eye has always been reduced. No complaints from the left eye. No family history of colobomas.
Eye examination: Visual acuity, right eye: 6/24 with + 1.5 D sph. + 0.5 D cyl. axis 100°; left eye: 6/6 with + 1.0 D sph. Slight horizontal nystagmus and exophoria. Anterior segments are normal. The right fundus shows incomplete coloboma of the optic disc and the choroid. Coarse pigmentation and depigmentation in the macular area. Sector-formed visual field defect extending from the blind spot. The left fundus is normal.
General examination showed nothing abnormal.

Figure 25. Right eye. Choroidal and retinal coloboma in the upper temporal quadrant.

The coloboma is bordered by some pigment. Optic disc is normal.

CLINICAL NOTE: Figure 25 is from a female, aged 24. Vision of her right eye has always been slightly reduced. No complaints from the left eye. No family history of colobomas.
Eye examination: Visual acuity, right eye: 6/9, unimproved by lenses; left eye: 6/6, emmetropia. Anterior segments are normal. The right fundus shows a large coloboma in the upper temporal quadrant, partially involving the macular area. Visual field defect corresponds to the coloboma. The left fundus is normal.
General examination showed nothing abnormal.

Figure 26. Left eye. Large coloboma of the choroid and retina in the lower half of the fundus. The optic disc is indicated by the entrance of the retinal vessels. Only a few retinal and choroidal vessels are seen in the colobomatous area.

CLINICAL NOTE: Figure 26 is from a female, aged 15. Her vision has always been defective in both eyes. No family history of colobomas.
Eye examination: Visual acuity, right eye: light perception; left eye: 6/60, unimproved by lenses. Anterior segments show iris colobomas below. Mature cataract on the right side. The left fundus shows large coloboma of the choroid and retina in the lower half of the globe. Visual field defect corresponds to the coloboma.
General examination showed nothing abnormal.

Figure 27. Right eye. Large coloboma of the choroid and retina in the lower half of the fundus. There is a staphyloma of the sclera in the circumpapillary area. Above, the coloboma is bordered by some pigment.

CLINICAL NOTE: Figure 27 is from a female, aged 31. Her vision has always been defective. Her father has coloboma of the iris, but her two children have no ocular defects.
Eye examination: Visual acuity, both eyes: 6/60 with − 5.0 D sph. Fine nystagmus and some divergent strabismus. In the lower part of both eyes there are colobomas of the iris, ciliary body, lens, choroid and retina. Upper halves of both visual fields are completely missing.
General examination showed nothing abnormal.

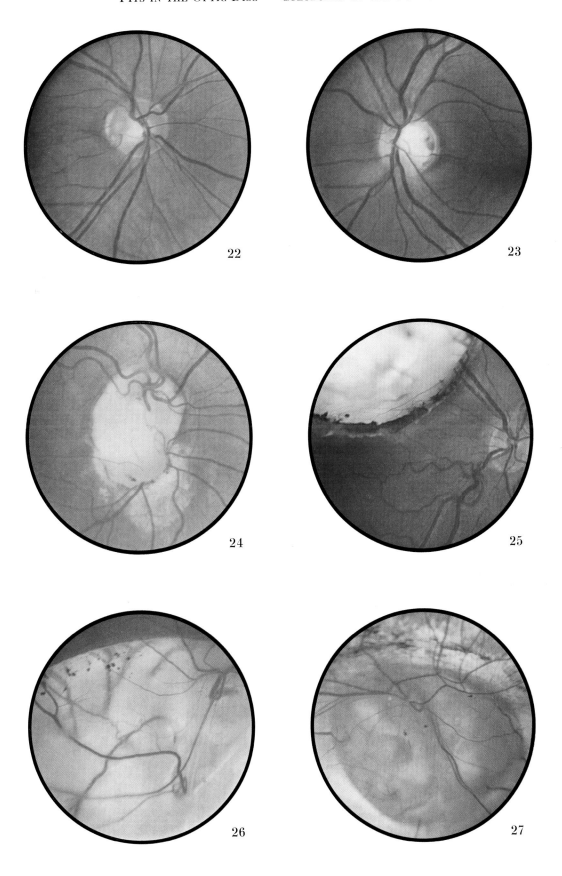

22

23

24

25

26

27

Figure 28. Left eye. Small, round, yellowish vitelliform cyst in the macular area. Optic disc and retinal vessels are normal.

CLINICAL NOTE: Figure 28 is from a male, aged 32. He has had psoriasis for some years. No ocular complaints.
Eye examination: Visual acuity, both eyes: 6/6, emmetropia. Anterior segments are normal. Right fundus is normal. In the left macular area there is a small vitelliform cyst. Paracentral scotoma corresponds to the macular cyst.
General examination showed psoriasis.

Figure 29. Left eye. Small, oval, yellowish vitelliform cyst in the macular area. Optic disc and retinal vessels are normal.

CLINICAL NOTE: Figure 29 is from a male, aged 37. Vision of the left eye slightly reduced for some years. No complaints from the right eye. No general symptoms.
Eye examination: Visual acuity, right eye: 6/6 with − 0.5 D sph. − 0.5 D cyl. axis 30°; left eye: 6/9 with − 1.0 D sph. + 2.0 D cyl. axis 85°. Anterior segments are normal. Right fundus is normal. In the left macular area there is a small vitelliform cyst. Paracentral scotoma corresponds to the macular cyst.
General examination showed nothing abnormal.

Figure 30. Left eye. Epipapillary membrane on the disc, ensheathing the retinal vessels for a short distance. Retinal vessels are normal. Central serous retinopathy is seen faintly.

CLINICAL NOTE: Figure 30 is from a female, aged 40. During the last week hazy vision of the left eye. No complaints from the right eye. No general symptoms.
Eye examination: Visual acuity, right eye: 6/6 with + 1.75 D sph.; left eye: 6/9 with + 1.5 D sph. Anterior segments are normal. Right fundus is normal. Epipapillary membrane on the left disc and central serous retinopathy. Small central scotoma for red light.
General examination showed nothing abnormal.

Figure 31. Right eye. Bergmeister's papilla. The optic disc is covered with a web of opaque tissue. Centrally there is a more solid white prominence projecting into the vitreous.

CLINICAL NOTE: Figure 31 is from a male, aged 8. No family history of visual disturbances. He developed right convergent strabismus at the age of one year. In spite of wearing correcting glasses, having a squint operation performed and afterwards receiving orthoptic training, vision remained defective in the right eye.
Eye examination: Visual acuity, right eye: counting fingers with + 5.5 D sph.; left eye: 6/6 with + 4.5 D sph. Right convergent strabismus of 10°. Anterior segments are normal. In the right fundus there is a Bergmeister papilla (unchanged for four years). The left fundus is normal.
General examination showed nothing abnormal.

Figure 32. Right eye. Persistent hyperplastic primary vitreous. A whitish veil of tissue covers the optic disc and projects far into the vitreous.

Figure 33. Same eye as figure 32, two years later. The whitish veil of tissue has diminished in size. It is now situated just prepapillary.

CLINICAL NOTE: Figures 32 and 33 are from a female, aged 9. She was born at term. The pregnancy had been normal. Vision of her right eye has always been defective.
Eye examination at the first admission: Visual acuity, right eye: 2/60, unimproved by lenses; left eye: 6/6 with + 1.0 D sph. Anterior segments are normal. In the right fundus there is persistent hyperplastic primary vitreous extending from the disc and ending as a small cord at the posterior pole of the lens. The left fundus is normal.
Eye examination, two years later: Visual acuity is unchanged. The prepapillary veil of fibrous tissue in the right eye has diminished in size, and is now lying just prepapillary.
General examination, including extensive blood studies, showed nothing abnormal.

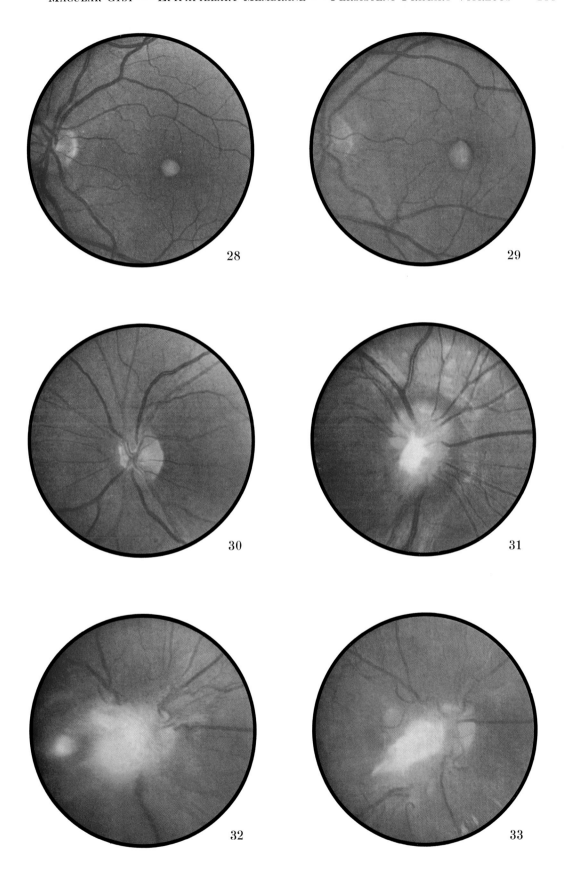

28

29

30

31

32

33

Figures 34 and 35. Right eye. Temporal and nasal part of the same fundus. Persistent hyperplastic primary vitreous. Whitish and grayish veils of fibrous tissue are lying in front of the retina, projecting far into the vitreous. Temporally, the fibrous tissue is attached to the retina by a pigmented footplate.

Figure 36. From the same eye as figures 34 and 35. Persistent hyaloid artery attached to the posterior lens capsule by a footplate.

CLINICAL NOTE: Figures 34—36 are from a male, aged 6. He was born at term. The pregnancy had been normal. Right divergent strabismus since birth.
Eye examination: Visual acuity, right eye: no light perception; left eye: 3/4.5 with + 2.0 D sph. Right divergent strabismus of 10°. Right eye of normal size. The eye presents persistent hyperplastic primary vitreous and persistent hyaloid artery. Left eye is normal.
General examination showed nothing abnormal.

Figure 37. Right eye. Retrolental fibroplasia. Part of grayish, annular retrolental fibrous mass is seen through the pupil.

Figure 38. From the same eye as figure 37. In the pupil, a grayish retrolental fibrous mass is seen below. Retinal vessels of the detached retina are seen above.

Figure 39. From the same eye as figures 37 and 38. Flat retinal detachment and dilated retinal vessels. Disc is partially hidden by vitreous haze. Nasally, the detached retina is most elevated.

CLINICAL NOTE: Figures 37—39 are from a five months old boy. His birth weight was 1,100 g, and his gestation age approximately 28 weeks. Because of his prematurity he was kept in an incubator and received oxygen therapy for about three weeks. About four weeks after removal from the incubator he developed retinal hemorrhages in both eyes. A month later the hemorrhages had disappeared, but instead grayish prominences were observed in both fundus peripheries. Still a month later, the right fundus showed an annular ring of retrolental fibrous tissue and total retinal detachment. The left vitreous was filled with a grayish mass of connective tissue.
General examination showed normal motor development.

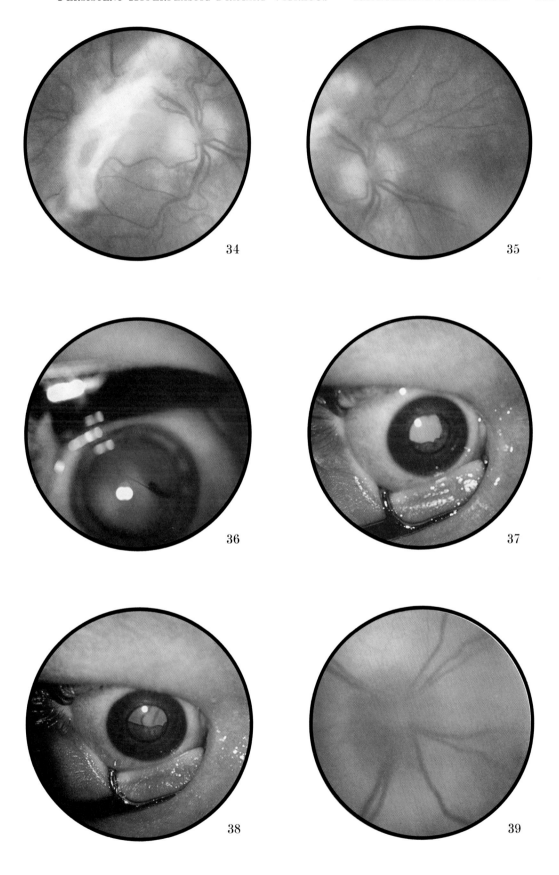

*Figure 40. Composite picture. Left eye. Fal-
ciform retinal detachment. From the optic
disc, which is partly hidden, an elevated
fold of retinal tissue extends to the lower
temporal fundus periphery. The retinal vessels do not as usual emerge from the disc
into the fundus. Only a few retinal vessels
extend from the retinal fold into the fundus. There is some scattered pigmentation
around the disc. Choroidal vessels are seen
plainly.*

CLINICAL NOTE: Figure 39 is from an eight
months old girl. Her birth weight was 1,080 g,
and her gestation age approximately 28 weeks.
Because of her prematurity she was kept in
an incubator and received oxygen therapy for
about three weeks. At the age of seven months,
the parents observed a grayish-white reflex
from the right pupil. She was admitted on suspicion of retinoblastoma.
Eye examination: Vision, both eyes: doubtful
light perception. Both eyes of normal size.
Right eye shows complete retrolental membrane formation. Ultrasonography showed no
retinal tumor, but condensed tissue behind the
lens. Left eye shows falciform retinal detachment with a broad elevated band of retinal tis-

sue in the lower temporal quadrant. There are
only few retinal vessels present, but choroidal
vessels are seen plainly.
General examination showed normal motor development.

*Figure 41. Composite picture. Left eye. Fal-
ciform retinal fold emerging from the optic
disc to the periphery of the lower temporal
quadrant. In the periphery, the fold is attached to the ciliary body. Retinal vessels
are normal.*

CLINICAL NOTE: Figure 41 is from a ten months
old girl. She was born at term. Her birth weight
was 3,750 g. Pregnancy had been normal. No
history of ocular diseases in the family. She
was admitted on suspicion of retinoblastoma.
Eye examination: Vision, both eyes: doubtful
light perception. Right divergent strabismus of
30°. The right eye is microphthalmic, the left
of normal size. Ciliary processes elongated in
both eyes. Right eye shows persistent hyperplastic primary vitreous. Ultrasonography
showed no retinal tumor. Left eye shows falciform retinal fold in the lower temporal quadrant.
General examination showed normal motor development.

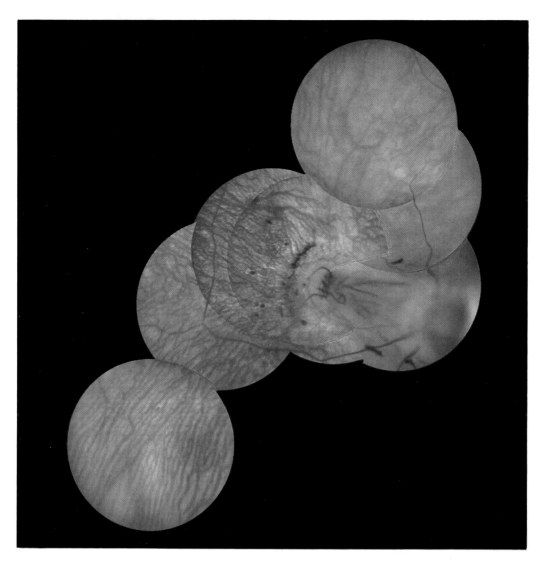

40

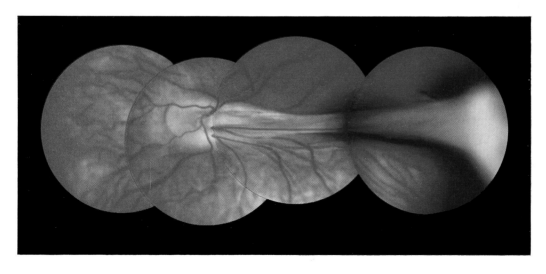

41

Figure 42. Left eye. Fundus in simple myopia, from a blond person. The macular area and its surroundings have a warm red color. Elsewhere, the fundus is lightly pigmented and choroidal vessels are seen plainly. The optic disc and retinal vessels are normal.

CLINICAL NOTE: Figure 42 is from the same patient as figure 474, a female, aged 11. No family history of myopia. She has had myopia since the age of eight years.
Eye examination: Visual acuity, right eye: 6/6 with − 2.25 D sph.; left eye: 6/6 with − 3.75 D sph. Anterior segments are normal. Both fundi are lightly pigmented except in and around the macular area. Scattered grouped pigmentation in both eyes.
General examination showed nothing abnormal.

Figures 43 and 44. Right and left eyes. Myopic conus seen as a whitish crescent at the temporal side of the disc. Disc and retinal vessels are normal.

CLINICAL NOTE: Figures 43 and 44 are from a male, aged 66. Simple myopia since childhood.
Eye examination: Visual acuity, both eyes: 6/6 with − 3.0 D sph. Anterior segments and fundi are normal, except for myopic conus.
General examination showed nothing abnormal.

Figure 45. Right eye. Large myopic conus seen as a whitish crescent at the temporal side of the disc. Disc and retinal vessels are normal.

CLINICAL NOTE: Figure 45 is from the same patient as figure 466, a male, aged 50. He and his five siblings have had progressive myopia since childhood. Six months ago he had retinal detachment in the right eye and was operated on with a good result.
Eye examination: Visual acuity, right eye: 6/18 with − 12.0 D sph.; left eye: 6/9 with − 8.5 D

sph. Anterior segments are normal. Some opacities in the right vitreous. Both fundi show myopic conus and some diffuse myopic atrophy. No retinal detachment. In the right fundus chorioretinal scars after diathermy operation. Visual field defect corresponds to the chorioretinal scars.
General examination showed nothing abnormal.

Figure 46. Left eye. Peripapillary atrophy in excessive myopia. The optic disc is normal and the choroidal vessels are seen plainly.

CLINICAL NOTE: Figure 46 is from a female, aged 53. Since childhood she has had progressive myopia. Four days ago she developed retinal detachment in the right eye.
Eye examination: Visual acuity, right eye: 6/36 with − 9.0 D sph.; left eye: 6/12 with − 9.0 D sph. − 2.0 D cyl. axis 165°. Anterior segments are normal. Right fundus shows retinal detachment with horseshoe-shaped tear in the upper temporal quadrant. Left fundus shows excessive myopia changes.
General examination showed hypertension. Blood pressure: 200/100 mm Hg. No proteinuria.

Figure 47. Right eye. Large peripapillary atrophy in excessive myopia. The optic disc margin is only seen faintly.

CLINICAL NOTE: Figure 47 is from a female, aged 76. No family history of myopia. Since childhood she has had progressive myopia. Two years ago she had a cataract extraction performed in the right eye.
Eye examination: Visual acuity, right eye: 6/36 with + 3.0 D sph.; left eye 3/24 with − 8.0 D sph. The right eye is aphakic, the left eye shows posterior cortical cataract. Severe myopic degeneration in both fundi.
General examination showed hypertension. Blood pressure: 210/110 mm Hg. No proteinuria.

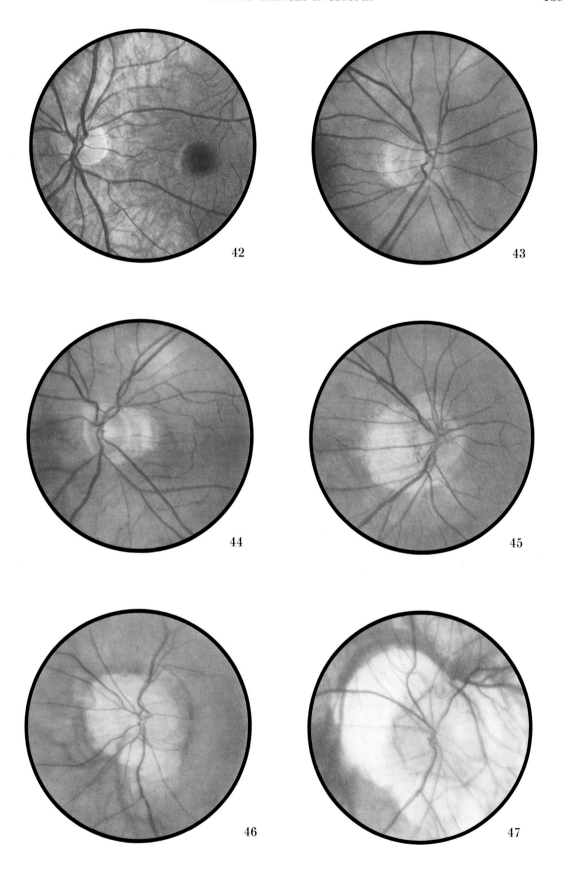

Figure 48. Left eye. Incipient development of Fuchs' spot in excessive myopia. There is slight macular edema and some punctate retinal hemorrhages in the edematous area.

Figure 49. From the same eye as Figure 48, a week later. Macular edema and retinal hemorrhages have increased in size. Subretinal hemorrhage is also present.

Figure 50. From the same eye as Figure 49, six weeks later. The macular edema is still increasing. The retinal and subretinal hemorrhages have nearly disappeared, and a pigmented scar is developing.

CLINICAL NOTE: Figures 48—50 are from a male, aged 30. He has had progressive myopia since childhood. Two days before the first eye examination he experienced a loss of central vision in his left eye.
Eye examination: Visual acuity, right eye: 6/12 with − 9.0 D sph. − 2.5 D cyl. axis 0°; left eye: 3/60 with − 7.5 D sph. − 1.0 D cyl. axis 0°. Anterior segments are normal. Right fundus is normal, without signs of excessive myopia. In the left macular area there is edema and some punctate retinal hemorrhages. Corresponding to the macular changes, there is a small central scotoma.
After a week the macular edema and retinal hemorrhages have increased in size and subretinal hemorrhage is also present.
Six weeks later, the macular edema is still increasing. The retinal and subretinal hemorrhages have nearly disappeared, and a pigmented scar is developing.
General examination showed nothing abnormal.

Figure 51. Right eye. Disseminated myopic atrophy around the disc and in the macular area. A pigmented spot, Fuchs' spot, is seen in the macula. The retinal arteries are narrow, the veins normal. The disc is normal.

CLINICAL NOTE: Figure 51 is from a female, aged 55. No family history of myopia. Since childhood she has had progressive myopia.

Eye examination: Visual acuity, right eye: 3/60 with − 12.0 D sph.; left eye: 6/18 with − 10.0 D sph. − 1.5 D cyl. axis 170°. Anterior segments are normal. Both fundi show disseminated myopic atrophy. Retinal arteries are narrow, the veins are normal. Fuchs' spot is present in the right macula. Visual fields show scattered defects in both fundi and central scotoma in the right eye.
General examination showed hypertension and some heart failure. Blood pressure: 215/110 mm Hg. No proteinuria.

Figure 52. Right eye. Excessive myopic fundus with peripapillary atrophy, and atrophies and scattered pigmentation in the macular area.

CLINICAL NOTE: Figure 52 is from a female, aged 25. No family history of myopia. She has had progressive myopia since childhood. Four years ago she developed central scotoma in the right eye. One week ago she experienced reduced central vision in the left eye.
Eye examination: Visual acuity, right eye: 1/24 with − 20.0 D sph.; left eye: 6/36 with − 12.0 D sph. Anterior segments are normal. Both fundi show excessive myopia changes with peripapillary atrophy. Atrophies and scattered pigmentations are seen in both macular areas. Visual field defects correspond to the fundal changes.
General examination showed nothing abnormal.

Figure 53. Right eye. Excessive myopic, quasi-albinotic fundus with temporal conus and a degenerative, whitish patch in the macular area.

CLINICAL NOTE: Figure 53 is from a male, aged 14. No family history of myopia. Since the age of 12 he has had progressive myopia and gradually reduced vision of the right eye.
Eye examination: Visual acuity, right eye: < 6/12 with − 14.0 D sph.; left eye: 6/6 with − 4.0 D sph. − 2.5 D cyl. axis 170°. Anterior segments are normal. Right fundus shows excessive myopia changes, pseudoalbinism and some macular degeneration. Left fundus is normal except for myopic conus.
General examination showed nothing abnormal.

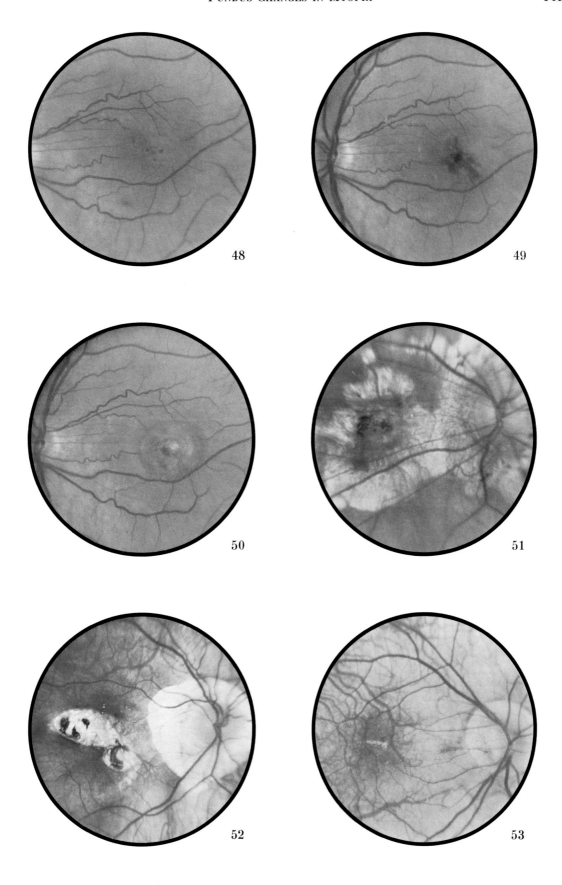

48

49

50

51

52

53

Figure 54. Right eye. Normal disc, seen centrally as a yellowish-pink, well-defined round area. The disc is slightly more red nasally than temporally. The retinal vessels and the fundus are normal.

CLINICAL NOTE: Figure 54 is from the same patient as figures 2 and 64, a male, aged 21. No general or ocular complaints.
Eye examination: Visual acuity, both eyes: 6/6 with + 1.5 D sph. Anterior segments are normal. Right fundus is normal. Left fundus shows large optic disc with conus and pigmentation temporally. Left blind spot slightly enlarged.
General examination showed nothing abnormal.

Figure 55. Right eye. Normal disc. The disc is slightly more red nasally than temporally. The retinal vessels and the fundus are normal.

CLINICAL NOTE: Figure 55 is from a male, aged 41. No general or ocular complaints.
Eye examination: Visual acuity, both eyes: 6/6 with − 0.5 D sph. Anterior segments are normal. Both fundi are normal.
General examination showed nothing abnormal.

Figure 56. Right eye. Normal optic disc and tessellated fundus. Retinal vessels are normal.

CLINICAL NOTE: Figure 56 is from a male, aged 41. No general or ocular complaints.
Eye examination: Visual acuity, both eyes: 6/6, emmetropia. Anterior segments and fundi are normal.
General examination showed nothing abnormal.

Figure 57. Right eye. Normal optic disc in a Negro. Retinal vessels are normal.

CLINICAL NOTE: Figure 57 is from the same patient as figure 4, a male, aged 30. No general or ocular complaints.
Eye examination: Visual acuity, both eyes: 6/6, emmetropia. Anterior segments and fundi are normal.
General examination showed nothing abnormal.

Figure 58. Right eye. Normal optic disc with temporal physiological excavation. The fundus and retinal vessels are normal.

CLINICAL NOTE: Figure 58 is from a female, aged 37. During the last half year some reduction of vision in the left eye. No complaints from the right eye. No general symptoms.
Eye examination: Visual acuity, right eye: 6/6 with + 1.5 D sph.; left eye: < 6/9 with + 1.5 D sph. Anterior segments and right fundus are normal. In the left fundus there is a juvenile macular degeneration with subretinal hemorrhage just above the fovea. Visual field defect corresponds to the fundal lesion.
General examination showed nothing abnormal.

Figure 59. Right eye. Central, deep physiological excavation of the optic disc. The central cup is whitish, while the surrounding part of the disc has retained its normal pink color. Fundus and retinal vessels are normal.

CLINICAL NOTE: Figure 59 is from a female, aged 18. No general or ocular complaints.
Eye examination: Visual acuity, both eyes: 6/6, emmetropia. Anterior segments and fundi are normal. Both discs show central, deep physiological cupping.
General examination showed nothing abnormal.

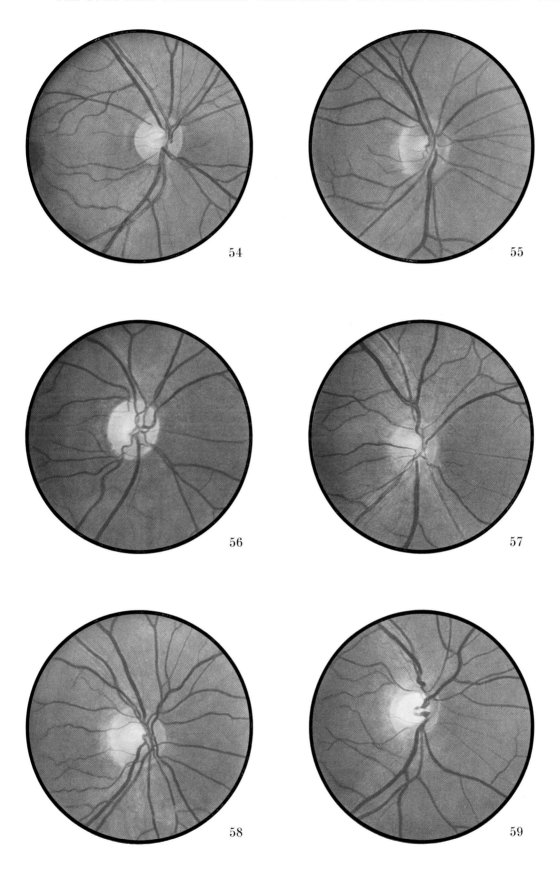

Figure 60. Right eye. Normal disc with large temporal physiological excavation. The disc is surrounded by a slight scleral ring. Fundus and retinal vessels are normal.

CLINICAL NOTE: Figure 60 is from a male, aged 39. He has had slightly reduced vision in both eyes for many years. No general symptoms.
Eye examination: Visual acuity, both eyes: 6/9 with + 0.75 D sph. + 0.75 D cyl. axis 90°. There is fine horizontal nystagmus, but otherwise eye movements are normal. Anterior segments and fundi are normal. Both discs show large temporal physiological cupping and a scleral ring.
General examination showed nothing abnormal.

Figure 61. Right eye. Hypoplasia of the disc and temporal conus. The disc is small and there is a whitish crescent at the temporal side of the disc.

CLINICAL NOTE: Figure 61 is from a female, aged 21. Disseminated lupus erythematosus was diagnosed two years ago. No ocular complaints.
Eye examination: Visual acuity, both eyes: 6/6 with − 2.5 D sph. Anterior segments are normal. The discs are small, but otherwise fundi are normal.
General examination showed disseminated lupus erythematosus.

Figure 62. Left eye. Small, pink optic disc. Normal physiological variation. Disc borders are well-defined. Temporally, there is a small whitish crescent. Retinal vessels are normal.

CLINICAL NOTE: Figure 62 is from a male, aged 21. No general or ocular complaints.
Eye examination: Visual acuity, both eyes: 6/6 with + 2.0 D sph. Anterior segments and fundi are normal. Both discs are small and more pink than usual.
General examination showed nothing abnormal.

Figure 63. Left eye. Large optic disc with conus formation nasally. Physiological variation.

CLINICAL NOTE: Figure 63 is from the same patient as figures 232—233, a female, aged 56. A week ago she observed some reduction of vision in the right eye. No general symptoms or complaints from the left eye.
Eye examination: Visual acuity, right eye: 6/12 with + 0.5 D cyl. axis 0°; left eye: 6/6 with + 0.5 D cyl. axis 0°. Anterior segments and intraocular tension are normal. Both fundi show moderate sclerosis of the retinal vessels and arteriovenous crossing phenomena. In the right fundus, there is an occlusion of the upper temporal retinal vein.
General examination showed nothing abnormal. Blood pressure: 140/80 mm Hg. No proteinuria.

Figure 64. Left eye. Large optic disc with conus formation and some pigmentation temporally. Physiological variation. Retinal vessels are normal.

CLINICAL NOTE: Figure 64 is from the same patient as figures 2 and 54, a male, aged 21. No general or ocular complaints.
Eye examination: Visual acuity, both eyes: 6/6 with + 1.5 D sph. Anterior segments are normal. Right fundus is normal. Left fundus shows large optic disc with conus and pigmentation temporally. Left blind spot slightly enlarged.
General examination showed nothing abnormal.

Figure 65. Left eye. Senile peripapillary atrophy. Retinal vessels are slightly narrowed.

CLINICAL NOTE: Figure 65 is from a male, aged 78. He was admitted for hypertrophia of the prostate. No ocular complaints.
Eye examination: Visual acuity, both eyes: 6/9, unimproved by lenses. Anterior segments show some posterior cortical cataract. Intraocular tension is normal. In both fundi, there is large senile peripapillary atrophy and some sclerosis of the retinal vessels.
General examination showed hypertrophia of the prostate. Blood pressure: 160/85 mm Hg. No proteinuria. Serum creatinine: 1.4 mg/100 ml.

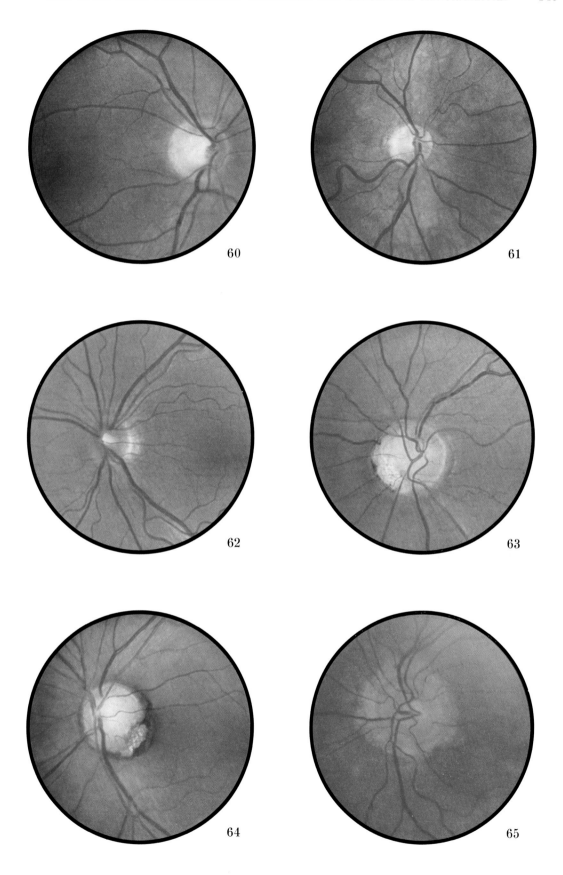

60

61

62

63

64

65

Figure 66. Left eye. Congenital variation of the optic disc. The disc is grayish-red and shows heavy pigment accumulation at the temporal side. Retinal vessels and fundus are normal.

CLINICAL NOTE: Figure 66 is from a male, aged 4. No family history of ocular disease. He has had left convergent strabismus since early infancy. No general symptoms.
Eye examination: Visual acuity, right eye: 3/4.5 with + 1.5 D sph.; left eye: light perception. He has left convergent strabismus of about 15°. Eye movements are normal. Anterior segments and right fundus are normal. The left disc is grayish-red and shows heavy accumulation of dark pigment temporally. Electroretinogram, right eye: normal; left eye: a-wave extinguished, b-wave diminished.
General examination showed nothing abnormal.

Figure 67. Right eye. Normal optic disc with accumulation of choroidal pigment temporally. A cilioretinal artery is present, and retinal vessels are normal.

CLINICAL NOTE: Figure 67 is from a female, aged 18. No general or ocular complaints.
Eye examination: Visual acuity, both eyes: 6/6, emmetropia. Anterior segments and fundi are normal. Incomplete choroidal ring formation at both discs.
General examination showed nothing abnormal.

Figure 68. Right eye. Large optic disc surrounded by a broad choroidal ring. Physiological variation. Retinal vessels and fundus are normal.

CLINICAL NOTE: Figure 68 is from a female, aged 17. No general or ocular complaints.
Eye examination: Visual acuity, both eyes: 6/6, emmetropia. Anterior segments and fundi are normal. Both discs are large and surrounded by a broad choroidal ring.
General examination showed nothing abnormal.

Figure 69. Right eye. The normal optic disc is surrounded by a broad zone of pigment, a choroidal ring. Choroidal vessels are seen plainly at the nasal side of the disc. Retinal vessels are normal.

CLINICAL NOTE: Figure 69 is from a female, aged 44. She has had simple myopia since childhood. No general symptoms.
Eye examination: Visual acuity, both eyes: 6/6 with − 5.5 D sph. Anterior segments are normal. In both fundi there is a broad choroidal ring. Choroidal vessels are seen plainly in the nasal quadrants.
General examination showed nothing abnormal.

Figure 70. Left eye. Normal optic disc surrounded by a yellowish-white scleral ring. Retinal vessels and fundus are normal.

CLINICAL NOTE: Figure 70 is from a male, aged 53. A year ago melanoma of the iris was diagnosed in the right eye. The tumor was removed locally, but recurred after nearly a year. The eye was enucleated, and histopathologic examination showed a malignant melanoma of mixed type in the iris. No complaints from the left eye. No general symptoms.
Eye examination: Right orbital cavity healed. Visual acuity, left eye: 6/6 with − 0.5 D sph. Anterior segment and fundus are normal. The disc is surrounded by a scleral ring.
General examination showed nothing abnormal.

Figure 71. Right eye. Normal optic disc surrounded by a yellowish-white scleral ring. Retinal vessels and fundus are normal.

CLINICAL NOTE: Figure 71 is from a female, aged 66. No ocular or general complaints.
Eye examination: Visual acuity, both eyes: 6/6 with + 1.5 D sph. Anterior segments and fundi are normal. Both discs are surrounded by a scleral ring.
General examination showed nothing abnormal.

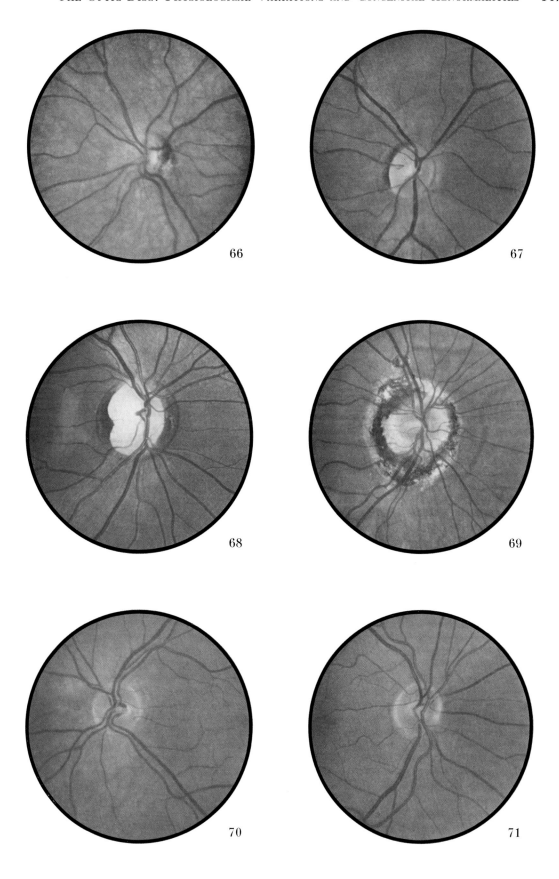

Figure 72. Left eye. Optic disc with yellow-ish-white nasal conus and inverted vascular trunk. The temporal part of the disc is slightly prominent. The retinal vessels appear in the temporal part of the disc and run nasally before bending into the lightly pigmented fundus.

CLINICAL NOTE: Figure 72 is from a male, aged 66. His vision has always been reduced in spite of wearing correcting glasses.
Eye examination: Visual acuity, right eye: 6/9 with + 4.0 D sph. + 1.0 D cyl. axis 0°; left eye: 6/18 with + 3.5 D sph. + 1.0 D cyl. axis 0°. Visual fields, intraocular tension and anterior segments are normal. In both fundi, the vascular trunks are inverted on the disc and nasal crescents are present.
General examination showed nothing abnormal.

Figure 73. Left eye. Optic disc with yellow-ish-white nasal conus and inverted vascular trunk. The retinal vessels appear in the temporal part of the disc and run nasally before bending into the lightly pigmented fundus.

CLINICAL NOTE: Figure 73 is from the same patient as figure 77, a male, aged 67. His vision has always been reduced in spite of wearing correcting glasses.
Eye examination: Visual acuity, right eye: 6/9 with − 1.5 D sph. − 1.0 D cyl. axis 10°; left eye: 6/9 with − 3.0 D sph. − 1.0 D cyl. axis 170°. Visual fields, intraocular tension and anterior segments are normal. In the right fundus there is an inferior conus. In the left fundus there is a nasal conus and inverted vascular trunk. Both fundi are lightly pigmented.
General examination showed nothing abnormal.

Figure 74. Left eye. Optic disc with yellow-ish-white nasal conus and inverted vascular trunk. The retinal vessels appear in the temporal part of the disc and run nasally before bending into the lightly pigmented fundus.

CLINICAL NOTE: Figure 74 is from a male, aged 47. No ocular complaints. Diabetes has just been demonstrated. It is regulated by diet only.
Eye examination: Visual acuity, right eye: 6/6 with + 1.0 D sph.; left eye: 6/6 with + 0.5 D cyl. axis 0°. Anterior segments, intraocular ten-

sion and visual fields are normal. In both fundi, the vascuar trunks are inverted on the disc and nasal crescents are present.
General examination showed diabetes without nephropathy or hypertension. Blood pressure: 140/80 mm Hg.

Figure 75. Left eye. Inferior conus. The retinal vessels emerge from the center of the pink, slightly elevated, oval disc. Below, there is a yellowish-white crescent.

CLINICAL NOTE: Figure 75 is from a male, aged 50. His vision has always been reduced, although he wears correcting glasses.
Eye examination: Visual acuity, right eye: 6/9 with − 3.25 D sph. − 2.75 D cyl. axis 90°; left eye: 6/12 with − 2.75 D sph. − 2.5 D cyl. axis 105°. Visual fields, intraocular tension and anterior segments are normal. Both fundi are normal apart from inferior conus formation.
General examination showed nothing abnormal.

Figure 76. Right eye. Optic disc with inferior conus formation. Retinal vessels are normal. Fundus slightly tessellated.

CLINICAL NOTE: Figure 76 is from a male, aged 55. No history of myopia in the family. He has had simple myopia since childhood. During the last week he has experienced a gradual loss of vision in the left eye. No complaints from the right eye.
Eye examination: Visual acuity, right eye: 6/9 with − 2.75 D sph. − 0.5 D cyl. axis 25°; left eye: hand movements with − 4.5 D sph. − 2.0 D cyl. axis 125°. Anterior segments and intraocular tension normal. The right fundus slightly tessellated. The disc shows inferior conus formation. In the left fundus, there is a total retinal detachment with a horseshoe-shaped tear in the upper temporal quadrant.
General examination showed nothing abnormal.

Figure 77. Right eye. Optic disc with inferior conus formation. The conus is rotated slightly nasally. Retinal vessels are normal. Fundus lightly pigmented nasally.

CLINICAL NOTE: Figure 77 is from the same patient as figure 73, a male, aged 67. His vision has always been reduced in spite of wearing correcting glasses.
For further clinical information, see clinical note to figure 73.

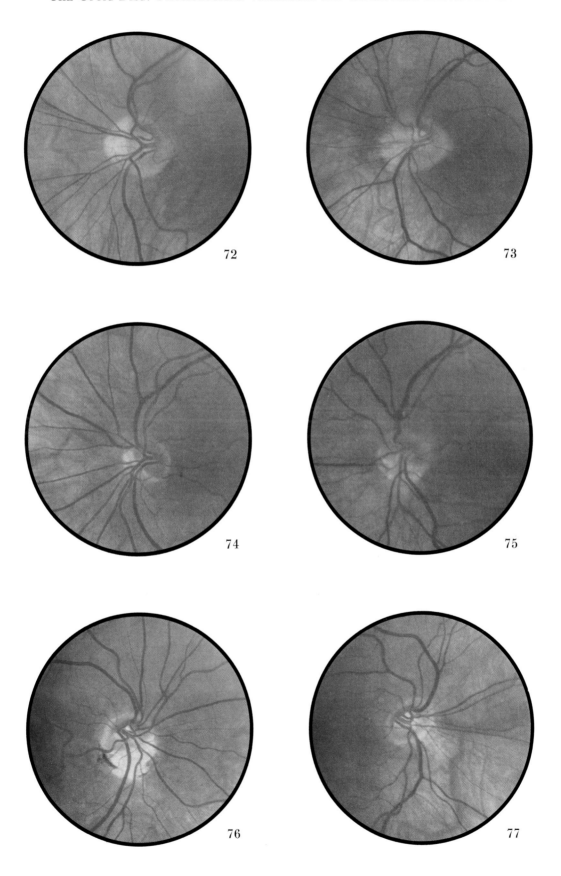

72

73

74

75

76

77

Figure 78. Right eye. Congenital anomaly of the optic disc. The disc is larger than normal, slightly prominent and covered by a delicate web of glial tissue. Retinal vessels and fundus are normal.

CLINICAL NOTE: Figure 78 is from a female, aged 7. No general or ocular complaints.
Eye examination: Visual acuity, both eyes: 3/4.5 without lenses. Anterior segments and left fundus are normal. The right disc shows a congenital malformation. The disc is enlarged, slightly elevated and covered by a delicate web of glial tissue.
General examination showed nothing abnormal.

Figure 79. Right eye. Pseudopapilledema. The disc margin is blurred nasally and the disc projects nasally for about one diopter. Retinal vessels are normal. No retinal hemorrhages or exudates.

CLINICAL NOTE: Figure 79 is from a female, aged 19. She has had myopia since school-age.
Eye examination: Visual acuity, both eyes: 6/6 with − 3.25 D sph. − 0.5 D cyl. axis 0°. Visual fields, intraocular tension and anterior segments are normal. Both optic discs show pseudopapilledema. The optic discs have remained unchanged for about four years.
General examination showed nothing abnormal.

Figure 80. Right eye. Pseudopapilledema and drusen of the disc. The disc margin is blurred and the disc projects about one diopter. Whitish drusen are seen in the tissue of the disc. Retinal vessels are normal. No retinal hemorrhages or exudates.

CLINICAL NOTE: Figure 80 is from the same patient as figure 88, a female, aged 13. At the age of six she had right convergent squint. Since then she has had amblyopia of the right eye. No general symptoms.
Eye examination: Visual acuity, right eye: 6/18, unimproved by lenses; left eye: 6/6, emmetropia. Intraocular tension and anterior segments are normal. Both discs show pseudopapilledema and drusen of the disc, but on the left disc there are also retinal hemorrhages. Both blind spots are slightly enlarged.
General examination, including neurological examination, carotid angiography, pneumoencephalography and electroencephalography, showed nothing abnormal.

Figure 81. Right eye. Pseudopapilledema and drusen of the disc. Disc margin is blurred and the optic disc projects about one diopter. Whitish drusen are seen in the tissue of the disc. Retinal vessels are normal. No retinal hemorrhages or exudates.

CLINICAL NOTE: Figure 81 is from a female, aged 13. Simple myopia since the age of eight years. No general symptoms.
Eye examination: Visual acuity, both eyes: 6/6 with − 1.5 D sph. Intraocular tension and anterior segments are normal. Both discs show pseudopapilledema and drusen of the disc (unchanged for two years), and both blind spots are slightly enlarged.
General examination showed nothing abnormal.

Figure 82. Left eye. Pseudopapilledema with drusen embedded in the optic nerve tissue. Retinal arteries narrowed, veins are normal. Fundus is lightly pigmented. No retinal hemorrhages or exudates.

CLINICAL NOTE: Figure 82 is from a female, aged 69. No ocular or general complaints.
Eye examination: Visual acuity, both eyes: 6/6 with + 1.5 D sph. Intraocular tension and anterior segments are normal. Fundi are lightly pigmented. There is hypertensive angiopathy with narrowing of retinal arteries and arteriovenous crossing phenomena. The right disc is normal. The left shows pseudopapilledema and drusen. Left blind spot slightly enlarged.
General examination showed essential hypertension. Blood pressure: 180/100 mm Hg. No proteinuria.

Figure 83. Right eye. Pseudopapilledema with drusen embedded in the optic nerve tissue. Retinal vessels and fundus are normal. No retinal hemorrhages or exudates.

CLINICAL NOTE: Figure 83 is from a female, aged 14. No general and ocular complaints.
Eye examination: Visual acuity, both eyes: 6/6 with + 0.5 D sph. + 0.5 D cyl. axis 0°. Intraocular tension, visual fields and anterior segments are normal. The right disc shows pseudopapilledema and drusen (unchanged through five years). Left disc is normal.
General examination showed nothing abnormal.

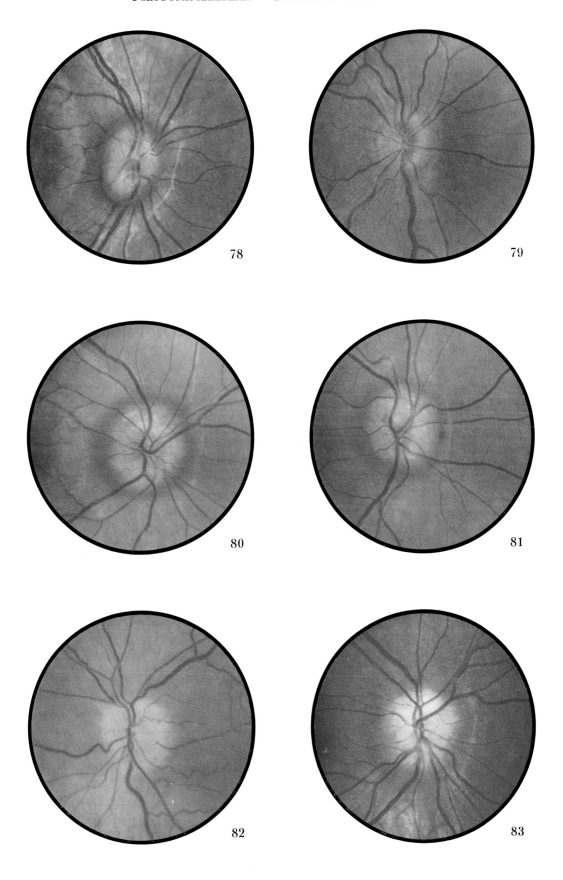

78

79

80

81

82

83

Figure 84. Right eye. Normal optic disc. Retinal arteries are normal, the veins are dilated.

Figure 85. The same eye as figure 84, four years later. Papilledema, early stage. The disc is reddened and projects slightly forwards. The disc margin is blurred and the disc is surrounded by some edema, partially obscuring the retinal vessels at the disc margin. The retinal veins are dilated and more tortuous. The retinal arteries are normal.

CLINICAL NOTE: Figures 84 and 85 are from the same patient as figures 144—157, a female, aged 21. No family history of cerebral or ocular diseases. She presents von Hippel-Lindau's syndrome. For further clinical information, see clinical note to figures 144—155.

Figure 86. Right eye. Papilledema, early stage. The disc is reddened and projects about one diopter. The disc margin is blurred and the disc surrounded by edema, partially obscuring the retinal vessels. Below, fine radiating light streaks indicate some retinal edema. The veins are dilated, the arteries are normal.

Figure 87. Left eye. From the same patient as figure 86. Papilledema, early stage. The papilledema is more advanced than in the right eye. The disc projects about two diopters, and fine radiating light streaks, indicating retinal edema, are seen above and below.

CLINICAL NOTE: Figures 86 and 87 are from a female, aged 44. During the last two years she has had some diffuse headache. Following a slight cranial trauma a month ago, the headache became progressive. A fortnight ago she had a convulsive attack, lasting some minutes. No ocular complaints.
Eye examination: Visual acuity, both eyes: 6/6 with + 1.0 D sph. Intraocular tension and anterior segments are normal. Both optic discs show some papilledema. No retinal hemorrhages or exudates. Both blind spots are enlarged, but otherwise no visual field defects.
General examination, including angiography, pneumoencephalography and electroencephalo-

graphy, aroused suspicion of a tumor in the left frontal region. Craniotomy revealed an ethmoidal meningioma, and the tumor was removed.

Figure 88. Left eye. Slight papilledema in a pseudopapilledema disc with drusen. Centrally, the disc is reddened, edematous and covered by small hemorrhages. Whitish drusen are seen in the disc tissue. The disc projects about one diopter. The disc margin is blurred, but the retinal vessels are not obscured at the disc margin. Retinal veins are slightly dilated, arteries are normal.

CLINICAL NOTE: Figure 88 is from the same patient as figure 80, a female, aged 13. At the age of six she had right convergent squint. Since then she has had amblyopia of the right eye. No general symptoms.
Eye examination: Visual acuity, right eye: 6/18, unimproved by lenses; left eye: 6/6 emmetropia. Intraocular tension and anterior segments are normal. Both discs show pseudopapilledema and drusen of the disc, but on the left disc there are some small hemorrhages and part of the disc is slightly edematous. Both blind spots are slightly enlarged.
General examination, including neurological examination, carotid angiography, pneumoencephalography and electroencephalography, showed nothing abnormal.

Figure 89. Right eye. Papilledema. The disc is hyperemic and projects about one diopter. Disc margin is blurred. The retinal veins are tortuous and congested, the arteries are normal. No hemorrhages or exudates.

CLINICAL NOTE: Figure 89 is from a male, aged 60. During the last month he complained of progressive headache and short attacks of hazy vision.
Eye examination: Visual acuity, right eye: 6/6 with + 3.0 D sph. + 1.0 D cyl. axis 100°; left eye: 6/6 with + 2.0 D sph. + 1.0 D cyl. axis 90°. Intraocular tension and anterior segments are normal. Both discs show papilledema projecting about one diopter. There are some retinal hemorrhages, but no exudates. Blind spots enlarged, but otherwise no visual field defects.
General examination, including neurological examination, aroused suspicion of a sphenoidal meningioma. Craniotomy confirmed the suspicion, and the meningioma was removed.

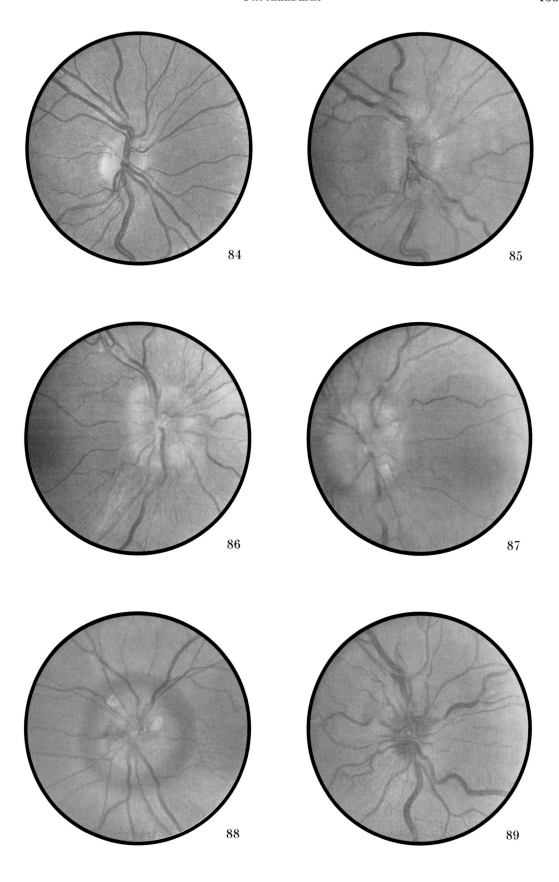

Figure 90. Left eye. Papilledema. The optic cup is filled and disc margin blurred. A few hemorrhages on the disc. Retinal veins only slightly congested.

Figure 91. Right eye. From the same patient as figure 90. Advanced papilledema. The disc projects two diopters. Woolly exudates cover the disc and streaky hemorrhages radiate from the disc into the retina. Retinal veins are congested.

CLINICAL NOTE: Figures 90 and 91 are from a male, aged 51. Three years ago, the left kidney was removed because of hypernephroma. After a slight cranial trauma three weeks ago he developed progressive headache and short attacks of hazy vision.
Eye examination: Visual acuity, right eye: 6/6 with + 1.5 D sph.; left eye: 6/6 with + 2.5 D sph. Intraocular tension and anterior segments are normal. The right disc shows advanced papilledema, the left moderate papilledema. Blind spots enlarged, but otherwise no visual field defects.
General examination, including neurological examination, angiography, electroencephalography and brain scanning, showed hypernephroma metastases in both hemispheres.

Figure 92. Right eye. Papilledema, advanced stage. The disc projects like a mushroom, about four diopters. There are numerous cotton-wool exudates. Hemorrhages radiate from the disc into the retina. The retinal veins are dilated and the arteries narrowed.

CLINICAL NOTE: Figure 92 is from a male, aged 70. Three months ago he had a cranial trauma and was unconscious for some minutes. Since then he has had slowly progressive headache starting in the frontal region and spreading to the occipital region. During the last week before admission, he developed progressive confusion, dullness and short attacks of hazy vision.
Eye examination: Visual acuity, both eyes: 6/6 with + 1.0 D sph. Anterior segments and intraocular tension are normal. The fundi show bilateral papilledema with woolly exudates and hemorrhages. Both blind spots enlarged.
General examination showed a dull and confused man with a stiff neck, but without pareses. Reflexes were normal. Blood pressure:

220/130 mm Hg. Bilateral carotid angiography showed bilateral subdural hematomas, which were removed surgically.

Figure 93. Left eye. Chronic papilledema in regression. The edematous disc is covered by a whitish veil, due to gliosis. Flame-shaped hemorrhages radiate from the disc into the fundus. Some retinal edema is seen at the temporal side of the disc.

CLINICAL NOTE: Figure 93 is from a male, aged 6. Two months ago he was operated on for mastoiditis on the right side. Soon afterwards he developed paralysis of the right oculomotor and trochlear nerves and presented bilateral papilledema, and thrombosis of the right jugular vein and cavernous sinus was diagnosed.
Eye examination a month later: Visual acuity, right eye: 4/18, unimproved by lenses; left eye: 4/4.5, emmetropia. The right eye presents oculomotor and trochlear nerve paralysis, but otherwise anterior segments are normal. Both discs present chronic papilledema and the right fundus also macular edema. Visual field cannot be recorded.
General examination showed thrombosis of the right jugular vein and cavernous sinus.

Figures 94 and 95. Right and left eyes. Chronic papilledema. Both discs are enlarged and pale due to edema and gliosis. On the right disc, a delicate network of dilated superficial capillaries is seen plainly. Retinal veins are congested. Both discs project about four diopters.

CLINICAL NOTE: Figures 94 and 95 are from a male, aged 39. As a child he had left convergent strabismus. Since childhood, he has had amblyopia of the left eye. Papilledema was diagnosed two years ago, but the cause was not found. During the last year progressive headache localized to the frontal regions.
Eye examination: Visual acuity, right eye: 6/6 with + 0.5 D sph.; left eye: 6/60, unimproved by lenses. Anterior segments are normal. Both optic discs present chronic papilledema with beginning atrophy. Blind spots enlarged and both visual fields contracted to 30°.
General examination, including neurological examination, aroused suspicion of a frontal tumor. Craniotomy revealed a glioma in the left frontal lobe.

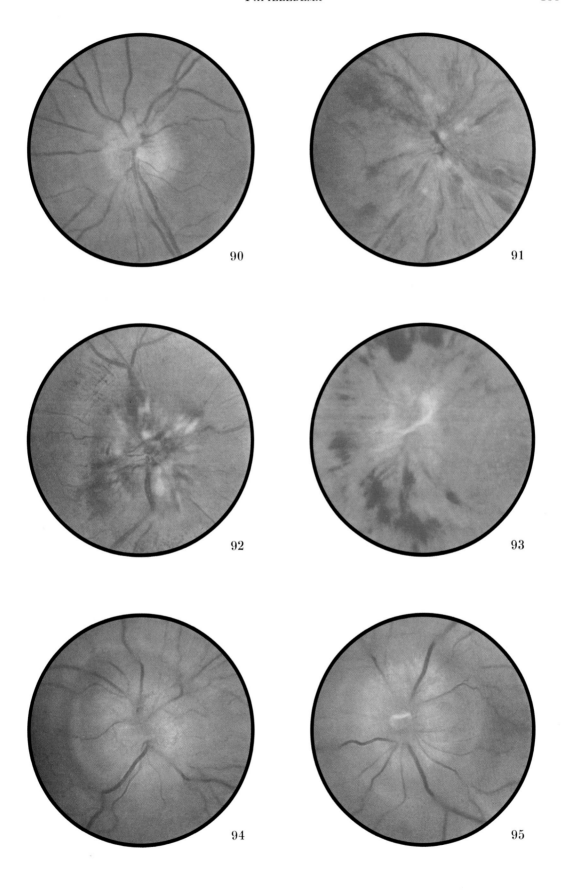

90

91

92

93

94

95

Figure 96. Right eye. Papilledema in hypertensive neuroretinopathy. The disc is edematous and projects about two diopters. There is some retinal edema. Retinal hemorrhages radiate from the disc. Retinal arteries are narrow, the veins are dilated.

CLINICAL NOTE: Figure 96 is from the same patient as figures 186—187, a male, aged 18. Six months ago he had an accident with his motorcycle. Shortly afterwards he developed hematuria and after some months a nearly total anuria and hypertension. He has been dialyzed with the artificial kidney at regular intervals since then.
Eye examination: Visual acuity, both eyes: 6/18, unimproved by lenses. Intraocular tension and anterior segments are normal. Both fundi present hypertensive neuroretinopathy with macular star formation.
General examination showed hypertension, proteinuria, uremia and hypochromic anemia. Blood pressure: 230/120 mm Hg. Serum creatine: 10.6 mg/100 ml. Hemoglobin: 8.6 g/100 ml.

Figure 97. Left eye. Papilledema in leukemia. The disc is swollen and projects about two diopters. At the disc, there are some cotton-wool exudates and streaky hemorrhages. There is also slight retinal edema. Retinal veins are dilated, arteries are narrowed.

CLINICAL NOTE: Figure 97 is from a male, aged 11. Granulocytic leukemia was diagnosed eight months ago. The last few months he has had severe headache and attacks of hazy vision.
Eye examination: Visual acuity, both eyes: 6/9 with + 1.0 D sph. Anterior segments are normal. Both discs present papilledema.
General examination showed a weak, anemic boy. Hemoglobin: 7.6 g/100 ml. Leucocytes: 34,000 per cu mm. Bone marrow examination and blood smears showed granulocytic leukemia. X-ray examination showed leukemic infiltration of bones all over the body. He died six weeks later.

Figure 98. Left eye. Chronic papilledema in macroglobulinemia. The disc is swollen, resembling a mushroom, and projects about four diopters. The disc is covered by a grayish-white veil, indicating some gliosis. Retinal veins are engorged and tortuous, the arteries are normal. Some small retinal hemorrhages are seen below and nasally.

CLINICAL NOTE: Figure 98 is from the same patient as figure 291, a female, aged 41. Macroglobulinemia was demonstrated five years ago. For further clinical information, see clinical note to figure 291.

Figure 99. Right eye. Papilledema in myelomatosis. The disc is swollen and projects about one diopter. There is a single splinter hemorrhage. Veins are engorged and tortuous. Arteries are normal. The fundus is pale, orange-red.

CLINICAL NOTE: Figure 99 is from the same patient as figures 285—287, a female, aged 51. Myelomatosis was recently diagnosed.
For further clinical information, see clinical note to figures 285—287.

Figure 100. Right eye. Chronic papilledema in neuroluetic infection. The disc is edematous, projecting about three diopters and surrounded by retinal edema. Retinal vessels are normal.

CLINICAL NOTE: Figure 100 is from a female, aged 39. Since childhood she has had right divergent strabismus and amblyopia. Fifteen years ago she had a luetic infection. The last few months she has experienced short attacks of hazy vision.
Eye examination: Visual acuity, right eye: 6/18, unimproved by lenses; left eye: 6/6, emmetropia. Right divergent strabismus of 10°. Eye movements are normal. Pupils do not react to light. Anterior segments are normal. Both fundi present papilledema and retinal edema. No retinal hemorrhages or exudates. Retinal vessels are normal.
General examination, including neurological examination and spinal fluid examination, showed evidence of neurolues.

Figure 101. Right eye. Slight papilledema due to a retrobulbar tumor. The optic cup is filled and vessels slightly obscured at the blurred disc margin. There is a single hemorrhage at the nasal side of the disc. Veins are slightly dilated, arteries are narrowed.

CLINICAL NOTE: Figure 101 is from a female, aged 48. During the last two years progressing exophthalmos of the right eye. No complaints from the left eye. No general symptoms.
Eye examination: Visual acuity, right eye: 6/9 with + 1.5 D sph.; left eye: 6/6 with + 0.5 D sph. Right eye is dislocated forwards and downwards. Motility reduced. Increased orbital resistance. Hertel: 23-16/95. Tumor is located behind the bulb. Probe-excision not possible. Anterior segments are normal. The right fundus presents papilledema and ridging of the retina in the posterior pole. Left fundus is normal. Right blind spot enlarged.
Five years later, exophthalmos is unchanged, but the right disc is now atrophic.
General examination showed nothing abnormal.

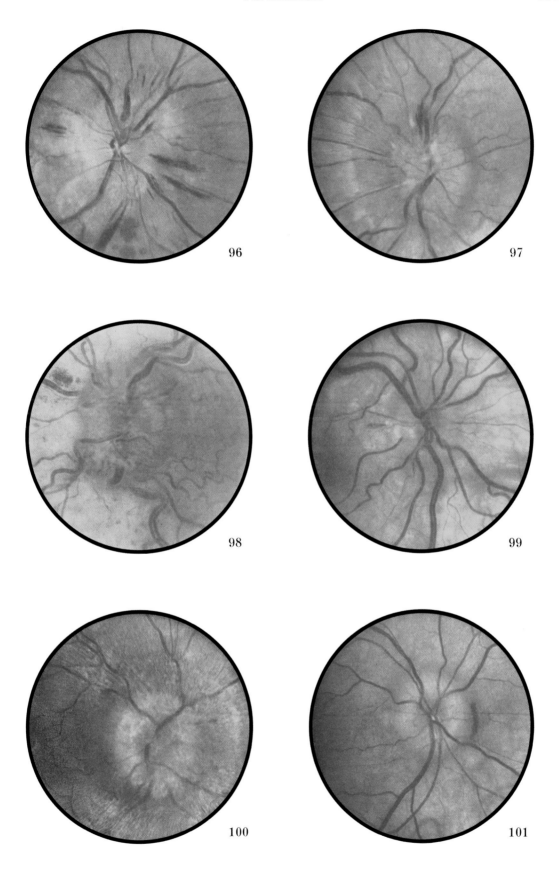

Figures 102 and 103. Right and left eyes. Pseudo Foster-Kennedy syndrome. The right disc shows chronic papilledema; the left disc is atrophic, pale, white, and shows slight cupping.

CLINICAL NOTE: Figures 102 and 103 are from a male, aged 49. Two years ago optic atrophy was demonstrated in the left eye. The last month he has had obscurations in the right eye.
Eye examination: Visual acuity, right eye: 6/6, emmetropia; left eye: < 6/6 with + 0.5 D sph. Intraocular tension and anterior segments are normal. The right disc presents chronic papilledema. The left disc is atrophic. Visual field, right eye: contracted to about 30°; left eye: contracted to 5°.
General examination, including neurologic examination, angiography and X-ray examination, aroused suspicion of chiasma syndrome. Explorative craniotomy showed adhesions between the chiasma and the arachnoid, but no tumor formation.

Figures 104 and 105. Right and left eyes. The right disc is normal. The left disc shows some pallor and cupping. Retinal vessels are normal.

CLINICAL NOTE: Figures 104 and 105 are from a male, aged 15. He has had headache for some years. Six months ago his vision was normal. Three months ago he experienced some reduction of vision in the left eye. During the last month he has had some obscurations.
Eye examination: Visual acuity, right eye: 6/6, emmetropia; left eye: hand movements, unimproved by lenses. Intraocular tension and anterior segments are normal. The right disc is normal, the left shows moderate atrophy. Visual field, right eye: defect in the upper temporal quadrant; left eye: large defect. There remains only a small intact area in the lower temporal quadrant.
General examination, including neurological examination, aroused suspicion of cranio-

pharyngioma. Craniotomy showed a large, inoperable craniopharyngioma. The patient died a fortnight after the operation.

Figure 106. Right eye. Optic nerve atrophy. The disc is pale, whitish and slightly cupped. Disc margin fairly distinct. Retinal vessels are normal and fundus lightly pigmented.

CLINICAL NOTE: Figure 106 is from a female, aged 21. Five years ago she had a cystic glioma removed from the left cerebellar hemisphere. Vision was already defective in both eyes before the operation.
Eye examination: Visual acuity, right eye: light perception; left eye: counting fingers. Unimproved by lenses. Right divergent strabismus of 30°. Some irregular nystagmus. Otherwise, eye movements are free. Both pupils react normally to light. Intraocular tension and anterior segments are normal. Both discs are atrophic. Retinal vessels are normal. Fundi lightly pigmented.
General examination, including neurological examination, showed sequelae after the removal of the cerebellar tumor.

Figure 107. Left eye. Optic nerve atrophy. The disc is pale, whitish and slightly cupped. Disc margin is fairly distinct. Retinal vessels are normal.

CLINICAL NOTE: Figure 107 is from a female, aged 19. During the last year she has had progressive headache. Some months ago she had a chromophobe adenoma of the pituitary gland removed. No visual complaints.
Eye examination: Visual acuity, right eye: 6/6 with − 0.5 D cyl. axis 90°; left eye: 6/9, unimproved by lenses. Intraocular tension and anterior segments are normal. Both discs are atrophic. Visual fields show bitemporal hemianopia.
General examination showed the patient in good condition. Her loss of pituitary function is well compensated by substitution therapy.

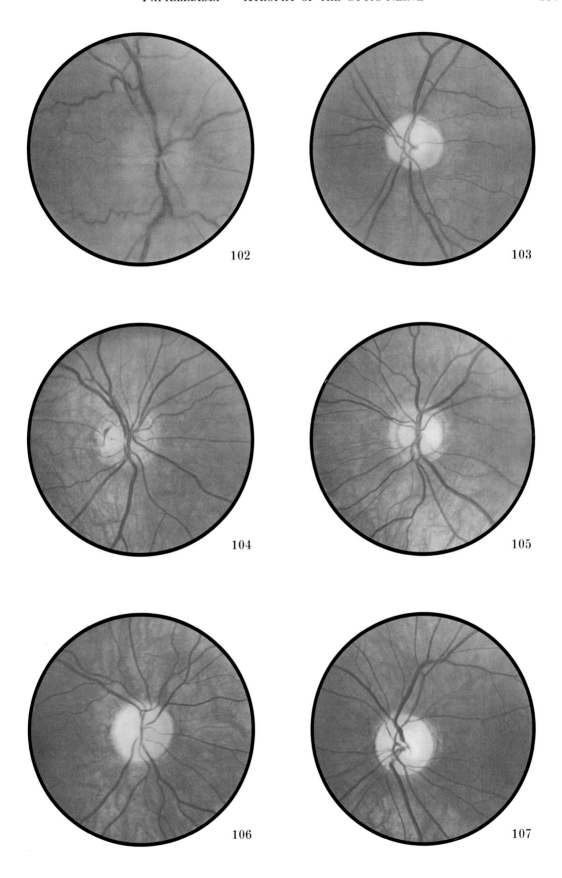

102

103

104

105

106

107

Figure 108. Left eye. Vascular optic atrophy. The disc is yellowish-white and slightly cupped. Temporally there is some peripapillary atrophy. Retinal vessels are very narrow. At the disc margin, the lower branch of the central retinal artery is covered by a whitish plaque. Some vessels show slight sheathing.

CLINICAL NOTE: Figure 108 is from a male, aged 66. Seven years ago he had transient blindness of the right eye. Six weeks ago he suddenly experienced a loss of vision in the left eye. During the last seven years he has had some heart failure.
Eye examination: Visual acuity, right eye: 6/18 with − 1.0 D sph. − 1.5 D cyl. axis 90°; left eye: no light perception. Anterior segments and intraocular tension normal. The right disc shows some temporal pallor. The retinal vessels are sclerotic. Visual field shows centrocecal scotoma. The left disc is totally atrophic and retinal vessels narrow.
General examination showed some heart failure. Electrocardiogram showed myocardial degeneration. Blood pressure: 140/90 mm Hg. Sedimentation rate: 19 mm/hour. Biopsy of the temporal artery was normal.

Figure 109. Left eye. Vascular optic atrophy. The disc is pale, yellowish-white and slightly cupped. Disc margin is ill-defined. Retinal arteries are very sclerotic, the veins somewhat dilated.

CLINICAL NOTE: Figure 109 is from a male, aged 58. Eight years ago gradually reduced vision in the left eye. One year ago gradually reduced vision in the right eye. Diabetes demonstrated a few months ago. No other general symptoms.
Eye examination: Visual acuity, right eye: 6/60 with + 3.0 D sph.; left eye: < 6/36 with + 3.0 D sph. Intraocular tension and anterior segments are normal. Both fundi show simple diabetic retinopathy, marked vascular sclerosis and optic atrophy. Visual fields show extensive defects, including central defects.
General examination showed diabetes without nephropathy. Blood pressure: 140/70 mm Hg. Sedimentation rate: 32 mm/hour. Hemoglobin: 12.8 g/100 ml. Biopsy of the temporal artery was normal. Muscle biopsy, however, showed heavy vascular and perivascular infiltration suspicious of periarteritis nodosa.

Figure 110. Right eye. Optic nerve atrophy. The disc is pale, whitish and slightly cupped. The disc margin is fairly distinct, but temporally there is some peripapillary atrophy. Retinal vessels slightly narrowed and the fundus has a tessellated appearance.

CLINICAL NOTE: Figure 110 is from a male, aged 44. Twenty-five years ago he had encephalomyelitis with transient paraplegia. The last five years progressive loss of vision. The last two years progressive spastic paraplegia.
Eye examination: Visual acuity, both eyes: 3/24. Unimproved by lenses. Intraocular tension and anterior segments are normal. Both optic discs are atrophic. Retinal vessels are narrowed and fundi tessellated. Visual fields show concentric contraction.
General examination, including neurological examination, showed severe spastic paraplegia of the lower limbs. Spinal fluid examination and electroencephalogram showed nothing abnormal. Wassermann reaction was negative. Blood pressure: 140/70 mm Hg.

Figure 111. Right eye. Optic atrophy in cranial dysostosis. The disc is pale, but not cupped. Disc margin is ill-defined. Retinal vessels are normal. Fundus sparsely pigmented.

CLINICAL NOTE: Figure 111 is from a male, aged 7. He has a cranial dysostosis (Crouzon's disease), but is otherwise healthy. Two years ago, chronic papilledema was observed in both eyes. He has no ocular complaints.
Eye examination: Visual acuity, both eyes: < 3/4.5 without lenses. He has some exophthalmos, but eye movements are normal. Anterior segments normal. Both discs show some atrophy. Visual fields contracted to about 30°.
General examination showed a boy with a cranial dysostosis (Crouzon's disease).

Figures 112 and 113. Right and left eyes. Hereditary optic atrophy. Both discs are pale, yellowish-white and slightly cupped. Retinal vessels are normal.

CLINICAL NOTE: Figures 112 and 113 are from a male, aged 59. Several cases of optic atrophy in the family. He has been weak-sighted since the age of seven years. No general symptoms.
Eye examination: Visual acuity, both eyes: 6/60 with + 2.5 D sph. Eye movements are normal. No nystagmus. Color vision defective. Large, bilateral centrocecal scotomas. Both discs show optic atrophy.
General examination showed nothing abnormal.

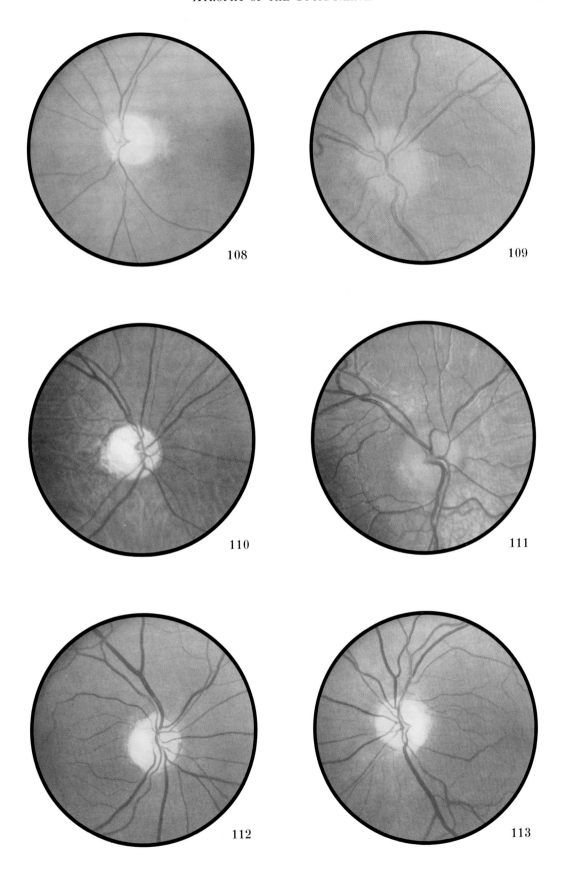

108

109

110

111

112

113

Figure 114. Left eye. Optic neuritis. The optic disc is swollen and ill-defined, and projects about one diopter. Streaky hemorrhages radiate from the disc. Retinal veins are engorged, the arteries are normal.

Figure 115. Same eye as figure 114, eight months later. Postneuritic optic atrophy. The disc is pale, yellowish-white and cupped. Disc margin is fairly distinct and bordered by a scleral ring. Retinal vessels are normal.

CLINICAL NOTE: Figures 114 and 115 are from the same patient as figure 240, a male, aged 41. During the last few days he has complained of hazy and gradually reduced vision in the left eye and left-sided retrobulbar pain. No general symptoms.
Eye examination: Visual acuity, right eye: 6/6 with − 0.5 D sph.; left eye: light perception. Intraocular tension and anterior segments are normal. The right fundus is normal. The left fundus shows optic neuritis associated with venous fullness, and retinal and preretinal hemorrhage. Central scotoma of about 30° in the left eye.
General examination, including neurological examination, showed nothing abnormal.
Vision in the left eye gradually increased to nearly normal level in the course of some months, but the disc became pale, atrophic and the visual field contracted to 30°.

Figure 116. Left eye. Postneuritic optic atrophy. The disc is pale, grayish-white and cupped. Disc margin is slightly irregular and bordered by a scleral ring. Retinal vessels are normal.

CLINICAL NOTE: Figure 116 is from a female, aged 53. Twenty years ago she had an optic neuritis in the left eye. No ocular or general complaints.
Eye examination: Visual acuity, right eye: 6/6 with + 1.0 D cyl. axis 135°; left eye: < 6/6 + 0.5 D cyl. axis 135°. Anterior segments and intraocular tension normal. Right fundus normal. Left disc shows postneuritic optic atrophy. Left visual field is slightly contracted.
General examination showed nothing abnormal.

Figure 117. Right eye. Postneuritic optic atrophy. The optic disc is pale, whitish and slightly cupped. Disc margin is fairly distinct, but temporally there is some peripapillary atrophy. Retinal vessels are normal.

CLINICAL NOTE: Figure 117 is from a female, aged 49. Ten years ago she had optic neuritis in the right eye. Since then vision in the right eye has decreased gradually. No complaints from the left eye. No general symptoms.
Eye examination: Visual acuity, right eye: no light perception; left eye: 6/6, emmetropia. Anterior segments and intraocular tension are normal. Right optic disc is atrophic. Left fundus is normal.
General examination showed nothing abnormal.

Figure 118. Left eye. Postneuritic optic atrophy. The disc is pale, whitish and cupped. The disc margin is fairly distinct. Myopic crescent is seen temporally. Retinal vessels are slightly narrowed and the fundus is lightly pigmented.

CLINICAL NOTE: Figure 118 is from a male, aged 13. He has been mentally retarded since early childhood. Reduced vision observed at the age of five years. At the same time toxoplasmosis reaction was highly positive (dye test positive in 1:1,250). Since then vision has shown progressive reduction.
Eye examination: Visual acuity, right eye: < 1/60 with − 5.0 D sph. − 3.0 D cyl. axis 10°; left eye: < 3/18 with − 4.0 D sph. − 2.0 D cyl. axis 170°. Right divergent squint of 20°. Fine irregular nystagmus. Visual fields cannot be recorded. Palpatory, intraocular tension is normal. Anterior segments are normal. Both optic discs are atrophic. Fundi are lightly pigmented and retinal vessels are narrowed.
General examination showed a mentally retarded boy. Pneumoencephalography showed cerebral atrophy. The electroencephalogram showed diffusely spread abnormal waves. The Sabin-Feldman dye test was positive in 1:250. Wassermann reaction was negative.

Figure 119. Left eye. Optic nerve atrophy after retrobulbar neuritis. Temporal sector-formed pallor of the disc. Temporally, there is some peripapillary atrophy. Retinal vessels are normal. Some colloid bodies are seen in the macular area.

CLINICAL NOTE: Figure 119 is from a female, aged 39. Ten years ago she had retrobulbar neuritis on the left side. No attacks since then. No general symptoms.
Eye examination: Visual acuity, right eye: 6/6, emmetropia; left eye: 6/12, unimproved by lenses. No nystagmus. Eye movements are normal. Anterior segments and intraocular tension are normal. Right fundus is normal. Left disc shows temporal pallor, and visual field shows centrocecal scotoma.
General examination showed no evidence of multiple sclerosis.

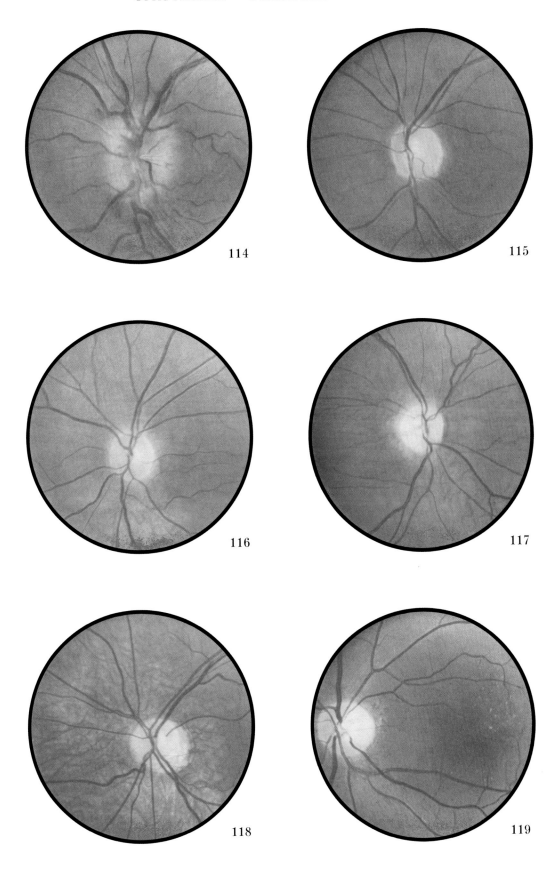

114

115

116

117

118

119

Figure 120. Right eye. Glaucomatous cupping of the optic disc in buphthalmos. The disc is pale, atrophic and deeply cupped. The retinal vessels are displaced nasally on the disc and bend sharply as they emerge from the disc into the retinal level. Retinal veins are tortuous and dilated, the arteries are normal.

CLINICAL NOTE: See clinical note to figure 161.

Figure 121. Right eye. Glaucomatous cupping of the optic disc in juvenile glaucoma. The disc is pale, atrophic and deeply cupped. Retinal vessels are displaced nasally on the disc.

CLINICAL NOTE: Figure 121 is from a male, aged 24. Glaucoma was demonstrated a fortnight ago. No general symptoms.
Eye examination: Visual acuity, right eye: 6/6 with − 6.5 D sph. − 1.0 D cyl. axis 90°; left eye: 6/6 with − 4.5 D sph. − 2.0 D cyl. axis 90°. Anterior segments, including gonioscopy, show nothing abnormal. Intraocular tension during local glaucoma treatment, both eyes: 16 mm Hg. Both discs present glaucomatous cupping. Visual fields are contracted to about 5°.
General examination showed nothing abnormal.

Figure 122. Left eye. Glaucomatous cupping of the optic disc. The disc is pale, atrophic and deeply cupped. Retinal vessels are displaced nasally on the disc.

CLINICAL NOTE: Figure 122 is from a male, aged 45. During the last few years several attacks of acute glaucoma in the left eye. No complaints from the right eye. No pain.
Eye examination: Visual acuity, right eye: 6/6 with + 2.75 D sph. + 0.5 D cyl. axis 90°; left eye: hand movements. Right anterior segment, fundus, visual field and intraocular tension are normal. Left anterior chamber is shallow, chamber angle closed, intraocular tension 36 mm Hg, visual field largely defective and optic disc atrophic and deeply cupped.
General examination showed nothing abnormal.

Figure 123. Left eye. Glaucomatous cupping of the optic disc. The disc is pale, atrophic and deeply cupped. Retinal vessels are displaced nasally on the disc. Peripapillary, there is a slight yellowish-white atrophic zone.

CLINICAL NOTE: Figure 123 is from a female, aged 58. Vision has gradually decreased during the last year, but she has not observed colored halos around lights, and has not had ocular pain.
Eye examination: Visual acuity, right eye: 6/9; left eye: 6/18. Unimproved by lenses. Anterior segments, including gonioscopy, show nothing abnormal. Intraocular tension during pilocarpin medication: 13—15 mm Hg. Both discs show deep glaucomatous cupping and atrophy. Visual fields are contracted to about 10°.
General examination showed nothing abnormal.

Figure 124. Left eye. Glaucomatous cupping of the optic disc and acute glaucoma attack. The deeply cupped optic disc is reddened and the retinal veins dilated during the acute glaucoma attack. Peripapillary, there is a pale atrophic zone.

CLINICAL NOTE: Figure 124 is from a male, aged 55. He has had glaucoma for some years, and was admitted during an acute glaucoma attack in the left eye.
Eye examination: Visual acuity, right eye: 6/6 with + 7.0 D sph.; left eye: 1/36 with + 7.0 D sph. Right anterior chamber is shallow. Chamber angle is narrow, but open. Intraocular tension during pilocarpin medication: 24 mm Hg. Fundus and visual field are normal. Left anterior chamber is shallow and chamber angle closed. Intraocular tension is 48 mm Hg. Disc is deeply cupped, but hyperemic. There are peripapillary atrophy and large visual field defect.
General examination showed nothing abnormal.

Figure 125. Right eye. Glaucomatous cupping of the optic disc in an aphakic eye. The disc is pale, grayish-white and deeply cupped. Retinal vessels are displaced nasally on the disc. Peripapillary, there is a whitish atrophic zone. In the periphery below, there is an atrophic area.

CLINICAL NOTE: Figure 125 is from a male, aged 42. At the age of 15 years he received a contusion of the right eye and developed a cataract. Ten years ago he was operated on for the cataract. Two years ago a glaucoma was demonstrated in the right eye. No complaints from the left eye.
Eye examination: Visual acuity, right eye: 2/60 with + 10.0 D sph. + 2.0 D cyl. axis 0°; left eye: 6/6, emmetropia. Right eye is aphakic. Chamber angle is open. Intraocular tension is 45 mm Hg. Disc is atrophic and deeply cupped. There is peripapillary atrophy and posttraumatic atrophy in the lower periphery. Visual field is contracted to about 5°. Left anterior segment, intraocular tension and fundus are normal.
General examination showed nothing abnormal.

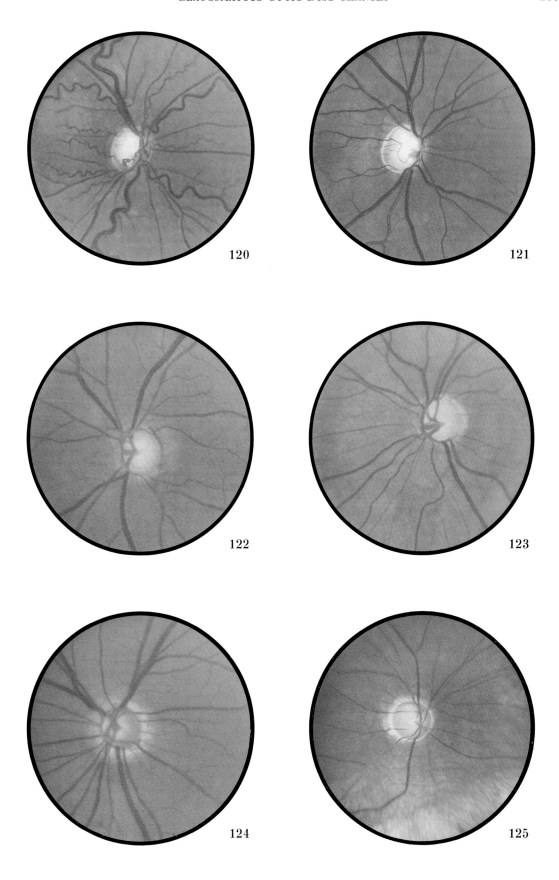

120

121

122

123

124

125

Figure 126. Left eye. Large cilioretinal artery. The cilioretinal artery appears separately in the temporal part of the disc, and supplies part of the macular area. Retinal vessels are normal.

CLINICAL NOTE: Figure 126 is from a female, aged 59. No ocular complaints.
Eye examination: Visual acuity, both eyes: 6/6 with + 1.0 D sph. Anterior segments are normal. The right fundus is normal. The left presents a cilioretinal artery.
General examination showed nothing abnormal.

Figure 127. Left eye. Two cilioretinal arteries supply the macular area. Optic disc and retinal vessels are normal.

CLINICAL NOTE: Figure 127 is from a female, aged 34. No ocular complaints.
Eye examination: Visual acuity, both eyes: 6/6, emmetropia. Anterior segments and right fundus are normal. The left fundus presents two cilioretinal arteries.
General examination showed nothing abnormal.

Figure 128. Left eye. Two cilioretinal arteries supply the macular area. The optic disc and retinal vessels are normal.

CLINICAL NOTE: Figure 128 is from the same patient as figure 211, a female, aged 31. At the age of 18 years she suddenly experienced a loss of vision in the right eye. Ophthalmoscopy showed occlusion of two cilioretinal arteries. No improvement of vision since then. No complaints from the left eye. No general symptoms.
Eye examination: Visual acuity, right eye: counting fingers; left eye: 6/6, emmetropia. Anterior segments are normal. Both fundi present cilioretinal arteries. The right macula presents some pigment changes, the left macula is normal. Retinal vessels are normal. Right visual field shows a defect corresponding to the previous occlusion of the cilioretinal arteries.
General examination showed nothing abnormal. Blood pressure: 140/80 mm Hg.

Figure 129. Right eye. The retinal arteries appear on the disc as three separate trunks. A small cilioretinal artery is also present. Optic disc and retinal vessels are normal.

CLINICAL NOTE: Figure 129 is from a male, aged 22. Diabetes demonstrated eight years ago.

Since then insulin treatment. Right convergent strabismus and amblyopia since the age of four years.
Eye examination: Visual acuity, right eye: 6/24, unimproved by lenses; left eye: 6/6 with + 1.0 D sph. Right convergent squint of about 10°. Eye movements are normal. Anterior segments and fundi normal. No signs of diabetic retinopathy. Retinal vessels appear as three separate trunks on both discs. Cilioretinal arteries are also present.
General examination showed diabetes without nephropathy or hypertension. Blood pressure: 125/65 mm Hg.

Figure 130. Left eye. Abnormal looping and twisting of the lower temporal retinal artery. The optic disc is normal.

CLINICAL NOTE: Figure 130 is from a female, aged 64. Diabetes demonstrated two years ago. Insulin treatment since then. No ocular complaints.
Eye examination: Visual acuity, right eye: 6/6 with + 1.5 D sph.; left eye: 6/6 with + 2.0 D sph. Anterior segments are normal. Both fundi present some vascular sclerosis, but no signs of diabetic retinopathy. In the left fundus the lower temporal artery shows some looping and twisting.
General examination showed diabetes. No nephropathy or hypertension. Blood pressure: 140/80 mm Hg.

Figure 131. Right eye. Abnormal tortuosity of retinal vessels in Sturge-Weber's syndrome.

CLINICAL NOTE: Figure 131 is from the same patient as figure 160, a female, aged 10. Since infancy she has had capillary angioma of the right side of the face, convulsions, left hemiplegia and has been mentally retarded. At the age of four years, craniotomy revealed a subdural hygroma and an angiomatous tumor in the right parietal lobe.
Eye examination: Visual acuity, both eyes: 3/4.5 with + 2.0 D sph. Anterior segments and intraocular tension normal. Visual fields cannot be recorded. In the right fundus retinal vessels are dilated and show many abnormal, anastomosing branches. A flat choroidal angioma is seen in the upper temporal quadrant. Left fundus is normal.
General examination showed mental retardation, capillary angioma of the right side of the face and left spastic hemiplegia. X-ray showed intracranial calcifications.

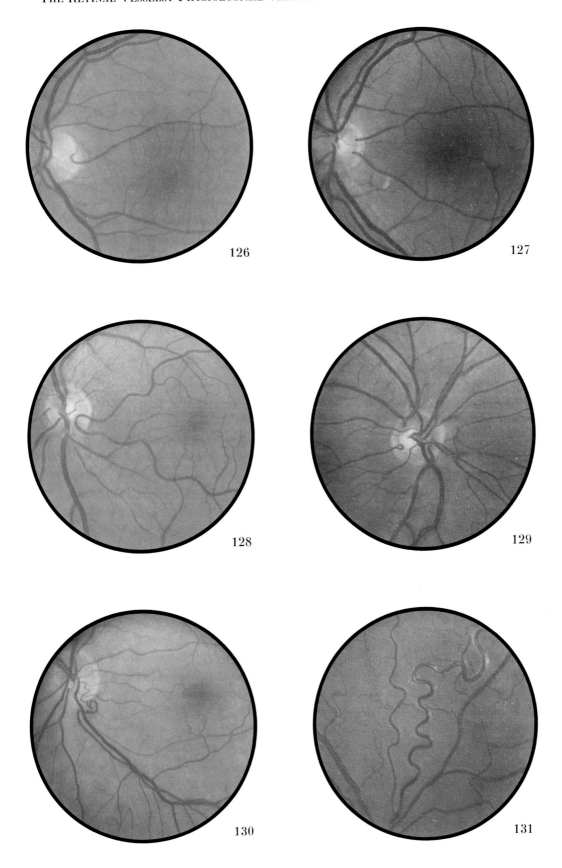

126

127

128

129

130

131

Figure 132. Right eye. Tortuosity of the retinal veins. The retinal veins are elongated and very tortuous. The retinal arteries are normal. The optic disc and fundus are normal.

CLINICAL NOTE: Figure 132 is from a male, aged 40. No general or ocular complaints.
Eye examination: Visual acuity, both eyes: 6/6 with − 4.0 D sph. Anterior segments are normal. In both fundi the veins are elongated and very tortuous. Retinal arteries, discs and fundi are normal.
General examination showed nothing abnormal.

Figure 133. Left eye. Tortuosity of the retinal vessels. Both arteries and veins are elongated and very tortuous. The fundus and optic disc are normal.

CLINICAL NOTE: Figure 133 is from a male, aged 37. No general or ocular complaints.
Eye examination: Visual acuity, both eyes: 6/6 with − 2.0 D sph. Anterior segments are normal. In both fundi the retinal vessels are elongated and very tortuous. The optic discs and fundi are normal.
General examination showed nothing abnormal.

Figure 134. Right eye. Tortuosity of the retinal veins in coarctation of the aorta. The retinal arteries, the optic disc and the fundus are normal.

CLINICAL NOTE: Figure 134 is from a male, aged 42. Six years ago he was operated on for a coarctation of the aorta. Now he has some heart failure and signs of stenosis of the aortic valve. No ocular complaints.
Eye examination: Visual acuity, both eyes: 6/6, emmetropia. Anterior segments are normal. Retinal veins are tortuous. Retinal arteries, optic discs and fundi are normal. No locomotion pulse.
General examination showed some heart failure and signs of stenosis of the aortic valve. Blood pressure: 110/90 mm Hg.
He was operated on again five years later, and died some days after the operation.

Figure 135. Right eye. Tortuosity of the retinal arteries and veins in coarctation of the aorta. The optic disc is normal. The fundus is slightly tessellated.

CLINICAL NOTE: Figure 135 is from a male, aged 41. One year ago he was operated on for co-
arctation of the aorta. He now presents slight signs of heart failure. No ocular complaints.
Eye examination: Visual acuity, both eyes: 6/6, emmetropia. Anterior segments are normal. Retinal vessels are tortuous. Retinal arteries slightly narrowed. The optic discs and fundi are normal. No locomotion pulse.
General examination showed some heart failure. Electrocardiogram showed some myocardial degeneration. Blood pressure: 150/80 mm Hg.

Figure 136. Right eye. Fundus changes in congenital heart disease with cyanosis. The optic disc is reddened and the margin blurred. The retinal veins are tortuous and dilated. The arteries are dark-red, and the veins and the fundus are cyanotic.

CLINICAL NOTE: Figure 136 is from a male, aged 18. Since early infancy he has had universal cyanosis. No signs of heart failure. No ocular complaints.
Eye examination: Visual acuity, both eyes: 6/9. Unimproved by lenses. Visual fields are normal. Slight bilateral anterior polar cataract. Both discs are reddened and their margins blurred. Retinal vessels are tortuous and dilated. The veins and fundi are cyanotic.
General examination showed universal cyanosis. Angiocardiogram showed congenital heart disease of Steno-Fallot type. Blood pressure: 120/90 mm Hg. Hemoglobin: 23.4 g/100 ml.

Figure 137. Right eye. Fundus changes in congenital heart disease with cyanosis. The optic disc is reddened, but the margin is distinct. Retinal vessels are tortuous. The veins are dilated and cyanotic. Fundus slightly tessellated.

CLINICAL NOTE: Figure 137 is from a female, aged 9. A sister died from congenital heart disease. At the age of three years she was operated on for congenital heart disease of Steno-Fallot type. Now she presents some heart failure and universal cyanosis. No ocular complaints.
Eye examination: Visual acuity, both eyes: 3/4.5 without lenses. Anterior segments are normal. Both discs are reddened, but disc margins are distinct. Retinal vessels are tortuous and the veins dilated and cyanotic. Fundi show some tessellation.
General examination showed a Greenlander with universal cyanosis. Angiocardiogram showed congenital heart disease of Steno-Fallot type. Blood pressure: 115/80 mm Hg. Hemoglobin: 21.2 g/100 ml.

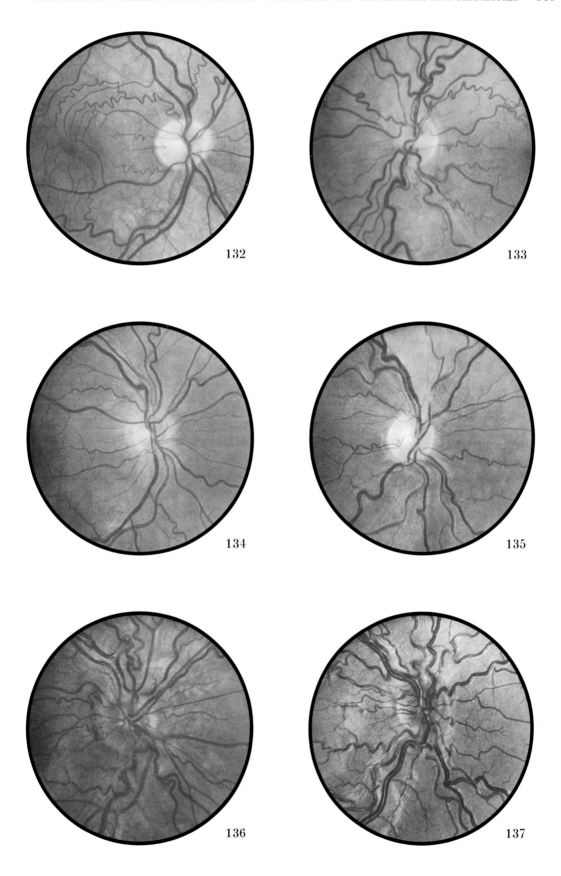

132

133

134

135

136

137

Figure 138. Right eye. Arteriovenous ana-stomosis with aneurysm formation at the temporal side of the optic disc. A cilioreti-nal artery is also present. The optic disc and the other retinal vessels are normal.

CLINICAL NOTE: Figure 138 is from a female, aged 48. No general or ocular complaints.
Eye examination: Visual acuity, both eyes: 6/6 with + 1.0 D sph. Anterior segments and fundi normal apart from arteriovenous aneurysm formation in the right fundus.
General examination showed nothing abnormal.

Figure 139. Right eye. Racemose heman-gioma of the retina. At the upper part of the optic disc there is a markedly dilated sausage-shaped vascular loop and partly hidden by this another vascular loop. In the lower temporal part of the disc there is a tortuous, possibly anastomosing vessel. Retinal vessels show some tortuosity.

CLINICAL NOTE: Figure 139 is from a male, aged 71. Ten years ago he had transient hazy vision and exophthalmos of the right eye. Since then no ocular complaints.
Eye examination: Visual acuity, right eye: 6/12 with − 1.5 D sph.; left eye: 6/6 with − 1.0 D sph. Eye movements are normal. No exoph-thalmos. Anterior segments, intraocular tension and visual fields are normal. At the right disc there is a racemose hemangioma. Retinal ves-sels show some tortuosity. Left fundus is nor-mal.
General examination, including neurological examination, carotid and vertebral angiogra-phy, showed nothing abnormal.

Figure 140. Right eye. Abnormally dilated retinal vessels. The optic disc and fundus are normal.

CLINICAL NOTE: Figure 140 is from a female, aged 52. Since infancy she has had a large capillary angioma in the right cheek and the right side of the tongue. The last ten years she has had right-sided exophthalmos in stooping position. After ligation of the right external carotid artery the angiomas disappeared, but intermittent exophthalmos was still present. No visual complaints.
Eye examination: Visual acuity, both eyes: 6/6 with + 1.0 D sph. No exophthalmos in upright position, but in stooping position the right eye

protrudes 7 mm. Eye movements are normal. Visual fields, intraocular tension and anterior segments are normal. In the right fundus, reti-nal vessels are abnormally dilated until the extreme periphery, but angiomas are not ob-served. The left fundus is normal.
General examination, including angiography, showed no signs of intracranial hemangioma.

Figures 141 and 142. Right eye. Congenital cavernous retinal hemangioma. A prereti-nal, grayish-white veil of fibrous tissue in the lower nasal quadrant is surrounded by pigment deposits and covered by numerous small and large red globules formed by ec-tasia of the small vessels. There are only a few hemorrhages.

CLINICAL NOTE: Figures 141 and 142 are from a female, aged 12. At the age of four years retinal hemangioma was observed in the right fundus. Although the lesion has remained nearly un-altered since then, vision in the right eye has decreased gradually. No complaints from the left eye.
Eye examination: Visual acuity, right eye: hand movements; left eye: 6/6, emmetropia. Inter-mittent right divergent strabismus. Anterior segments are normal. In the right fundus at about 5 o'clock, there is a circumscribed area containing a whitish fibrous veil surrounded by pigment deposits and covered by numerous small and large red vascular globules. The left fundus is normal.
General examination, including neurological examination, showed nothing abnormal.

Figure 143. Right eye. Congenital cavernous retinal hemangioma. A grayish-white area in the lower nasal fundus periphery is al-most covered by small and large red vascu-lar globules. Only few hemorrhages.

CLINICAL NOTE: Figure 143 is from a female, aged 21. A year ago she observed some muscae volitantes and a retinal hemangioma was found in the right eye. The lesion has remained un-altered. No visual disturbances.
Eye examination: Visual acuity, both eyes: 6/6, emmetropia. Anterior segments and intraocular tension are normal. In the right fundus there is a circumscribed hemangioma of the retina at about 5 o'clock, and a corresponding visual field defect. Left fundus is normal.
General examination showed nothing abnormal.

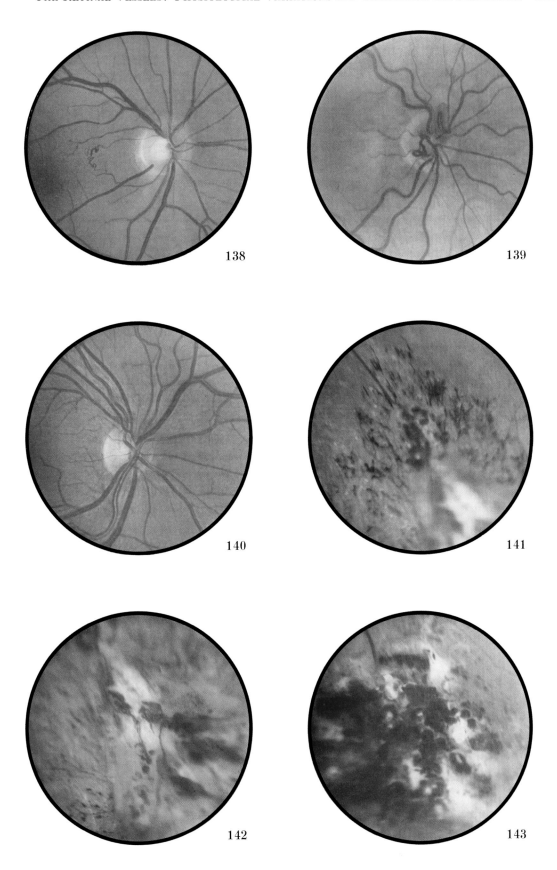

Figure 144. Left eye. Angiomatosis of the retina. There is a prepapillary whitish mass of tissue projecting about three diopters. The lower temporal vein is tortuous and dilated.

Figures 145—147. From the same eye as figure 144, ten months later. Angiomas are developing at the upper and lower border of the whitish prepapillary mass. Retinal veins are very dilated and tortuous. In the upper temporal quadrant there is an angiomatous tumor, supplied by a single retinal artery and vein, and surrounded by extensive, dense yellowish exudate.

Figures 148 and 149. From the same eye as figures 144—147, nine months later. Total retinal detachment. The extensive, dense yellowish exudate is still present.

CLINICAL NOTE: Figures 144—149 are from the same patient as figures 84—85 and 150—157, a female, aged 21. She has always been weak-sighted in the left eye. Five years ago she developed left divergent strabismus.

Eye examination at first admission: Visual acuity, right eye: 6/6, emmetropia; left eye: hand movements. The left eye diverges about 10°. Intraocular tension and anterior segments are normal. The right fundus is normal. In the left fundus there is a prepapillary mass of whitish tissue.

Ten months later angiomatous tumors had developed at the disc and in the upper temporal quadrant. Extensive, dense yellowish exudate surrounds the angiomas.

Nine months later, she developed painful glaucoma and total retinal detachment. The eye was enucleated and histopathological examination showed angiomatosis of the retina and total retinal detachment.

A few months later angiomatous tumors were observed in the right eye. During the next year these tumors enlarged slowly and dense exudates developed. Light-coagulation was performed with good result.

Nearly three years later she developed signs of a cerebellar tumor, and a cerebellar angioreticuloma was removed.

A year later, her vision decreased and the fundal lesions showed severe progression.

Shortly afterwards, she developed papilledema and signs of intracranial tumor growth. Craniotomy showed recurrence of the cerebellar tumor. She died shortly after the operation.

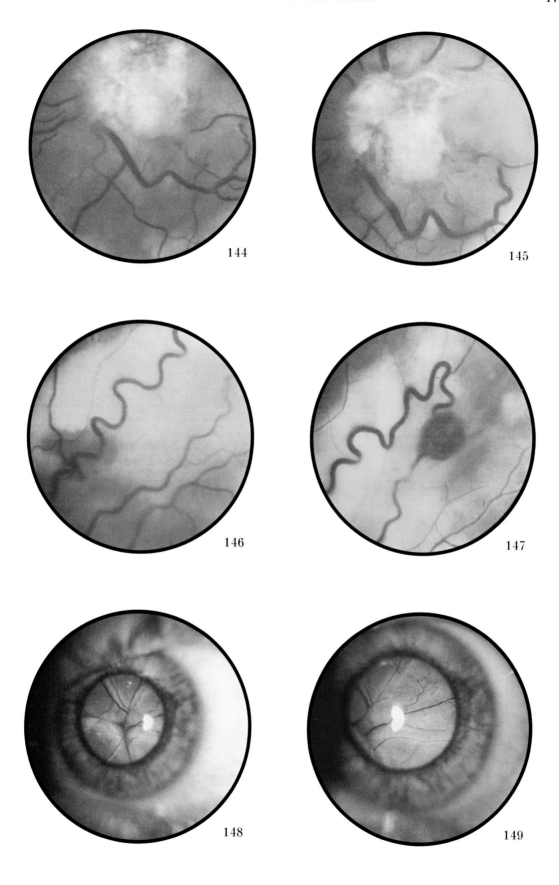

144

145

146

147

148

149

Figures 150—153. Right eye. Angiomatosis of the retina. The pictures show the development of two angiomatous tumors during a period of one year. Both tumors are supplied by a single artery and vein. Yellowish retinal exudate formation shows a steady progression.

Figures 154—155. Same eye as figures 150—153. Progressive formation of dense yellowish-white exudate during a period of about one year.

CLINICAL NOTE: Figures 150—155 are from the same patient as figures 84—85, 144—149 and 156—157, a female, aged 21. She has always been weak-sighted in the left eye. Five years ago she developed left divergent strabismus. *Eye examination* at first admission: Visual acuity, right eye: 6/6, emmetropia; left eye: hand movements. The left eye diverges about 10°. Intraocular tension and anterior segments are normal. The right fundus is normal. In the left fundus there is a prepapillary mass of whitish tissue.

Ten months later angiomatous tumors had developed at the disc and in the upper temporal quadrant. Extensive, dense yellowish exudate surrounds the angiomas.

Nine months later, she developed painful glaucoma and total retinal detachment. The eye was enucleated and histopathological examination showed angiomatosis of the retina and total retinal detachment.

A few months later angiomatous tumors were observed in the right eye. During the next year these tumors enlarged slowly and dense exudates developed. Light-coagulation was performed with good result.

Nearly three years later she developed signs of a cerebellar tumor, and a cerebellar angioreticuloma was removed.

A year later, her vision decreased and the fundal lesions showed severe progression.

Shortly afterwards, she developed papilledema and signs of intracranial tumor growth. Craniotomy showed recurrence of the cerebellar tumor. She died shortly after the operation.

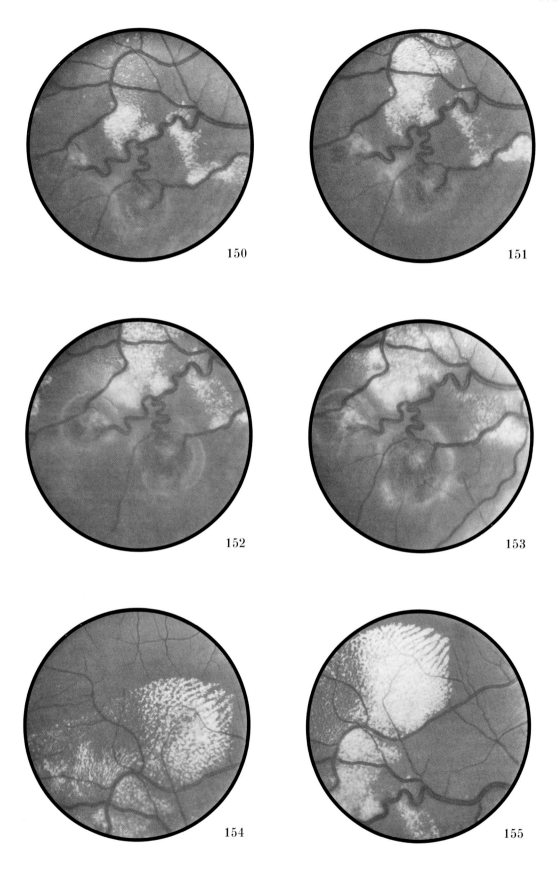

150

151

152

153

154

155

Figure 156. Same eye as figure 155, three years later. The dense yellowish-white exudate has increased in size and now fills a large part of the macular area.

Figure 157. Same eye as figures 150—156. Angiomatous tumor in the upper nasal quadrant of the eye. The tumor is whitish and it is supplied by a single retinal artery and vein.

Clinical note: Figures 156—157 are from the same patient as figures 84—85 and 144—155, a female, aged 21. She presents von Hippel-Lindau's syndrome. For further clinical information, see clinical note to figures 144—155.

Figure 158. Right eye. Tuberous sclerosis. There is a circumscribed yellowish-white, mulberry-like tumor below the disc. The surface is lobulated and the tumor projects about four diopters. Optic disc and retinal vessels are normal.

Figure 159. Same eye as figure 158. Tuberous sclerosis. A small ill-defined, grayish-white elevated nodule partly hides some of the retinal vessels in the upper temporal quadrant.

Clinical note: Figures 158 and 159 are from a female, aged 46. She has been mentally retarded since infancy. No ocular complaints.
Eye examination: Visual acuity, both eyes: 4/4.5 without lenses. Anterior segments are normal. At the right disc there is a mulberry-like whitish tumor. Some grayish-white, slightly elevated nodules are seen elsewhere in both fundi.
General examination showed a mentally retarded woman with cutaneous manifestations of tuberous sclerosis.

Figure 160. Right eye. Sturge-Weber's syndrome. Choroidal angioma seen as an ill-defined yellowish-orange area in the fun- dus. Retinal vessels are tortuous and show abnormal anastomoses.

Clinical note: Figure 160 is from the same patient as figure 131, a female, aged 10. Since infancy she has had capillary angioma of the right side of the face, convulsions, left hemiplegia and has been mentally retarded. At the age of four years, a craniotomy revealed a subdural hygroma and an angiomatous tumor in the right parietal lobe.
Eye examination: Visual acuity, both eyes: 3/4.5 with + 2.0 D sph. Anterior segments and intraocular tension normal. Visual fields cannot be recorded. In the right fundus retinal vessels are dilated and show many abnormal, anastomosing branches. A flat choriodal angioma is seen in the upper temporal quadrant. Left fundus is normal.
General examination showed mental retardation, capillary angioma of the right side of the face and left spastic hemiplegia. X-ray showed intracranial calcifications.

Figure 161. Left eye. Sturge-Weber's syndrome. The optic disc is glaucomatous excavated and atrophic. Retinal veins are tortuous. In the bends of some of the veins, there are ill-defined, small, rounded yellowish choroidal angiomas.

Clinical note: Figure 161 is from the same patient as figure 120, a male, aged 13. He has a Sturge-Weber syndrome with bilateral capillary angiomas of the face, bilateral buphthalmos and mental retardation. No convulsions. Glaucoma operation was performed on the left eye two years ago. Since then intraocular tension in that eye has been normal, but vision has decreased.
Eye examination: Visual acuity, right eye: 6/12 with − 1.75 D sph.; left eye: 6/36 with − 3.0 D sph. Both eyes are buphthalmic. Intraocular tension, right eye: 48 mm; left eye: 22 mm. Left eye shows sequelae after glaucoma operation. Both fundi show some choriodal angiomas, tortuosity of the retinal veins and glaucomatous optic atrophy. Visual fields show large ring-shaped scotomas.
General examination showed a boy with a typical Sturge-Weber syndrome.

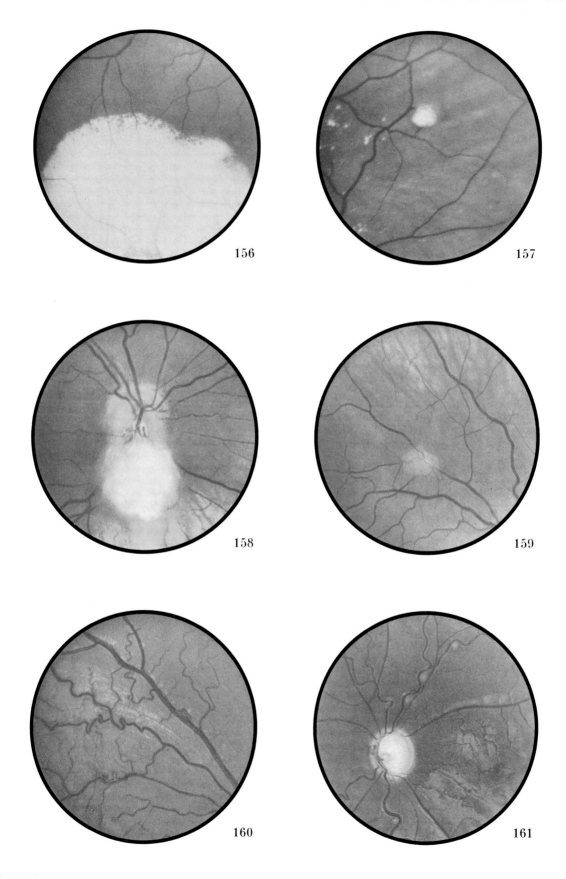

Figure 162. Right eye. Slight sclerosis of the retinal vessels. The retinal arteries are slightly narrowed and the axial reflex is broad (copper-wire artery). Slight arteriovenous crossing phenomena are present. The retinal veins appear nearly normal. The disc and fundus are normal.

CLINICAL NOTE: Figure 162 is from a male, aged 60. A week ago he had a cerebral episode with some expressive aphasia and paresis of the right upper limb. The condition has been stationary since then. No ocular complaints.
Eye examination: Visual acuity, both eyes: 6/6 with + 1.0 D sph. Anterior segments are normal. Both fundi show some sclerosis of the retinal vessels.
General examination showed some aphasia, right facial nerve palsy and some weakness of the right upper limb. Carotid angiography showed vascular sclerosis, and the electrocardiogram myocardial degeneration. Blood pressure: 125/80 mm Hg. No proteinuria.

Figure 163. Right eye. Moderate sclerosis of the retinal vessels with typical arteriovenous crossing phenomena.

CLINICAL NOTE: Figure 163 is from a female, aged 70. No ocular or general complaints.
Eye examination: Visual acuity, both eyes: 6/6 with + 1.5 D sph. Anterior segments are normal. Both fundi show moderate sclerosis of the retinal vessels. The optic discs and maculae are normal.
General examination showed nothing abnormal. Blood pressure: 140/90 mm Hg.

Figure 164. Right eye. Moderate sclerosis of the retinal vessels. The retinal arteries appear straighter than normal, are slightly narrowed and show a broad axial reflex. The retinal veins show slight irregular tortuosities. An arteriovenous crossing phenomenon is present at the crossing between the upper temporal artery and vein. The disc and fundus are normal.

Figure 165. Same eye as figure 164 (15°). Arteriovenous crossing phenomenon. At the crossing between the artery and vein, the vein is kinked and slightly obscured on both sides of the crossing by the sclerosed artery.

CLINICAL NOTE: Figures 164 and 165 are from a female, aged 67. A fortnight ago she suddenly felt reduction of vision in the left eye. No complaints from the right eye.
Eye examination: Visual acuity, right eye: 6/9; left eye: 6/60. Unimproved by lenses. Incipient cataract on both sides. The right fundus shows moderate sclerosis of the retinal vessels. The left fundus is obscured by a vitreous hemorrhage.
General examination showed nothing abnormal. Blood pressure: 150/90 mm Hg.

Figure 166. Left eye (15°). Arteriovenous crossing phenomenon. The vein shows some nicking as it crosses underneath the artery. The vein is slightly irregular in caliber, and the artery is narrow.

Figure 167. Right eye (15°). From the same patient as figure 166. Arteriovenous crossing phenomena. At the upper arteriovenous crossing, the vein shows an apparent tapering on each side of the artery, and at the lower, the vein shows tapering and an S-formed bend. The artery is slightly narrowed and the axial reflex is broad.

CLINICAL NOTE: Figures 166 and 167 are from a male, aged 55. Diabetes demonstrated one year ago. Insulin treatment since then. No ocular complaints.
Eye examination: Visual acuity, both eyes: 6/6, emmetropia. Anterior segments are normal. In both fundi, the retinal vessels present moderate sclerosis. No diabetic retinopathy.
General examination showed diabetes without nephropathy or hypertension. X-ray examination showed calcifications in the arteries of the lower limbs. Blood pressure: 120/80 mm Hg.

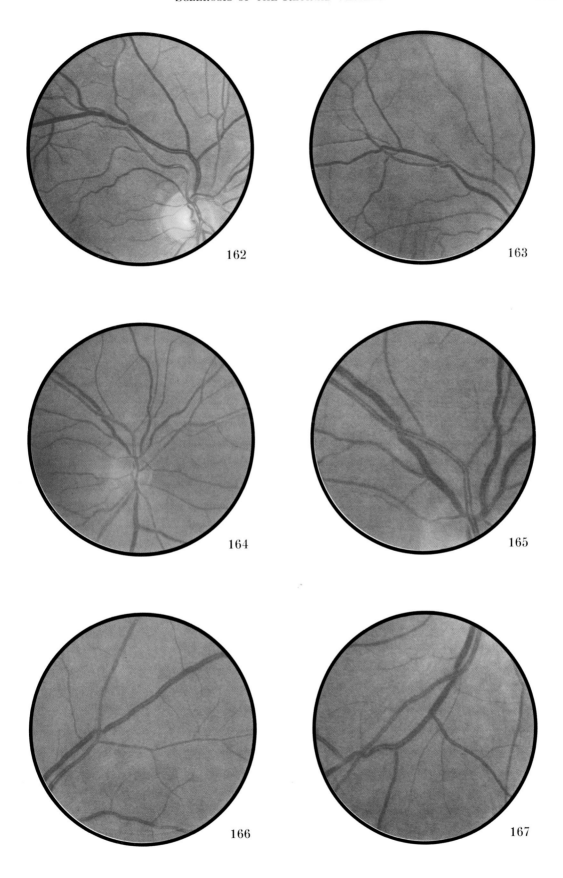

Figure 168. Right eye. Hypertensive angio-pathy without vascular sclerosis. The reti-nal arteries are narrowed and slightly ir-regular in caliber. The retinal veins are normal. The optic disc and fundus are nor-mal.

Clinical note: Figure 168 is from a female, aged 19. She is eight months pregnant. Hyper-tension demonstrated a month ago. No ocular complaints.
Eye examination: Visual acuity, both eyes: 6/6, emmetropia. Anterior segments are normal. Both fundi present hypertensive angiopathy without vascular sclerosis.
General examination showed a pregnant wo-man with hypertension. Blood pressure: 160/100 mm Hg.
After delivery blood pressure and fundi were normalized.

Figure 169. Left eye. Hypertensive angio-pathy without vascular sclerosis. The reti-nal arteries are slightly narrowed and ir-regular in caliber. The retinal veins are normal. The optic disc and fundus are nor-mal.

Clinical note: Figure 169 is from a female, aged 33. She is nine months pregnant and has had hypertension and proteinuria the last two months. No ocular complaints.
Eye examination: Visual acuity, both eyes: 6/6 with − 0.5 D sph. Anterior segments are nor-mal. Both fundi present hypertensive angio-pathy without vascular sclerosis.
General examination showed a pregnant wom-an with hypertension. Blood pressure: 160/110 mm Hg. Proteinuria: 0.1—0.2 g/24 hours. Serum creatinine: 0.8 mg/100 ml.

Figure 170. Right eye. Normal retinal ves-sels during antihypertensive treatment. Disc and fundus are normal.

Figure 171. From the same eye as figure 170, two years later, during exacerbation of

hypertension. All retinal arteries are now constricted and the retinal veins also show some narrowing.

Clinical note: Figures 170—171 are from the same patient as figures 192—197, a female, aged 14. Nearly four years ago she developed convulsive attacks. On admission acute glome-rulonephritis was demonstrated. Vision was slightly blurred.
Eye examination in the acute stage: Visual acu-ity, both eyes: 6/9. Unimproved by lenses. Vis-ual fields show paracentral scotomas. Anterior segments are normal. Both fundi present hy-pertensive neuroretinopathy with macular star formation.
General examination showed acute glomerulo-nephritis. Blood pressure: 200/140 mm Hg.
On antihypertensive treatment the hyperten-sion was well regulated and the general state improved gradually. Fundi were normalized and vision became normal.
During the last few months severe hyperten-sion (175/140 mm Hg) has developed in spite of antihypertensive therapy and she is now uremic.
Eye examination, four years after the first ex-amination: Visual acuity, both eyes: 6/6, em-metropia. Anterior segments are normal. Both fundi present hypertensive angiopathy.
Two months later she died in uremia.

Figures 172 and 173. Right and left eyes. Hypertensive angiopathy with retinal ede-ma. The retinal arteries are very narrow and in some places nearly hidden by reti-nal edema. The retinal veins and the optic discs are normal.

Clinical note: Figures 172 and 173 are from a female, aged 20. She has had hypertension with hypertensive crises for some years. No ocular complaints.
Eye examination: Visual acuity, both eyes: 6/6 with + 0.5 D sph. Anterior segments are nor-mal. Both fundi present hypertensive angio-pathy with retinal edema.
General examination revealed a pheochromo-cytoma, which was removed. Blood pressure: 240/170 mm Hg.

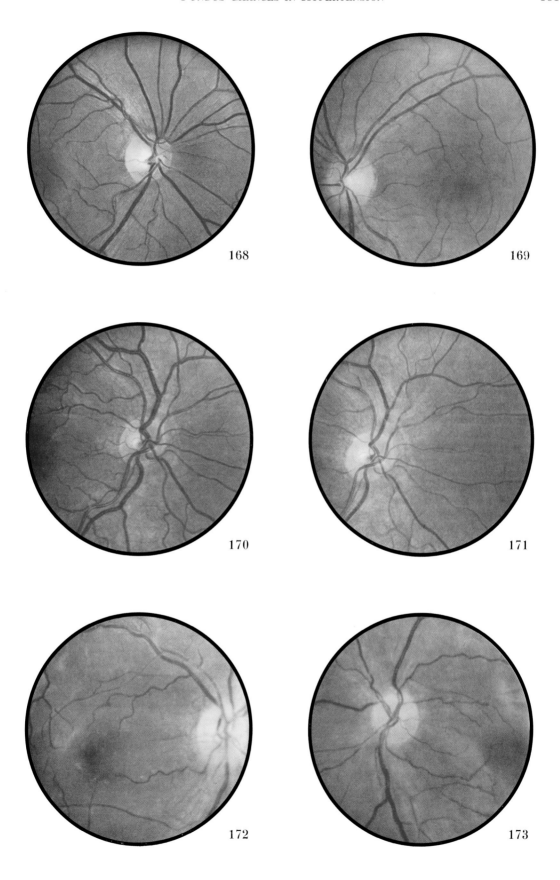

168

169

170

171

172

173

Figure 174. Right eye. Hypertensive angio-pathy with vascular sclerosis. Retinal arteries are narrowed. They show caliber variations and broad axial reflex. Arteriovenous crossing phenomena are seen above and below. Some of the veins are tortuous. The optic disc and fundus are normal.

CLINICAL NOTE: Figure 174 is from a male, aged 52. He has had hypertension with hypertensive crises for some years. No ocular complaints.
Eye examination: Visual acuity, both eyes: 6/6, emmetropia. Anterior segments are normal. In both fundi, the vessels show hypertensive angiopathy with vascular sclerosis.
General examination revealed a pheochromocytoma, which was removed surgically. Blood pressure: 220/130 mm Hg.

Figures 175 and 176. Right and left eyes. Hypertensive angiopathy with vascular sclerosis. The retinal arteries are narrowed and show marked caliber variations. Arteriovenous crossing phenomena are seen in both fundi. The optic discs and fundi are normal.

CLINICAL NOTE: Figures 175 and 176 are from a male, aged 55. He has had essential hypertension for several years. No ocular complaints.
Eye examination: Visual acuity, both eyes: 6/6 with + 2.0 D sph. Anterior segments are normal. Both fundi present hypertensive angiopathy with vascular sclerosis.
General examination showed hypertension. Blood pressure: 180/120 mm Hg. No proteinuria. Serum creatinine: 1.6 mg/100 ml.

Figure 177. Right eye. Hypertensive retinopathy. The retinal vessels are tortuous. The retinal arteries are narrow and irregular in caliber. The veins are slightly dilated. There are superficial, flame-shaped retinal hemorrhages and some whitish cotton-wool exudates. The disc is reddened, but disc margin is distinct.

CLINICAL NOTE: Figure 177 is from a female, aged 53. Severe hypertension demonstrated five years ago. She has received antihypertensive treatment since then. The last few months, there has been hypertensive encephalopathy and sensation of flickers of light in both visual fields, but no reduction of vision.

Eye examination: Visual acuity, both eyes: 6/6, emmetropia. Anterior segments and visual fields are normal. Both fundi show hypertensive retinopathy.
General examination showed severe hypertension and slight proteinuria. Blood pressure: 220/140 mm Hg. Proteinuria: 0.2—0.6 g/24 hours. Serum creatinine: 1.0 mg/100 ml.

Figure 178. Right eye. Hypertensive retinopathy. The retinal arteries are narrow. Peripapillary, there are some hard exudates and a single flame-shaped hemorrhage. The optic disc is normal.

CLINICAL NOTE: Figure 178 is from the same patient as figure 182, a male, aged 27. Twelve years ago he developed acute glomerulonephritis and hypertension. He has received antihypertensive treatment the last six years. During the last five years he has developed uremia. No ocular complaints.
Eye examination: Visual acuity, both eyes: 6/6 with + 1.5 D sph. Anterior segments and visual fields are normal. Both fundi present hypertensive retinopathy and a macular star.
General examination showed chronic glomerulonephritis and uremia. Blood pressure: 170/115 mm Hg. Hemoglobin: 8.1 g/100 ml. Proteinuria: 0.4—0.8 g/24 hours. Serum creatinine: 9.9 mg/100 ml.

Figure 179. Right eye. Hypertensive retinopathy. The retinal arteries are slightly narrowed and irregular in caliber. There are several whitish cotton-wool exudates and a single retinal hemorrhage. The optic disc is normal.

CLINICAL NOTE: Figure 179 is from the same patient as figures 180 and 181, a male, aged 47. Six years ago he developed acute glomerulonephritis and hypertension. The last two years he has been dialyzed with the artificial kidney at regular intervals. No ocular complaints.
Eye examination: Visual acuity, both eyes: 6/6 with + 1.0 D sph. Calcareous deposits are seen at the limbus of both corneae and in the subconjunctival tissue. Both fundi present hypertensive retinopathy.
General examination showed chronic glomerulonephritis and uremia. Blood pressure: 190/110 mm Hg. Hemoglobin: 9.2 g/100 ml. Proteinuria: 0.6—0.8 g/24 hours. Serum creatinine: 6.5—11.0 mg/100 ml.

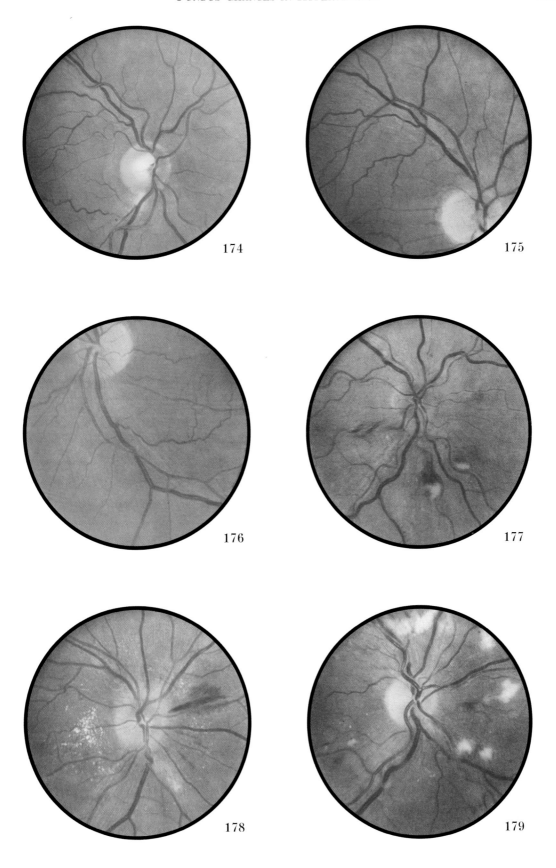

174

175

176

177

178

179

Figure 180. Right eye (15°). Hypertensive retinopathy. The retinal artery is heavily sclerosed and there is a marked arteriovenous crossing phenomenon. Cotton-wool exudates and a retinal hemorrhage are also present.

Figure 181. Same eye as figure 180 (15°), two months later. The vascular changes are unaltered. The cotton-wool exudates are markedly diminished in size and retinal hemorrhage has nearly disappeared.

CLINICAL NOTE: Figures 180 and 181 are from the same patient as figure 179, a male, aged 47. Six years ago he developed acute glomerulonephritis and hypertension. The last two years he has been dialyzed with the artificial kidney at regular intervals. No ocular complaints.
Eye examination: Visual acuity, both eyes: 6/6 with + 1.0 D sph. Calcareous deposits are seen at the limbus of both corneae and in the subconjunctival tissue. Both fundi present hypertensive retinopathy.
General examination showed chronic glomerulonephritis and uremia. Blood pressure: 190/110 mm Hg. Hemoglobin: 9.2 g/100 ml. Proteinuria: 0.6—0.8 g/24 hours. Serum creatinine: 6.5—11.0 mg/100 ml.

Figure 182. Left eye. Slight macular star formation in hypertensive retinopathy. The macular star is composed of whitish exudates radiating from the fovea. No hemorrhages in the macular area.

CLINICAL NOTE: Figure 182 is from the same patient as figure 178, a male, aged 27. Twelve years ago he developed acute glomerulonephritis and hypertension. He has received antihypertensive treatment the last six years. During the last five years he has developed uremia. No ocular complaints.
Eye examination: Visual acuity, both eyes: 6/6 with + 1.5 D sph. Anterior segments and visual fields are normal. Both fundi present hypertensive retinopathy and a macular star.
General examination showed chronic glomerulonephritis and uremia. Blood pressure: 170/

115 mm Hg. Hemoglobin: 8.1 g/100 ml. Proteinuria: 0.4—0.8 g/24 hours. Serum creatinine: 9.9 mg/100 ml.

Figures 183 and 184. Right and left eyes. Pronounced macular star formation in hypertensive retinopathy. The macular stars are formed by dense whitish exudates radiating from the fovea. Cotton-wool exudates are also present. Retinal arteries are narrow. The optic discs are normal.

CLINICAL NOTE: Figures 183 and 184 are from a female, aged 41. She has had hypertension for many years. During the last few months vision had gradually decreased in both eyes.
Eye examination: Visual acuity, both eyes: 6/60 with − 2.0 D cyl. axis 0°. Anterior segments are normal. Both fundi present macular star formation, retinal hemorrhages and cotton-wool exudates. The retinal arteries are narrow, irregular in caliber and there are arteriovenous crossing phenomena.
General examination showed hypertension. Blood pressure: 195/100 mm Hg. No proteinuria. Serum creatinine: 0.8 mg/100 ml.

Figure 185. Right eye. Hypertensive neuroretinopathy. The optic disc is edematous with blurred margin. Retinal arteries are narrow, the veins dilated. There are several cotton-wool exudates and a few small retinal hemorrhages. In the macular area there is a macular star.

CLINICAL NOTE: Figure 185 is from a female, aged 48. The last four months she has developed signs of severe hypertension and heart failure during hypertensive crises. The last month reduced vision in both eyes.
Eye examination: Visual acuity, both eyes: 2/60. Unimproved by lenses. Anterior segments are normal. Both fundi present neuroretinopathy with macular star formation.
General examination showed evidence of a pheochromocytoma, but operation was not performed because she had recurrent episodes of small pulmonary embolisms. Blood pressure: 230/160 mm Hg. Electrocardiogram showed myocardial degeneration.

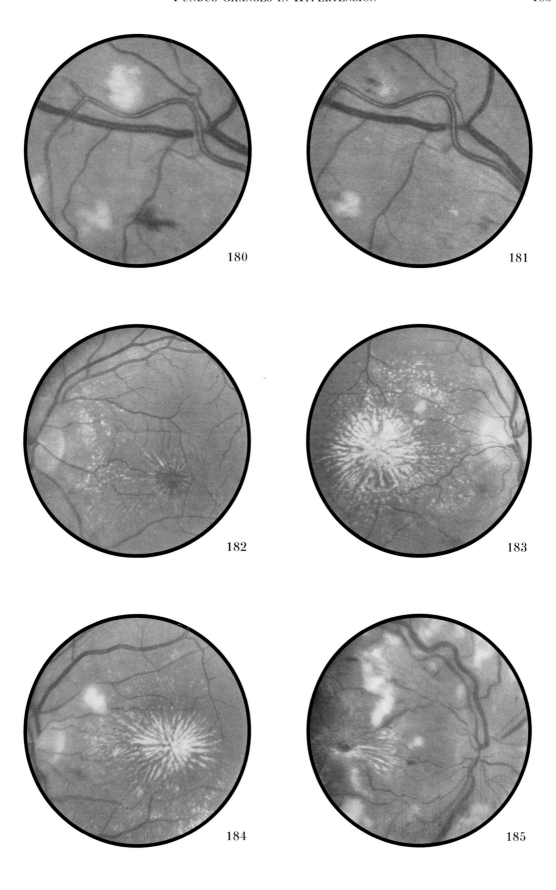

180

181

182

183

184

185

Figure 186. Right eye. Hypertensive neuro-retinopathy. The optic disc is swollen and the margin blurred. Retinal arteries are narrow and the veins slightly dilated. Retinal hemorrhages are seen radiating from the disc. Around the disc and in the macular area there are some exudates.

Figure 187. Same eye as figure 186, three weeks later. The fundus changes have progressed markedly.

CLINICAL NOTE: Figures 186 and 187 are from the same patient as figure 96, a male, aged 18. Six months ago he had an accident with his motorcycle. Shortly afterwards he developed hematuria and after some months a nearly total anuria and hypertension. He has been dialyzed with the artificial kidney at regular intervals since then.
Eye examination: Visual acuity, both eyes: 6/18, unimproved by lenses. Intraocular tension and anterior segments are normal. Both fundi present hypertensive neuroretinopathy with macular star formation.
General examination showed hypertension, proteinuria, uremia and hypochromic anemia. Blood pressure: 230/120 mm Hg. Serum creatinine: 10.6 mg/100 ml. Hemoglobin: 8.6 g/100 ml.

Figure 188. Right eye. Hypertensive neuro-retinopathy. The disc is swollen and the margin blurred. Some pallor and whitish streaks are seen around the disc, indicating a retinal edema. Retinal arteries are narrow and the veins slightly dilated. There are streaky retinal hemorrhages and some cotton-wool exudates.

Figure 189. Same eye as figure 188, seventeen months later. Papilledema has subsided, leaving slight peripapillary atrophy. The retinal arteries are still narrow and vary in caliber. Their axial reflex is wide. The veins are of normal caliber. A single arteriovenous crossing phenomenon is seen below. Retinal hemorrhages and exudates have disappeared.

CLINICAL NOTE: Figures 188 and 189 are from a male, aged 43. After a throat infection some months ago he developed acute glomerulonephritis and vision was blurred.
Eye examination in the acute stage: Visual acuity, right eye: 6/24 with +4.0 D sph.; left eye: 6/18 with +4.0 D sph. Anterior segments are normal. Both fundi show hypertensive neuro-retinopathy.

General examination showed acute glomerulonephritis. Blood pressure: 230/125 mm Hg.
The general state improved and vision became normal on antihypertensive treatment.
Eye examination, 17 months after the first examination: Visual acuity, both eyes: 6/6 with +4.0 D sph. Both fundi show hypertensive angiopathy with vascular sclerosis.
General examination showed chronic glomerulonephritis with reduced kidney function. Blood pressure: 160/100 mm Hg. Creatinine clearance: 18 ml/min.

Figure 190. Right eye. Sequelae after hypertensive neuroretinopathy. The retinal arteries are slightly narrowed and vary in caliber. The axial reflex is wide. In the macular area there are numerous small white hard exudates. The optic disc is normal.

CLINICAL NOTE: Figure 190 is from a female, aged 19. Since the age of two years she has had recurrent episodes of hematuria. During the last few years she has developed uremia and hypertension. She is now dialyzed with the artificial kidney at regular intervals. She presented neuroretinopathy one year ago. No ocular complaints now.
Eye examination: Visual acuity, both eyes: 6/6, emmetropia. Calcareous deposits are seen at the limbus of both corneae. Both fundi show hypertensive angiopathy with vascular sclerosis and small hard exudates in the macular areas.
General examination showed nearly total anuria, uremia and hypertension. Blood pressure: 160/110 mm Hg. Serum creatinine: 2.0—14.1 mg/100 ml.

Figure 191. Right eye. Sequelae after advanced hypertensive retinopathy. There are areas of pigmentation and depigmentation following fundal hemorrhage.

CLINICAL NOTE: Figure 191 is from a female, aged 22. Chronic pyelonephritis and hypertension was demonstrated three years ago. Since then she has received antihypertensive treatment. Two years ago blurred vision. Since then vision has been slightly reduced.
Eye examination: Visual acuity, both eyes: 6/12. Unimproved by lenses. Anterior segments are normal. Both fundi present hypertensive angiopathy with vascular sclerosis and sequelae after extensive retinal hemorrhages.
General examination, including renal aortography, showed bilateral chronic pyelonephritis. Blood pressure: 180/130 mm Hg. Proteinuria: 2.0 g/24 hours. Serum creatinine: 3.0 mg/100 ml. Hemoglobin: 9.4 g/100 ml.

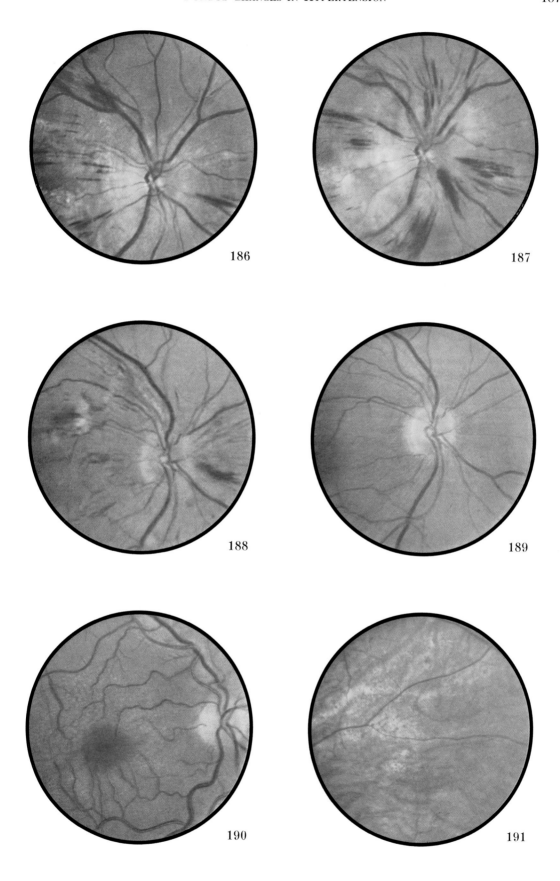

186

187

188

189

190

191

Figure 192. Right eye. Hypertensive neuro-retinopathy. The optic disc is swollen and the margin blurred. There is diffuse retinal edema, a single retinal hemorrhage and two cotton-wool exudates. A macular star radiates from the fovea.

Figure 193. Same eye as figure 192, three weeks later. Retinal edema is in regression. Retinal hemorrhage and cotton-wool exudates have disappeared. Macular star is unchanged. The optic disc is still swollen.

Figure 194. Same eye as figure 193, a week later. Retinal edema has disappeared. Papilledema is in regression. Macular star has diminished in size.

Figure 195. Same eye as figure 194, four months later. Papilledema has disappeared. There are only small remnants of the macular star. Retinal arteries are still narrow and the veins dilated.

Figure 196. Same eye as figure 195, thirteen months later. The hypertensive fundus changes have nearly disappeared. In the macular area there is some patchy atrophy. The retinal vessels are normal. The fundus has assumed its normal color.

Figure 197. Same eye as figure 196, twenty-eight months later, during exacerbation of hypertension. Retinal vessels, and especially the arteries are narrowed. The arteries show also some caliber variation. The fundus has assumed a more pale color.

CLINICAL NOTE: Figures 192—197 are from the same patient as figures 170—171, a female, aged 14. Nearly four years ago she developed convulsive attacks. On admission acute glomerulonephritis was demonstrated. Vision was slightly blurred.
Eye examination in the acute stage: Visual acuity, both eyes: 6/9. Unimproved by lenses. Visual fields show paracentral scotomas. Anterior segments are normal. Both fundi present hypertensive neuroretinopathy with macular star formation.
General examination showed acute glomerulonephritis. Blood pressure: 200/140 mm Hg.
On antihypertensive treatment the hypertension was well regulated and the general state improved gradually. Fundi were normalized and vision became normal.
During the last few months severe hypertension (175/140 mm Hg) has developed in spite of antihypertensive therapy and she is now uremic.
Eye examination, four years after the first examination: Visual acuity, both eyes: 6/6, emmetropia. Anterior segments are normal. Both fundi present hypertensive angiopathy.
Two months later she died in uremia.

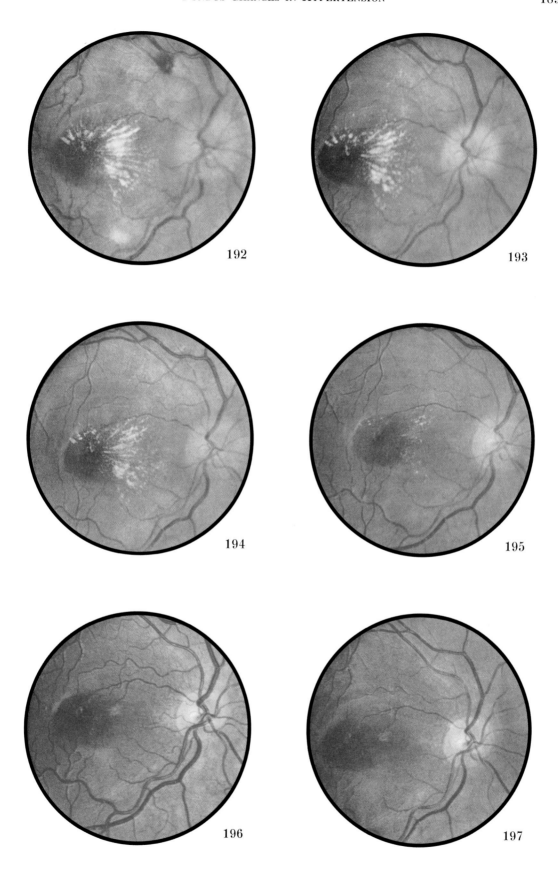

192

193

194

195

196

197

Figure 198. Right eye. Occlusion of the central retinal artery, acute stage. The fundus is pale, edematous and the fovea is seen as a "cherry-red" spot. Retinal vessels are of normal caliber. The disc is pale.

Figure 199. Same eye as figure 198, two months later. The retinal edema has disappeared except in an area surrounding the fovea. The disc is pale, atrophic and the retinal vessels narrow. There is a slight myopic crescent at the temporal side of the disc. Choroidal vessels are seen plainly above and below the optic disc.

CLINICAL NOTE: Figures 198 and 199 are from a male, aged 18. After a cranial trauma three years ago he has had severe headache. A carotid angiography was performed on the right side two days ago, and following this he experienced loss of vision in the right eye.
Eye examination in the acute stage: Visual acuity, right eye: light perception; left eye: 6/6 with − 5.5 D sph. Anterior segments are normal. The right fundus shows occlusion of the central retinal artery, the left is normal.
General examination aroused suspicion of schizophrenia. Blood pressure: 120/80 mm Hg. Sedimentation rate: 4 mm/hour.
Eye examination two months later: Visual acuity is unchanged. Retinal edema has nearly disappeared. Disc and retinal vessels are atrophic.

Figure 200. Right eye. Occlusion of the central retinal artery, acute stage. The fundus is pale, edematous and the fovea is seen as a dark-red spot. Retinal vessels are narrow, and the disc margin blurred.

Figure 201. Same eye as figure 200, ten days later. The retinal edema is in regression, but the "cherry-red" spot in the fovea is still present. Disc margin is now distinct.

CLINICAL NOTE: Figures 200 and 201 are from a female, aged 48. During the last year she has had several attacks of hazy vision in the right eye. Three days ago she experienced a sudden loss of vision in the right eye. No complaints from the left eye. No general symptoms.
Eye examination, acute stage: Visual acuity, right eye: light perception; left eye: 6/6 with + 3.5 D sph. Anterior segments are normal. The right fundus presents occlusion of the central retinal artery with retinal edema and a "cherry-red" spot in the macula. The left fundus shows some vascular sclerosis.
General examination showed nothing abnormal. Blood pressure: 160/80 mm Hg. Sedimentation rate: 22 mm/hour. Temporal artery biopsy was normal.
Eye examination, ten days later: Vision unaltered. The retinal edema in the right fundus is in regression.

Figures 202 and 203. Same right eye. Occlusion of the central retinal artery, acute stage. The fundus is pale, edematous and the fovea is seen as a red-brown spot. In the upper temporal vessels, the blood column is broken up into segments because of the reduced blood flow. The movement of the blood stream is seen by comparing the two pictures.

CLINICAL NOTE: Figures 202 and 203 are from a male, aged 62. He has had hypertension for several years. One year ago he had a coronary occlusion. The day before the examination he experienced a sudden loss of vision in the right eye and the day of the examination he developed a new coronary occlusion.
Eye examination: Visual acuity, right eye: light perception; left eye: 6/6, emmetropia. Anterior segments are normal. The right fundus presents an occlusion of the central retinal artery. The left fundus presents hypertensive angiopathy with vascular sclerosis.
General examination showed coronary occlusion and hypertension. Blood pressure: 220/130 —150/90 mm Hg. Sedimentation rate: 15—66—36 mm/hour.

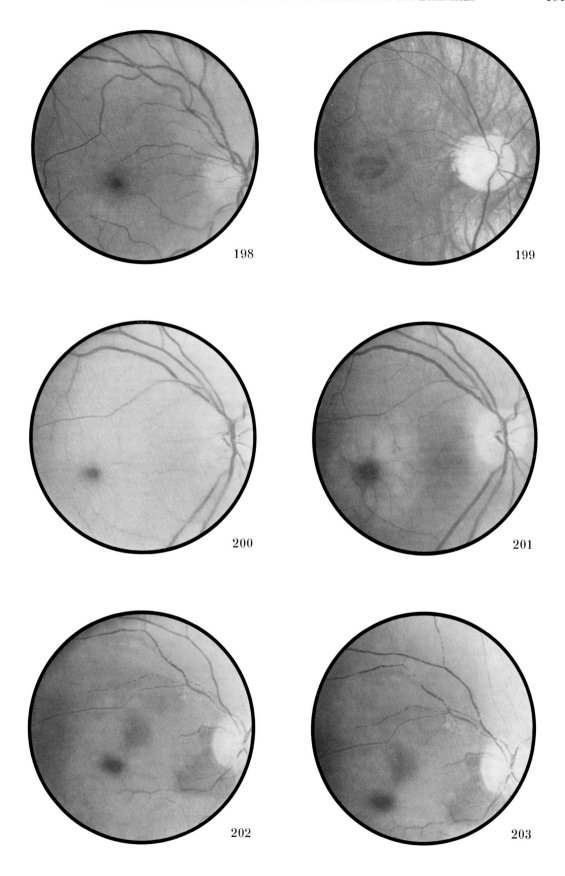

198

199

200

201

202

203

Figure 204. Right eye. Occlusion of the central retinal artery, acute stage. The fundus is pale, edematous and the fovea is seen as a dark-red spot. A small area supplied by the cilioretinal vessels is normal. Disc and retinal vessels appear normal.

CLINICAL NOTE: Figure 204 is from a male, aged 15. A week ago he received a kick against his right eye. Following this accident he experienced a loss of vision in the right eye. No complaints from the left eye.
Eye examination: Visual acuity, right eye: light perception; left eye: 6/6, emmetropia. He presents a hematoma around the right eye, which is enophthalmic due to an orbital fracture. Anterior segments are normal. The right fundus shows an occlusion of the central retinal artery, the left is normal.
General examination showed nothing abnormal.

Figure 205. Left eye. Occlusion of the central retinal artery, acute stage. The macular area is pale, edematous and the fovea is seen as a dark-red spot. Retinal arteries are slightly narrowed, the veins normal. The disc is edematous and the margin is blurred.

Figure 206. Same eye as figure 205, three weeks later. Central edema has nearly disappeared and disc margin is now distinct.

Figure 207. Same eye as figure 206, two months later. The central edema has disappeared, but the macular area now presents slight degenerative changes. The disc shows slight pallor, and retinal arteries are narrow.

CLINICAL NOTE: Figures 205—207 are from a female, aged 33. During the last few months she has had several episodes of hazy vision in the left eye. A week ago she experienced an abrupt loss of vision in the left eye.
Eye examination in the acute stage: Visual acuity, right eye: 6/6, emmetropia; left eye: hand movements. Anterior segments are normal. The right fundus is normal, the left presents an occlusion of the central retinal artery.
General examination showed a seven months pregnant woman without hypertension or nephropathy. Blood pressure: 125/70 mm Hg.

Eye examination, two months later: Visual acuity unchanged. Right fundus normal. In the left fundus, retinal edema has disappeared. Some macular degeneration is developing.

Figure 208. Right eye. Occlusion of the central retinal artery, late stage. The retinal arteries are very narrow. They show changes in caliber and some sheathing. The veins are narrow and the optic disc is pale, atrophic, yellowish-white.

CLINICAL NOTE: Figure 208 is from a female, aged 66. She has had essential hypertension for many years. One year ago she experienced abrupt loss of vision in the right eye. No complaints from the left eye.
Eye examination: Visual acuity, right eye: hand movements; left eye: 6/6 with + 2.0 D sph. Anterior segments are normal. The right fundus presents sequelae after occlusion of the central retinal artery. The left fundus shows hypertensive angiopathy with vascular sclerosis.
General examination showed essential hypertension. Blood pressure: 190/110 mm Hg.

Figure 209. Left eye. Occlusion of the central retinal artery, late stage. The retinal arteries are very narrow and accompanied by white sheaths, which at some places hide the arteries. The veins are slightly irregular in caliber. The disc is atrophic and surrounded by a grayish zone. There are numerous discrete and confluent yellowish-white exudates in the fundus.

CLINICAL NOTE: Figure 209 is from a female, aged 40. Hypertension was demonstrated six years ago. No ocular complaints until three months ago, when she experienced abrupt loss of vision in the left eye.
Eye examination: Visual acuity, right eye: 6/9 with + 1.0 D sph.; left eye: no light perception. Left pupil does not react to direct light stimulation. Otherwise anterior segments are normal. The right fundus shows hypertensive angiopathy with vascular sclerosis. The left shows the sequelae after occlusion of the central retinal artery.
General examination showed hypertension and reduced kidney function. Blood pressure: 210/120 mm Hg. Serum creatinine: 2.9 mg/100 ml and creatinine clearance: 23 ml/min. No proteinuria.

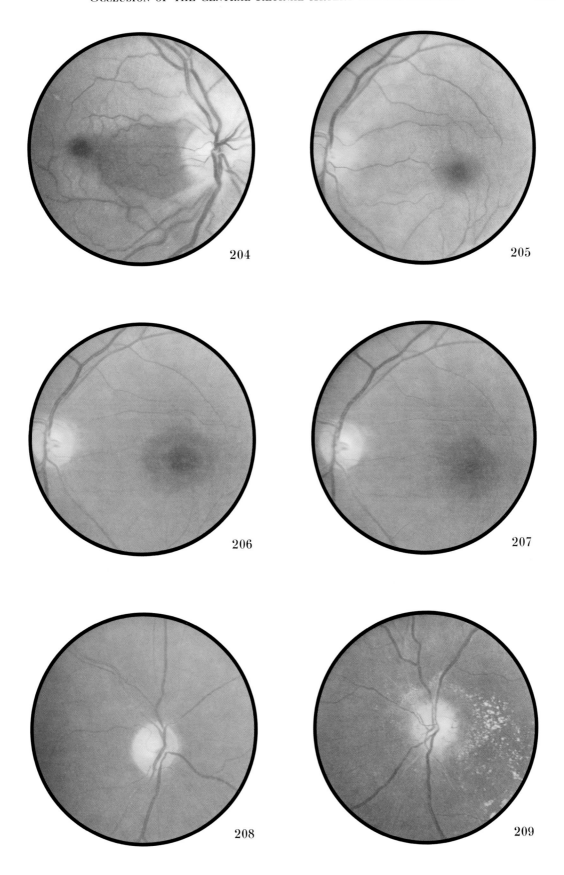

204

205

206

207

208

209

Figure 210. Left eye. Occlusion of the central retinal artery and the presence of a cilioretinal artery. That part of the fundus supplied by the cilioretinal artery is normal in color. The remaining part of the fundus is pale, edematous. The retinal arteries are narrow and partly obscured by retinal edema. The disc is normal.

CLINICAL NOTE: Figure 210 is from a male, aged 76. Hypertension demonstrated many years ago. Four days ago he had several attacks of hazy vision in the left eye. Two days ago he experienced an abrupt loss of vision in the left eye.
Eye examination: Visual acuity, right eye: 6/6, emmetropia; left eye: 6/18 with − 0.5 D sph. Anterior segments are normal. The right fundus shows some vascular sclerosis. The left shows occlusion of the central retinal artery, but an area supplied by a cilioretinal artery is normal. Left visual field is contracted to an area of about 2 to 3° centrally.
General examination showed generalized arteriosclerosis and essential hypertension. Blood pressure: 180/110 mm Hg. No proteinuria.

Figure 211. Right eye. Sequelae after occlusion of cilioretinal artery. The macula appears slightly granular with fine depigmentation and pigmentation.

CLINICAL NOTE: Figure 211 is from the same patient as figure 128, a female, aged 31. At the age of 18 years she suddenly experienced a loss of vision in the right eye. Ophthalmoscopy showed occlusion of two cilioretinal arteries. No improvement of vision since then. No complaints from the left eye. No general symptoms.
Eye examination: Visual acuity, right eye: counting fingers; left eye: 6/6, emmetropia. Anterior segments are normal. Both fundi present cilioretinal arteries. The right macula presents some pigment changes, the left macula is normal. Retinal vessels are normal. Right visual field shows a defect corresponding to the previous occlusion of the cilioretinal arteries.
General examination showed nothing abnormal. Blood pressure: 140/80 mm Hg.

Figure 212. Right eye. Retinal artery branch occlusion, acute stage. The area supplied by the lower temporal retinal artery is pale, edematous and the artery is narrow and partly hidden by edema.

Figure 213. Same eye as figure 212, six months later. The retinal edema has subsided. The retinal artery is still narrow and shows fine irregularities in caliber.

CLINICAL NOTE: Figures 212 and 213 are from a female, aged 27. She has been healthy until a week ago when she experienced a shadow in front of the left eye. Two days ago she experienced a similar shadow in front of the right eye.
Eye examination in the acute stage: Visual acuity, both eyes: 6/6 with − 1.0 D sph. Anterior segments are normal. Both fundi present occlusion of the lower temporal retinal artery, and visual field defects correspond to the lesions.
Eye examination, six months later: The affected retinal arteries show irregularities in caliber, but fundi look normal. Visual field defects are unchanged.
General examination, including blood studies, showed nothing abnormal. Blood pressure: 120/80 mm Hg.

Figure 214. Right eye. Retinal artery branch occlusion, acute stage. Whitish plaque is seen at the first branching of the lower temporal retinal artery. The area supplied by this artery is pale, edematous and the artery narrow.

Figure 215. Same eye as figure 214, five months later. The retinal edema has disappeared, but a whitish plaque is still seen at the bifurcation of the artery.

CLINICAL NOTE: Figures 214 and 215 are from a female, aged 59. She has had hypertension for many years. The day of the examination she suddenly experienced a shadow in front of the right eye. No complaints from the left eye.
Eye examination in the acute stage: Visual acuity, both eyes: 6/6, emmetropia. Anterior segments are normal. The right fundus shows retinal artery branch occlusion, and a whitish plaque is seen at the site of the occlusion. Visual field defect corresponds to the lesion. Left fundus shows hypertensive angiopathy with some vascular sclerosis.
Eye examination, five months later: A whitish plaque is still present at the bifurcation of the lower temporal retinal artery. The fundus looks normal, but visual field defect is unchanged.
General examination showed carotid insufficiency and hypertension. Blood pressure: 180/100 mm Hg.

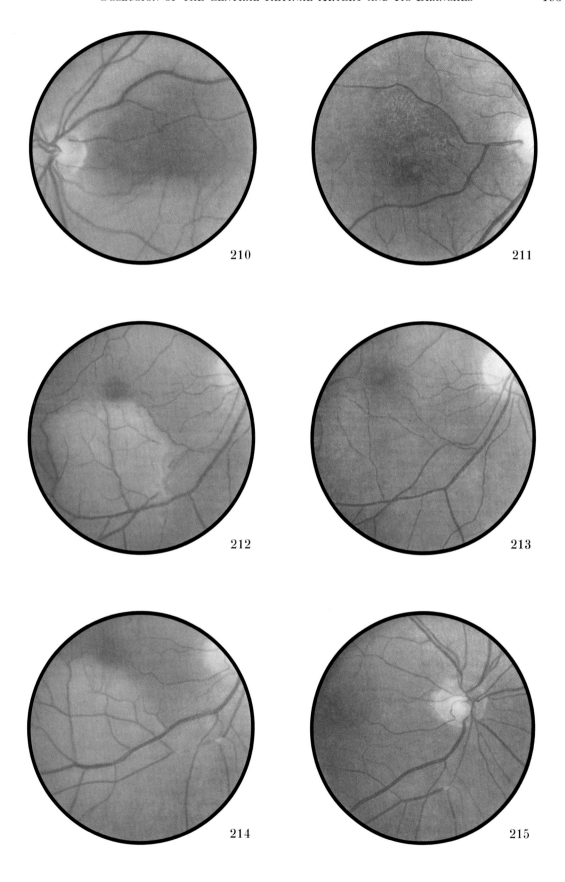

210

211

212

213

214

215

Figure 216. Left eye. Old occlusion of two branches of the central retinal artery. The first part of the upper nasal retinal artery is occluded and converted into a fibrous string, but the peripheral part is open and is seen to communicate with the lower nasal retinal artery. The upper temporal artery is left as a slightly visible small coil between the abnormal loops of the central part of the upper temporal vein.

CLINICAL NOTE: Figure 216 is from a male, aged 57. An occlusion of the upper retinal arteries in the left eye was observed nine years ago, but he had no visual complaints.
Eye examination: Visual acuity: 6/9 with − 1.0 D sph.; left eye: 6/6 with − 1.0 D sph. Anterior segments are normal. Right fundus is normal. Left fundus shows the sequelae after branch artery occlusion.
General examination showed nothing abnormal. Blood pressure: 140/90 mm Hg.

Figure 217. Left eye (15°). Old occlusion of a retinal artery. The occluded artery is seen as a whitish string. A network of new-formed vessels extends from the vein and overlies the occluded artery. A few retinal hemorrhages and hard exudates are also seen.

CLINICAL NOTE: Figure 217 is from a male, aged 55. Diabetes was demonstrated 16 years ago. Since then insulin treatment. Diabetic retinopathy observed one year ago.
Eye examination: Visual acuity, right eye: < 6/6 with + 1.0 D sph.; left eye: 4/60 with + 1.0 D sph. Anterior segments are normal. Both fundi present simple diabetic retinopathy. In the left fundus there is an old branch artery occlusion.
General examination showed diabetes with nephropathy. Proteinuria: 0.4—0.7 g/24 hours. Serum creatinine: 1.17 mg/100 ml. Blood pressure: 140/90 mm Hg.

Figure 218. Left eye. Atheromatous plaque at the bifurcation of the lower retinal artery. Retinal vessels slightly sclerotic. The optic disc is normal.

CLINICAL NOTE: Figure 218 is from a male, aged 64. Two years ago he had a coronary occlusion.

The last year vision has gradually been reduced in both eyes.
Eye examination: Visual acuity, right eye: 1/60 with + 1.0 D sph.; left eye: 6/24 with + 2.0 D sph. Anterior segments are normal. Both fundi present some vascular sclerosis and senile macular degeneration. An atheromatous plaque is seen in the left lower retinal artery.
General examination showed generalized arteriosclerosis. Blood pressure: 140/100 mm Hg.

Figure 219. Right eye. Sheathing of the lower temporal retinal artery.

CLINICAL NOTE: Figure 219 is from a male, aged 60. Hypertension was demonstrated about five years ago. Since then he has received antihypertensive treatment. The last six months he has had several short attacks of loss of vision in the right eye. Since the last attack one week ago, vision has remained defective in the right eye.
Eye examination: Visual acuity, right eye: light perception; left eye: 6/6, emmetropia. Anterior segments are normal. In the right fundus, the retinal arteries are narrow and ensheathed at many places. The disc is atrophic. The left fundus shows some vascular sclerosis.
General examination, including angiography, showed carotid insufficiency on the right side. Blood pressure: 160/100 mm Hg.

Figures 220 and 221. Same left eye. Sequelae after branch artery occlusion. The upper temporal artery is occluded and the corresponding vein is ensheathed. In the perimacular area anastomoses have developed between the upper and lower retinal vessels.

CLINICAL NOTE: Figures 220 and 221 are from a female, aged 51. Two years ago she suddenly experienced a shadow in the left visual field, and a retinal artery branch occlusion was observed. One year ago severe hypertension was demonstrated.
Eye examination: Visual acuity, right eye: 6/6 with + 2.0 D sph.; left eye: 6/9 with + 1.5 D sph. Anterior segments are normal. The right fundus presents hypertensive angiopathy with vascular sclerosis. The left fundus presents sequelae after branch artery occlusion and a corresponding visual field defect.
General examination showed hypertension. Blood pressure: 215/140 mm Hg.

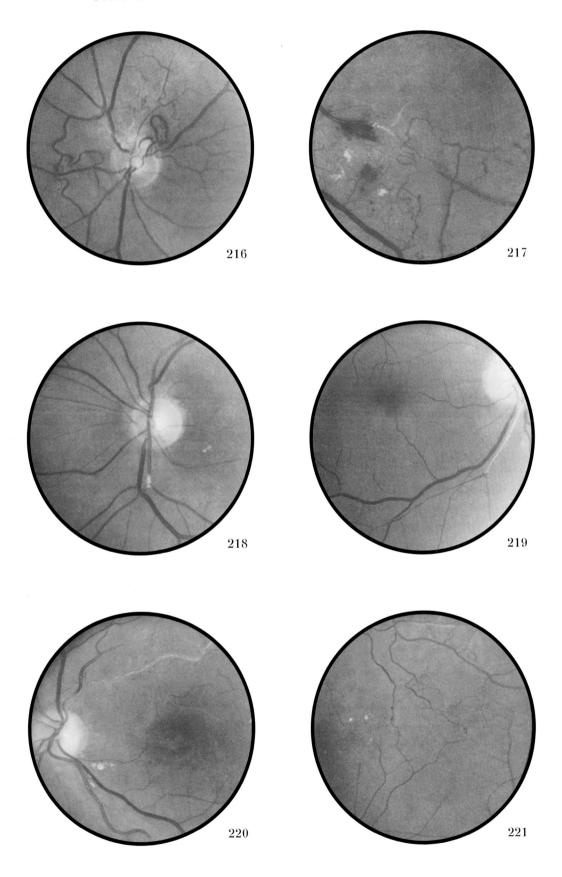

216

217

218

219

220

221

Figures 222 and 223. Right and left eyes. Bilateral occlusion of the central retinal vein, acute stage. The disc is swollen and the margin blurred. Flame-shaped retinal hemorrhages radiate from the disc. Cotton-wool exudates are also present.

CLINICAL NOTE: Figures 222 and 223 are from a male, aged 36. Diabetes demonstrated 18 years ago. Insulin treatment since then. During the last two years he has developed hypertension and nephropathy. Two months ago rapid loss of vision in both eyes.
Eye examination: Visual acuity, right eye: 1/60 with − 1.0 D sph.; left eye: 6/36 with − 1.0 D sph. Anterior segments and intraocular tension are normal. Both fundi present central vein occlusion and simple diabetic retinopathy.
General examination showed diabetes with nephropathy. Blood pressure: 200/120 mm Hg. Proteinuria: 6.0—11.5 g/24 hours. Serum creatinine: 4.8 mg/100 ml.

Figure 224. Left eye. Occlusion of the central retinal vein. The disc is swollen and the margin blurred. Flame-shaped hemorrhages and cotton-wool exudates surround the disc. The retinal veins are engorged and tortuous.

CLINICAL NOTE: Figure 224 is from a female, aged 23. Three weeks ago she observed a gradual loss of vision in the left eye. No complaints from the right eye. No general symptoms.
Eye examination: Visual acuity, right eye: 6/6, emmetropia; left eye: 1/60, unimproved by lenses. Anterior segments and intraocular tension are normal. The right fundus is normal. The left presents a central vein occlusion.
General examination, including blood studies, showed nothing abnormal. Blood pressure: 130/85 mm Hg.

Figure 225. Left eye. Central retinal vein occlusion, acute stage. The disc is swollen

and the margin blurred. Retinal hemorrhages and cotton-wool exudates surround the disc. Retinal veins are dilated and tortuous. Retinal arteries are narrow.

Figure 226. Same eye as figure 225, four months later. Retinal veins have decreased in size and show some sheathing. The arteries are still narrow. Retinal hemorrhages are more diffuse. Cotton-wool exudates have disappeared. The papilledema has disappeared, and a tuft of new-formed vessels lies in front of the disc. Fine veils of preretinal connective tissue have developed.

Figure 227. Same eye as figure 226, six years later. The retinal vessels are narrow. Preretinal connective tissue is more extensive. The prepapillary tuft of new-formed vessels has remained unchanged. There are no hemorrhages but hard exudates in the macular area.

CLINICAL NOTE: Figures 225—227 are from a female, aged 77. She has had essential hypertension for many years. About six years ago she observed a gradual reduction of vision in the left eye. No general symptoms or complaints from the right eye.
Eye examination, acute stage: Visual acuity, right eye: 6/6, emmetropia; left eye: 2/60. The right fundus shows hypertensive angiopathy with vascular sclerosis. The left presents a central vein occlusion.
Eye examination, six years later: Right eye: 6/9; left eye: hand movements. Unimproved by lenses. Incipient cataract in both eyes. Intraocular tension is normal. The right fundus is unchanged. The left fundus presents the sequelae after central vein occlusion.
General examination showed hypertension. Blood pressure: 170/100 mm Hg. No proteinuria.

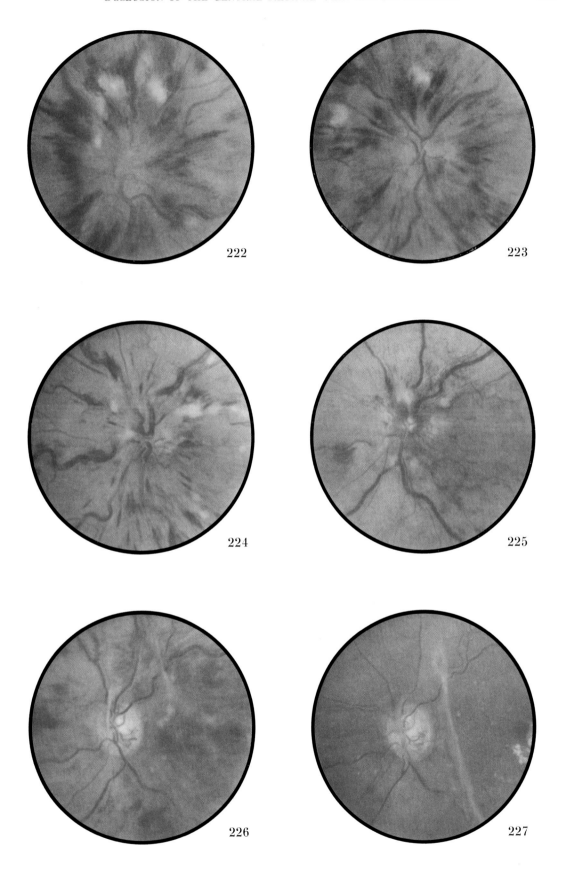

222

223

224

225

226

227

Figure 228. Right eye. Commencing multiple retinal branch vein occlusions. The retinal veins are dilated and tortuous, and there are several small retinal hemorrhages.

Figure 229. Same eye as figure 228, a week later. The fundus now presents the typical picture of multiple branch vein occlusions.

CLINICAL NOTE: Figures 228 and 229 are from a male, aged 76. His vision has been reduced in the left eye for many years. Two days ago, vision in the right eye was reduced gradually. No general symptoms.
Eye examination: Visual acuity, both eyes: 6/36 with + 2.0 D sph. Bilateral incipient cataract. Intraocular tension, right eye: 27 mm; left eye: 18 mm. Both fundi present senile macular degeneration. The right fundus shows commencing multiple branch vein occlusions.
A week later, he presented typical hemorrhagic glaucoma in the right eye and multiple branch vein occlusions.
General examination showed hypertension. Blood pressure: 210/110 mm Hg.

Figure 230. Right eye. Commencing retinal branch vein occlusion. The disc is swollen and the disc margin blurred. The lower retinal vein is engorged. An abnormal retinal vessel emerges from the lower retinal vessels into the upper part of the fundus.

CLINICAL NOTE: Figure 230 is from a female, aged 60. She has had hypertension for many years. No visual complaints.
Eye examination: Visual acuity, both eyes: 6/6, emmetropia. Anterior segments and intraocular tension are normal. The right fundus presents a commencing retinal branch vein occlusion. The left fundus shows hypertensive angiopathy with vascular sclerosis.

A fortnight later she presented a typical branch vein occlusion in the right fundus.
General examination showed hypertension. Blood pressure: 180/100 mm Hg.

Figure 231. Left eye. Retinal branch vein occlusion, acute stage. The venous occlusion is situated at the crossing between the lower temporal artery and vein. Retinal hemorrhages and cotton-wool exudates are seen in the area drained by the vein.

CLINICAL NOTE: Figure 231 is from a male, aged 54. Ten days ago he experienced reduction of vision in the left eye. No general symptoms.
Eye examination: Visual acuity, right eye: 6/6 with + 2.0 D sph.; left eye: 6/18 with + 1.75 D sph. Anterior segments and intraocular tension normal. The right fundus is normal. The left presents a branch vein occlusion.
General examination, including blood studies, showed nothing abnormal. Blood pressure: 140/90 mm Hg.

Figures 232 and 233. Same right eye. Retinal branch vein occlusion. Peripheral to the occlusion there are flame-shaped retinal hemorrhages and cotton-wool exudates.

CLINICAL NOTE: Figures 232 and 233 are from the same patient as figure 63, a female, aged 56. A week ago she observed some reduction of vision in the right eye. No general symptoms or complaints from the left eye.
Eye examination: Visual acuity, right eye: 6/12 with + 0.5 D cyl. axis 0°; left eye: 6/6 with + 0.5 D cyl. axis 0°. Anterior segments and intraocular tension are normal. Both fundi show moderate sclerosis of the retinal vessels and arteriovenous crossing phenomena. In the right fundus, there is an occlusion of the upper temporal retinal vein.
General examination showed nothing abnormal. Blood pressure: 140/80 mm Hg. No proteinuria.

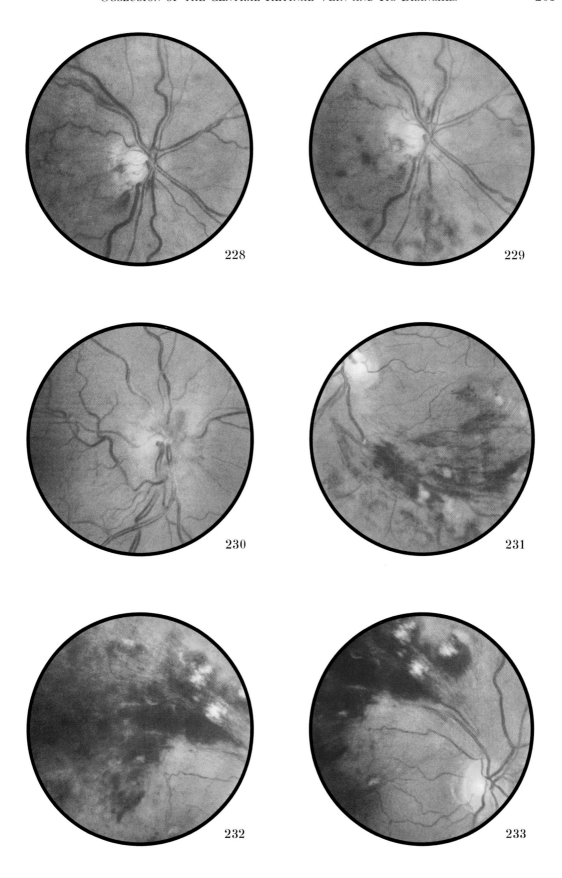

Figure 234. Right eye (15°). Old retinal branch vein occlusion. The vein is tapered at the arteriovenous crossing. Peripheral to the crossing there are numerous punctate retinal hemorrhages and microaneurysms.

CLINICAL NOTE: Figure 234 is from a male, aged 56. He has always been healthy and has not had ocular complaints.
Eye examination: Visual acuity, both eyes: 6/6 with + 1.0 D sph. Anterior segments and intraocular tension are normal. The right fundus shows sequelae after branch vein occlusion. Retinal vessels in both fundi present moderate sclerosis.
General examination showed nothing abnormal. Blood pressure: 130/80 mm Hg.

Figure 235. Right eye. Old retinal branch vein occlusion. The vein has been occluded near the disc. Centrally, the vein is narrow, irregular and sheathed. The peripheral part is dilated and tortuous. Above, a rete mirabile of new-formed vessels extends from the vein. The accompanying artery is sheathed at the disc.

CLINICAL NOTE: Figure 235 is from a female, aged 54. She has had hypertension for several years, and antihypertensive treatment has been given the last two years. Branch vein occlusion observed one year ago.
Eye examination: Visual acuity, right eye: 6/9 with − 0.5 D sph. + 2.5 D cyl. axis 115°; left eye: 6/9 with + 2.0 D cyl. axis 70°. Intraocular tension is normal. Both lenses show incipient cataract. There is hypertensive retinopathy, and the right fundus presents an old branch vein occlusion.
General examination showed essential hypertension. Blood pressure: 150/120 mm Hg.

Figures 236—238. Same right eye. Old retinal branch vein occlusion. At the disc, there is a small tuft of new-formed vessels and several small retinal hemorrhages. The peripheral part of the lower temporal vein is ensheathed. A small rete mirabile and some microaneurysms are seen below the fovea. In the perimacular area both arteries and veins are totally ensheathed.

CLINICAL NOTE: Figures 236—238 are from a male, aged 60. He has had hypertension for many years. One year ago branch vein occlusion was observed in the right eye.
Eye examination: Visual acuity, both eyes: 6/9 with + 2.0 D sph. Anterior segments and intraocular tension are normal. The right fundus shows an old branch vein occlusion, and the left hypertensive retinopathy.
General examination showed hypertension. Blood pressure: 220/115 mm Hg.

Figure 239. Left eye. Old branch vein occlusion. In the perimacular area, there are numerous retinal hemorrhages and microaneurysms. In the periphery, the retinal vessels are totally ensheathed.

CLINICAL NOTE: Figure 239 is from a male, aged 44. A collagenosis was diagnosed two years ago. Since then he has had recurrent vitreous hemorrhages in the right eye and recurrent branch vein occlusions in the left eye.
Eye examination: Visual acuity, right eye: 6/18 with + 1.0 D sph.; left eye: < 6/6 with + 1.5 D sph. Anterior segments and intraocular tension are normal. The right vitreous shows opacities and in the fundus retinal vessels are totally ensheathed temporally. New-formed vessels are seen on the disc. The left fundus presents old branch vein occlusion and heavy ensheathing of the retinal vessels temporally. Both visual fields show large defects nasally.
General examination, including blood studies, showed a collagenosis and hypercoagulability of the blood. Blood pressure: 145/85 mm Hg.

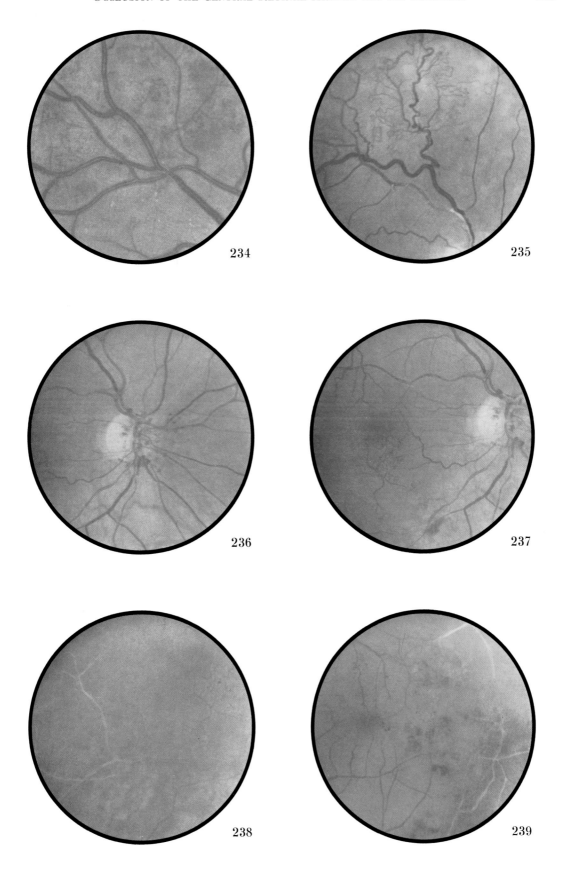

234

235

236

237

238

239

Figure 240. Left eye. Large preretinal hemorrhage. The upper border is horizontal, the lower convex and fairly distinct. The lower margin is bordered by a zone of diffuse retinal hemorrhage.

CLINICAL NOTE: Figure 240 is from the same patient as figures 114 and 115, a male, aged 41. During the last few days he complained of hazy and gradually reduced vision in the left eye and left-sided retrobulbar pain. No general symptoms.
Eye examination: Visual acuity, right eye: 6/6 with − 0.5 D sph.; left eye: light perception. Intraocular tension and anterior segments are normal. The right fundus is normal. The left fundus shows optic neuritis associated with venous fullness, and retinal and preretinal hemorrhage. Central scotoma of about 30° in the left eye.
General examination, including neurological examination, showed nothing abnormal.
Vision in the left eye gradually increased to nearly normal level in the course of some months, but the disc became pale, atrophic and the visual field contracted to 30°.

Figure 241. Right eye. Large preretinal hemorrhage in the macular area. The upper border is nearly horizontal, the lower border convex and distinct.

Figure 242. Same eye as figure 241, nine weeks later. The preretinal hemorrhage is in absorption.

Figure 243. Same eye as figure 242, five weeks later. The hemorrhage has disappeared. Some fibrin and slight edema are still seen in the foveal region.

CLINICAL NOTE: Figures 241—243 are from a male, aged 25. He has been healthy until five months ago when he suddenly experienced a loss of vision in the right eye.
Eye examination, in the acute stage: Visual acuity, right eye: hand movements; left eye: 6/6, emmetropia. Anterior segments are normal. In the right fundus there is a large preretinal hemorrhage in the macular area, and in the left fundus there are some scattered retinal hemorrhages. Retinal vessels appear normal.

The hemorrhages were absorbed in the course of five months and vision returned to normal. *General examination,* including blood studies, showed nothing abnormal. Blood pressure: 120/70 mm Hg.

Figure 244. Right eye. Preretinal and subretinal hemorrhage in the macular area. The central part of the subretinal hemorrhage is slate-gray, the peripheral part is red. The preretinal hemorrhage is dark red.

CLINICAL NOTE: Figure 244 is from a female, aged 59. Five years ago she experienced a sudden loss of vision in the left eye. A preretinal and a vitreous hemorrhage were observed. Two days ago she experienced a loss of vision in the right eye. No general symptoms.
Eye examination: Visual acuity, right eye: 1/24; left eye: hand movements. Unimproved by lenses. Anterior segments and intraocular tension are normal. In the right macular area there is a large subretinal and preretinal hemorrhage. The left macular area presents disciform macular degeneration. The retinal vessels show hypertensive angiopathy with vascular sclerosis.
General examination showed severe hypertension. Blood pressure: 280/180 mm Hg. No proteinuria.

Figure 245. Right eye. Subretinal, retinal and preretinal hemorrhages. Dark slate-gray subretinal hemorrhages are seen in the macular area and below the disc. Retinal hemorrhages are also present in the same area. Below, there is a preretinal hemorrhage extending into the vitreous.

CLINICAL NOTE: Figure 245 is from a female, aged 45. A fortnight ago she experienced a sudden loss of vision in the right eye. No general symptoms.
Eye examination: Visual acuity, right eye: 1/24; left eye: 6/6 with − 1.25 D sph. Anterior segments are normal. In the right fundus subretinal, retinal and preretinal hemorrhages involve the macula and the lower part of the fundus. Below, the preretinal hemorrhage extends into the vitreous. Left fundus is normal. Retinal vessels appear normal.
General examination, including blood studies, showed nothing abnormal. Blood pressure: 100/70 mm Hg.

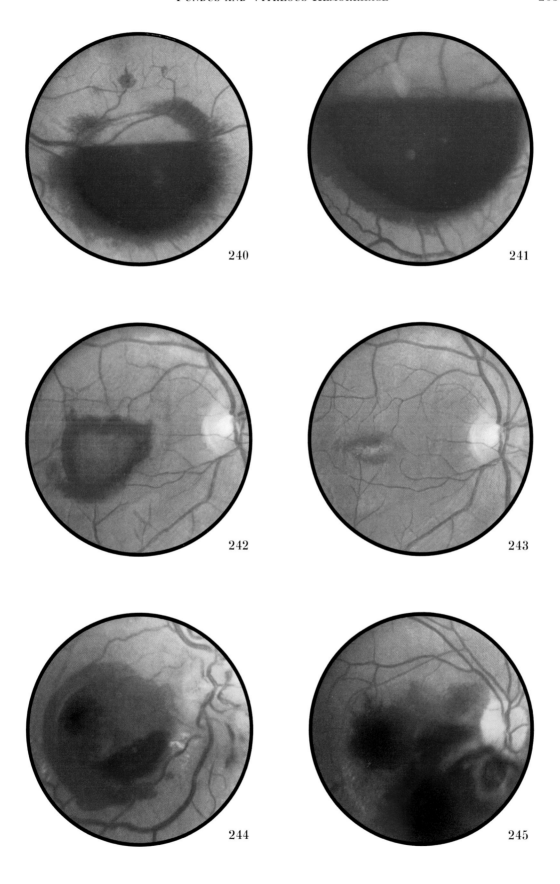

Figure 246. Right eye. Simple diabetic reti-nopathy in a young diabetic, early stage. In the macular area there are some micro-aneurysms seen as punctate, round, red dots and a few small retinal hemorrhages and hard exudates.

Figure 247. Left eye. From the same patient as figure 246. Diabetic retinopathy in this eye is slightly more advanced, presenting numerous microaneurysms, small retinal hemorrhages and small hard exudates.

CLINICAL NOTE: Figures 246 and 247 are from a male, aged 31. Diabetes demonstrated 12 years ago. Insulin treatment since then. Retinopathy observed one year ago.
Eye examination: Visual acuity, both eyes: 6/6, emmetropia. Anterior segments are normal. Both fundi present simple diabetic retinopathy. *General examination* showed diabetes without nephropathy. Blood pressure: 125/70 mm Hg.

Figure 248. Right eye. Simple diabetic reti-nopathy in a young diabetic. In the macu-lar area there are numerous confluent hard exudates and a few microaneurysms.

CLINICAL NOTE: Figure 248 is from a female, aged 28. Diabetes demonstrated 25 years ago. Insulin treatment since then. Retinopathy ob-served one year ago.
Eye examination: Visual acuity, both eyes: 6/6, emmetropia. Anterior segments are normal. Both fundi present simple diabetic retinopathy. *General examination* showed diabetes without nephropathy. Blood pressure: 120/80 mm Hg.

Figure 249. Left eye. Simple diabetic retino-pathy in an old diabetic. In the macular area there are numerous sharply outlined, irregular, small and large, yellowish-white exudates, tending to coalesce. In between the exudates there are several microaneu-rysms and small retinal hemorrhages.

CLINICAL NOTE: Figure 249 is from a male, aged 65. Diabetes demonstrated 11 years ago. Re-ceived insulin treatment during the last ten years. Retinopathy observed two years ago. Vision gradually reduced during the last two years.

Eye examination: Visual acuity, right eye: < 6/18; left eye: < 6/24. Unimproved by lenses. Anterior segments are normal. Both fundi pre-sent simple diabetic retinopathy, dominated by hard exudates. There is also moderate vascular sclerosis.
General examination showed diabetes without nephropathy. Blood pressure: 150/90 mm Hg.

Figure 250. Left eye. Simple retinopathy in a young diabetic. Besides some microaneu-rysms, small retinal hemorrhages and hard exudates in the macular area, there is a whitish cotton-wool exudate above the ma-cula. The upper temporal vein is very di-lated. Retinal arteries appear normal.

CLINICAL NOTE: Figure 250 is from the same pa-tient as figure 264, a female, aged 23. Diabetes demonstrated 13 years ago. Insulin treatment since then. No ocular complaints.
Eye examination: Visual acuity, right eye: 6/6 with − 1.0 sph.; left eye: 6/6 with − 1.5 D sph. Anterior segments are normal. The right fundus presents proliferative diabetic retino-pathy with new-formed preretinal vessels, reti-nal hemorrhages and microaneurysms. The left fundus shows simple diabetic retinopathy.
General examination showed diabetes without nephropathy. Blood pressure: 130/80 mm Hg.

Figure 251. Left eye. Rubeosis of the retina in diabetic retinopathy. Retinal capillaries show diffuse dilatation. There are numer-ous small retinal hemorrhages and micro-aneurysms. There is slight edema of the macula. Above the macula there is a cotton-wool exudate.

CLINICAL NOTE: Figure 251 is from a female, aged 20. Diabetes demonstrated ten years ago. Insulin treatment since then. Progressive reti-nopathy observed during pregnancy. She is now four months pregnant.
Eye examination: Visual acuity, right eye: 6/6, emmetropia; left eye: 6/9, unimproved by lenses. Anterior segments are normal. Both fundi show diabetic retinopathy with rubeosis of the fundi.
General examination showed a four months pregnant woman with diabetes. No nephro-pathy. Blood pressure: 140/80 mm Hg.
Legal abortion was performed.

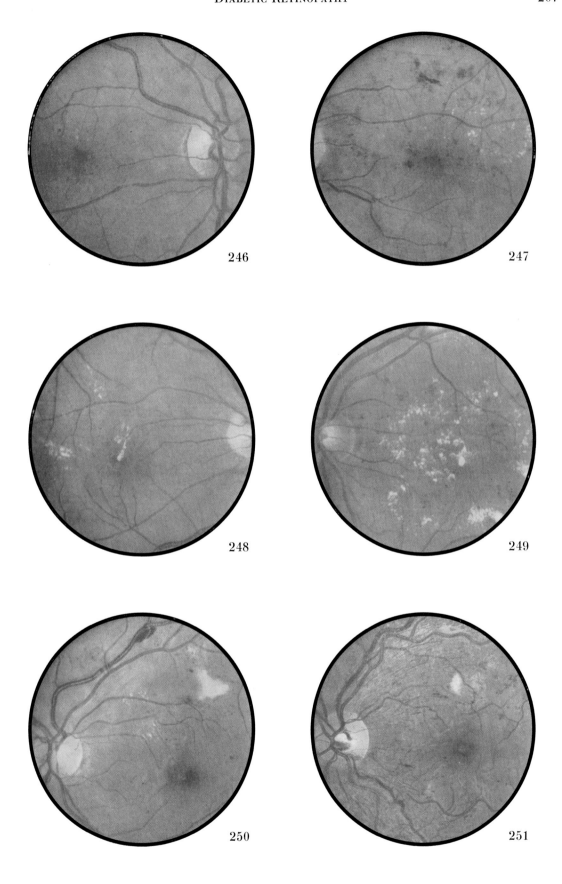

246

247

248

249

250

251

Figure 252. Left eye. Sheathing of retinal vessels in diabetic retinopathy. In the fundus periphery the veins are heavily ensheathed.

CLINICAL NOTE: Figure 252 is from a male, aged 34. Diabetes demonstrated 18 years ago. Insulin treatment since then. Retinopathy observed three years ago. Two years ago he had a vitreous hemorrhage in the right eye.
Eye examination: Visual acuity, right eye: < 6/60 with − 5.0 D sph.; left eye: 6/12 with − 5.0 D sph. Anterior segments are normal. The right fundus shows proliferative diabetic retinopathy and opacities in the vitreous. The left fundus presents simple diabetic retinopathy with heavy sheathing of several of the retinal vessels.
General examination showed diabetes without nephropathy. Blood pressure: 110/80 mm Hg.

Figure 253. Left eye. Heavy sheathing of retinal vessels in diabetic retinopathy. The retinal arteries are converted into white strands (pipe-stem sheathing). Sheathing of the veins is not as advanced. The fundus shows some patchy atrophy.

CLINICAL NOTE: Figure 253 is from a male, aged 30. Diabetes demonstrated 23 years ago. Since then insulin treatment. The last few years vision has been gradually reduced in both eyes.
Eye examination: Visual acuity, right eye: 3/24 with − 1.0 D sph.; left eye: hand movements. Anterior segments are normal. Both fundi present retinal degeneration, but only few microaneurysms and retinal hemorrhages. The retinal vessels show pronounced sheathing and the discs some atrophy.
General examination showed diabetes with nephropathy, uremia and hypertension. Proteinuria: 6—10 g/24 hours. Serum creatinine: 3.2 mg/100 ml. Blood pressure: 205/120 mm Hg.

Figure 254. Right eye (15°). Advanced phlebopathy in diabetic retinopathy. The veins are of very uneven caliber, showing varicose and globular dilatations.

CLINICAL NOTE: See clinical note to figure 267.

Figure 255. Right eye. Preretinal hemorrhage. The upper border of the hemorrhage is horizontal, while the lower margin is slightly convex.

CLINICAL NOTE: Figure 255 is from a male, aged 51. Diabetes demonstrated 28 years ago. Insulin treatment since then. Retinopathy observed seven years ago. Small proliferative vessels observed five years ago. Since then episodes of hazy vision.
Eye examination: Visual acuity, right eye: 6/6 with − 1.0 D sph.; left eye: < 6/6 with − 1.0 D sph. Anterior segments are normal. Both fundi present commencing proliferative retinopathy and some preretinal hemorrhages.
General examination showed diabetes without nephropathy. Blood pressure: 130/70 mm Hg.

Figure 256. Left eye. Vitreous detachment. The vitreous is detached above the clearcut curved line. The retrovitreal space is filled with hemorrhagic fluid. The disc is blurred and the fundus pale. Some newformed vessels are also present.

CLINICAL NOTE: Figure 256 is from a female, aged 26. Diabetes demonstrated 18 years ago. Insulin treatment since then. Retinopathy and nephropathy observed six years ago. Two months ago she experienced a loss of vision in both eyes.
Eye examination: Visual acuity, right eye: 6/60; left eye: 1/60. Unimproved by lenses. Bilateral incipient cataract. Both fundi show proliferative diabetic retinopathy, and in the left eye there is a large vitreous detachment.
General examination showed diabetes with nephropathy and hypertension. Proteinuria: 6.5—11 g/24 hours. Serum creatinine: 2.8 mg/100 ml. Blood pressure: 170/110 mm Hg.

Figure 257. Right eye. Degenerative changes in the hyaloid membrane. In some places the hyaloid membrane is converted into white patches and irregular lines of fibrous tissue.

CLINICAL NOTE: Figure 257 is from a female, aged 33. Diabetes demonstrated 26 years ago. Insulin treatment since then. The last six years gradual loss of vision in the right eye.
Eye examination: Visual acuity, right eye: 1/60; left eye: 6/6, emmetropia. Anterior segments are normal. The right fundus presents extensive proliferative retinopathy with preretinal veils of connective tissue and degenerative changes in the hyaloid membrane. The left fundus shows commencing proliferative retinopathy.
General examination showed diabetes with nephropathy. Proteinuria: 0.6—1.2 g/24 hours. Serum creatinine: 1.2 mg/100 ml. Blood pressure: 120/80 mm Hg.

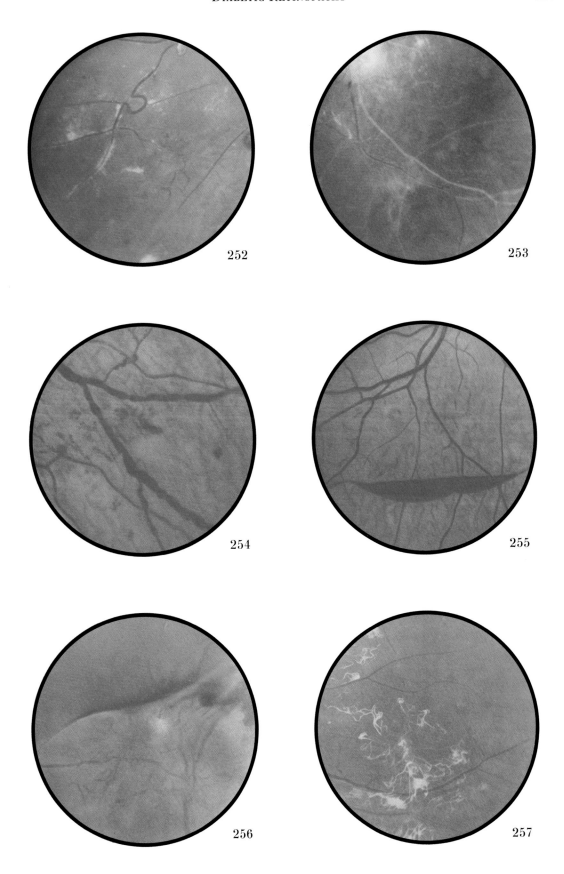

252

253

254

255

256

257

Figure 258. Right eye. Preretinal hemorrhage with extension into the vitreous.

CLINICAL NOTE: Figure 258 is from the same patient as figure 261, a male, aged 47. Diabetes was demonstrated 16 years ago. Insulin treatment was abolished after five years and instead he received oral anti-diabetic medication. Two years ago, however, insulin was needed again. Retinopathy was observed two years ago. Since then vision has decreased gradually.
Eye examination: Visual acuity, right eye: 6/60; left eye: 6/12. Unimproved by lenses. Anterior segments are normal. The right fundus shows proliferative retinopathy together with large preretinal and some vitreous hemorrhage. The left fundus presents fan-shaped prepapillary neovascularization and scattered hemorrhages and exudates.
General examination showed diabetes without nephropathy. Blood pressure: 160/105 mm Hg.

Figure 259. Left eye. Vitreous hemorrhage. Hemorrhagic clots are floating around in the vitreous. Outlines of disc and retinal vessels are seen faintly.

CLINICAL NOTE: Figure 259 is from a male, aged 56. Diabetes demonstrated 22 years ago. Since then insulin treatment. Retinopathy observed two years ago, and nephropathy one year ago. The last two years recurrent vitreous hemorrhages in the left eye.
Eye examination: Visual acuity, right eye: 6/6, emmetropia; left eye: 6/9, unimproved by lenses. Anterior segments are normal. Both fundi present proliferative retinopathy. Some vitreous hemorrhage in the left eye.
General examination showed diabetes with nephropathy. Proteinuria: 2.0—3.4 g/24 hours. Serum creatinine: 1.1 mg/100 ml. Blood pressure: 160/85 mm Hg.

Figure 260. Right eye. Proliferative diabetic retinopathy with a small prepapillary tuft of new-formed vessels. Retinal arteries are narrow, veins are dilated. Microaneurysms and small retinal hemorrhages are also present.

CLINICAL NOTE: Figure 260 is from a male, aged 45. Diabetes demonstrated 20 years ago. Insulin treatment since then. Some bilateral reduction of vision the last year.
Eye examination: Visual acuity, right eye: 6/12; left eye: 6/18. Unimproved by lenses. Anterior segments are normal. Both fundi present proliferative retinopathy with prepapillary tufts of new-formed vessels and numerous retinal hemorrhages.
General examination showed diabetes without nephropathy. Blood pressure: 130/80 mm Hg.

Figure 261. Left eye. Proliferative diabetic retinopathy with fan-shaped prepapillary neovascularization.

CLINICAL NOTE: Figure 261 is from the same patient as figure 258, a male, aged 47. Diabetes was demonstrated 16 years ago. Insulin treatment was abolished after five years and instead he received oral anti-diabetic medication. Two years ago, however, insulin was needed again. Retinopathy was observed two years ago. Since then vision has decreased gradually. For further clinical information, see clinical note to figure 258.

Figures 262 and 263. Same left eye. Proliferative diabetic retinopathy with extensive fan-shaped preretinal network of new-formed vessels. The vascular proliferations leave the macula free.

CLINICAL NOTE: Figures 262 and 263 are from a male, aged 33. Diabetes demonstrated 18 years ago. Retinopathy and nephropathy observed two years ago, when he experienced a sudden loss of vision in the right eye. Since then some muscae volitantes in the left eye.
Eye examination: Visual acuity, right eye: 1/24; left eye: 6/6, emmetropia. Anterior segments are normal. Right fundus is obscured by vitreous hemorrhage. The left fundus shows proliferative retinopathy.
General examination showed diabetes with nephropathy. Proteinuria: 0.4—1.0 g/24 hours. Serum creatinine: 1.0 mg/100 ml. Blood pressure: 130/90 mm Hg.

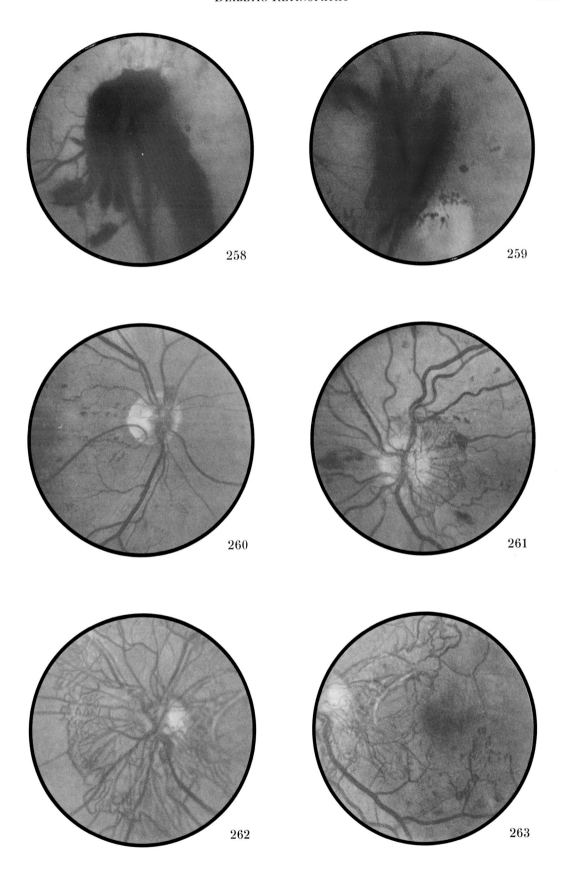

258

259

260

261

262

263

Figure 264. Right eye. Proliferative diabetic retinopathy. Numerous new-formed preretinal vascular loops are seen above and below the macula.

CLINICAL NOTE: Figure 264 is from the same patient as figure 250, a female, aged 23. Diabetes was demonstrated 13 years ago. Insulin treatment since then. No ocular complaints.
Eye examination: Visual acuity, right eye: 6/6 with − 1.0 sph.; left eye: 6/6 with − 1.5 D sph. Anterior segments are normal. The right fundus presents proliferative diabetic retinopathy with new-formed preretinal vessels, retinal hemorrhages and microaneurysms. The left fundus shows simple diabetic retinopathy.
General examination showed diabetes without nephropathy. Blood pressure: 130/80 mm Hg.

Figure 265. Right eye. Proliferative diabetic retinopathy. There is a large prepapillary proliferation containing fibrous tissue and new-formed vessels. The proliferation is bordered by some hemorrhages.

CLINICAL NOTE: Figure 265 is from a male, aged 53. Diabetes demonstrated 27 years ago. Insulin treatment since then. Retinopathy observed three years ago, when he developed a vitreous hemorrhage in the left eye.
Eye examination: Visual acuity, right eye: 6/6, emmetropia; left eye: hand movements. Anterior segments are normal. The right fundus presents proliferative retinopathy with large prepapillary proliferation, the left fundus is obscured by vitreous hemorrhage.
General examination showed diabetes without nephropathy. Blood pressure: 120/75 mm Hg.

Figure 266. Right eye. Proliferative diabetic retinopathy. Large vascular proliferation with scanty fibrous tissue projects far into the vitreous.

CLINICAL NOTE: Figure 266 is from a female, aged 46. Diabetes demonstrated 15 years ago. Insulin treatment since then. Retinopathy was observed four years ago. The last year reduced vision in both eyes.
Eye examination: Visual acuity, right eye: 6/12; left eye: 6/60. Unimproved by lenses. Anterior segments are normal. In the right fundus there is a large vascular proliferation extending from the disc. The left fundus is obscured by vitreous haze and connective tissue veils.

General examination showed diabetes without nephropathy. Blood pressure: 140/80 mm Hg.

Figure 267. Right eye (15°). Proliferative diabetic retinopathy. A delicate meshwork of new-formed vessels lies just preretinally in the fundus periphery.

CLINICAL NOTE: Figure 267 is from the same patient as figure 254, a male, aged 23. Diabetes demonstrated 14 years ago. Insulin treatment since then. Nephropathy observed two years ago. The last few months vision in both eyes has been reduced.
Eye examination: Visual acuity, right eye: 6/18; left eye: 6/12. Unimproved by lenses. Anterior segments are normal. Both fundi present proliferative diabetic retinopathy with fan-shaped preretinal neovascularization and marked phlebopathy.
General examination showed diabetes with nephropathy. Proteinuria: 2.4—8.0 g/24 hours. Serum creatinine: 1.5 mg/100 ml. Blood pressure: 120/90 mm Hg.

Figure 268. Left eye (15°). Proliferative diabetic retinopathy. A fan-shaped meshwork of preretinal new-formed vessels is seen in the fundus periphery.

CLINICAL NOTE: Figure 268 is from a male, aged 32. Diabetes demonstrated 20 years ago. Insulin treatment since then. Retinopathy observed three years ago. Two years ago he experienced a sudden loss of vision in the right eye. Since then gradual reduction of vision in the left eye.
Eye examination: Visual acuity, right eye: hand movements; left eye: 6/18, unimproved by lenses. Anterior segments are normal. Right fundus obscured by a vitreous hemorrhage. Left fundus shows proliferative retinopathy with many tufts of new-formed preretinal vessels all over the fundus.
General examination showed diabetes without nephropathy. Blood pressure: 125/75 mm Hg.

Figure 269. Right eye. Proliferative diabetic retinopathy. Extensive preretinal fibrous veil in the nasal fundus periphery.

CLINICAL NOTE: See clinical note to figures 273—275.

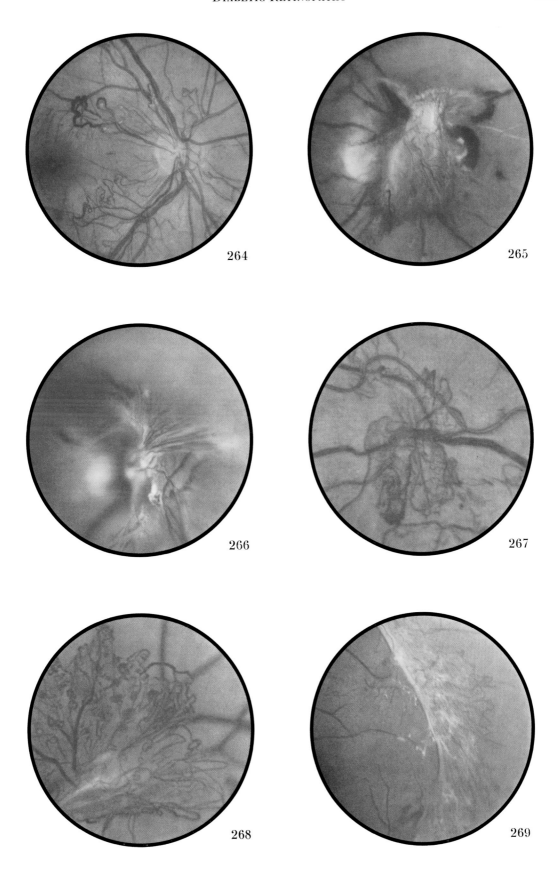

264

265

266

267

268

269

Figure 270. Right eye. Proliferative diabetic retinopathy. Preretinal mass of fibrous tissue containing numerous small new-formed vessels.

CLINICAL NOTE: Figure 270 is from a female, aged 34. Diabetes demonstrated 26 years ago. Insulin treatment since then. Retinopathy observed two years ago. The last few months recurrent attacks of loss of vision in the left eye.
Eye examination: Visual acuity, right eye: 6/6, emmetropia; left eye: hand movements. Anterior segments are normal. Both fundi present proliferative retinopathy and the left also a retinal detachment.
General examination showed diabetes without nephropathy. Blood pressure: 110/70 mm Hg.

Figures 271 and 272. Same right eye. Proliferative diabetic retinopathy. Preretinal whitish veil of fibrous tissue covers the disc and a large part of the fundus.

CLINICAL NOTE: Figures 271 and 272 are from a male, aged 35. Diabetes demonstrated 20 years ago. Insulin treatment since then. Retinopathy observed in both eyes ten years ago. Three years ago vitreous hemorrhage developed in the right eye. During the last year some reduction of vision in the left eye.
Eye examination: Visual acuity, right eye: 2/60; left eye: 6/12. Unimproved by lenses. Anterior segments are normal. Both fundi present proliferative retinopathy. In the right fundus there are extensive preretinal veils of fibrous tissue. In the left fundus there are several tufts of new-formed vessels.

General examination showed diabetes and nephropathy. Proteinuria: 1.5—3.1 g/24 hours. Serum creatinine: 3.5 mg/100 ml. Blood pressure: 130/80 mm Hg.

Figures 273 and 274. Same right eye. Proliferative diabetic retinopathy with retinal detachment. The proliferative tissue is seen on top of the detached retina, causing traction on the retina.

Figure 275. Same eye as figures 273 and 274. Retinal tear partly covered and surrounded by hemorrhage. Detachment folds are seen above.

CLINICAL NOTE: Figures 273—275 are from the same patient as figure 269, a male, aged 36. Diabetes demonstrated 27 years ago. Insulin treatment since then. Three years ago proliferative retinopathy was observed in both eyes. A fortnight ago he experienced a loss of vision in the right eye.
Eye examination: Visual acuity, right eye: hand movements temporally; left eye: < 6/6 with + 2.5 D cyl. axis 90°. Anterior segments and intraocular tension are normal. The right fundus shows proliferative retinopathy with extensive fibrous tissue formation and retinal detachment in both temporal quadrants. A retinal tear is seen at 10 o'clock. The left fundus presents also proliferative retinopathy.
General examination showed diabetes without nephropathy. Blood pressure: 160/85 mm Hg.

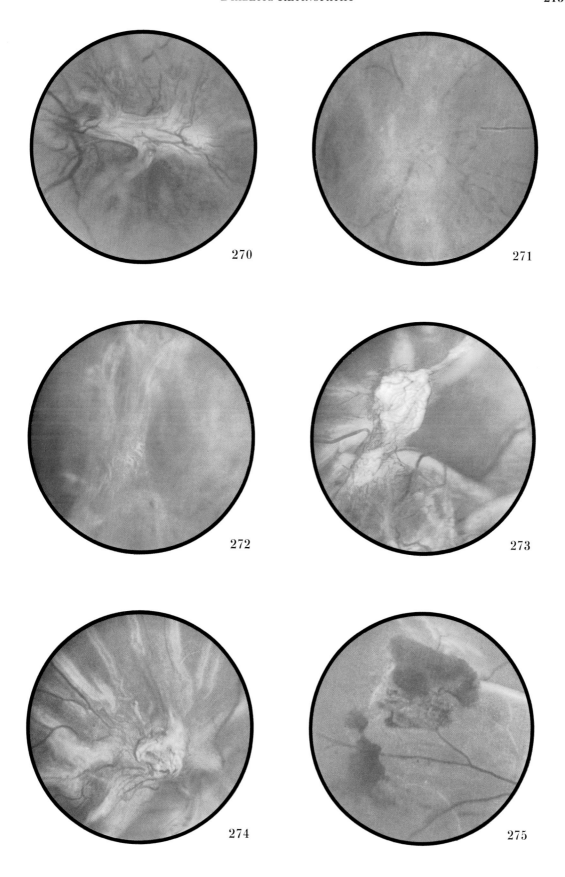

270

271

272

273

274

275

Figures 276 and 277. Same right eye. Lipemia retinalis. The fundus is pale and the retinal vessels have a nearly salmon-pink color. Both arteries and veins show a wide axial reflex. A vitreous haze is responsible for the slight blurring of the fundus.

CLINICAL NOTE: Figures 276 and 277 are from a male, aged 44. During the last year he has developed typical universal lipemic xanthomatosis together with some neurological symptoms. On admission diabetes was demonstrated.
Eye examination: Visual acuity, both eyes: 6/9, unimproved by lenses. Anterior segments are normal. There is pronounced bilateral vitreous haze. Both fundi are pale. The retinal vessels are salmon-pink and their axial reflex is wide. No diabetic retinopathy.
General examination showed universal lipemic xanthomatosis and diabetes. Serum cholesterol: 797 mg/100 ml. No proteinuria. Blood pressure: 140/90 mm Hg.

Figures 278 and 279. Right and left eyes. Retinopathy in anemia. Flame-shaped retinal hemorrhages and some cotton-wool exudates are seen in both fundi.

CLINICAL NOTE: Figures 278 and 279 are from a male, aged 64. During the last six months he has been very tired, anemic and has had no appetite. No visual complaints.

Eye examination: Visual acuity, both eyes: 6/6, emmetropia. Anterior segments are normal. Both fundi present retinopathy with flame-shaped hemorrhages and cotton-wool exudates. *General examination* showed severe hypochromic anemia. Hemoglobin raised from 3.6 to 11.3 g/100 ml after several blood transfusions. White blood cells: 600 → 2,700 per cu mm, with 60 per cent leucocytes and 32 per cent lymphocytes. Blood pressure: 140/95 mm Hg.

Figures 280 and 281. Right and left eyes. Fundus changes in polycythemia. The retinal vessels, the optic discs and the fundi have assumed a darker red color than normal.

CLINICAL NOTE: Figures 280 and 281 are from a male, aged 67. Four years ago polycythemia vera was diagnosed. No ocular complaints.
Eye examination: Visual acuity, right eye: < 6/6 with + 1.0 D sph. + 0.5 D cyl. axis 15°; left eye: 6/9 with + 1.0 D sph. + 0.5 D cyl. axis 0°. The conjunctival vessels are engorged. Anterior segments are normal. In both fundi, the retinal vessels, optic disc and fundus have assumed a darker red color than normal. No hemorrhages or exudates.
General examination showed a patient with congested facies, some dyspnea and heart failure. Hemoglobin: 21.2 g/100 ml. Red blood cells: 8.2 mill/cu mm. Sedimentation rate: < 1 mm/hour. Blood pressure: 200/100 mm Hg. Slight proteinuria. No glycosuria.

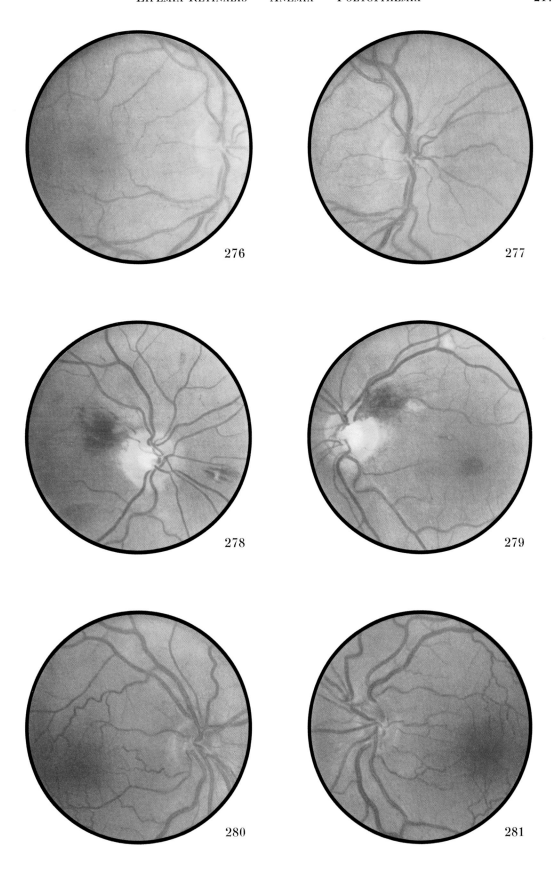

Figures 282 and 283. Right and left eyes. Fundus changes in leukemia, consisting of flame-shaped retinal hemorrhages. Some of the hemorrhages have a fluffy whitish center. Discs and retinal vessels are normal.

CLINICAL NOTE: Figures 282 and 283 are from a female, aged 58. A month ago she developed acute myeloblastic leukemia. No visual complaints.
Eye examination: Visual acuity, both eyes: 6/6, emmetropia. Anterior segments are normal. Both fundi present retinal hemorrhages, some of them having a fluffy, whitish center.
General examination showed an anemic patient with enlargement of spleen and lymph nodes. Hemoglobin: 6.1 g/100 ml. Sedimentation rate: 112 mm/hour. Bone marrow showed 86 per cent myeloblasts, 4 per cent myelocytes, 8 per cent lymphocytes, 2 per cent plasma cells. White blood cells: 8,000 per cu mm.

Figure 284. Right eye. Fundus changes in myelomatosis. The fundus presents retinal hemorrhages and fluffy exudates. The optic disc and retinal vessels are normal.

CLINICAL NOTE: Figure 284 is from a male, aged 51. During the last year he has become very tired, anemic, lost weight and has had no appetite. No visual complaints.
Eye examination: Visual acuity, both eyes: 6/6 with + 0.5 D sph. Anterior segments are normal. Both fundi present retinal hemorrhages and fluffy exudates.
General examination showed myelomatosis. Hemoglobin: 8.6 g/100 ml. Sedimentation rate: 148 mm/hour. Bone marrow showed myelomatosis. Urine showed Bence-Jones protein. Blood pressure: 130/80 mm Hg.

Figure 285. Right eye. Fundus changes in myelomatosis associated with paraproteinemia. The fundus is pale, orange-red. The disc is swollen. The retinal veins are engorged and tortuous, the arteries are normal. There are some small retinal hemorrhages.

Figure 286. Left eye. From the same patient as figure 285. The disc is swollen. Retinal veins are engorged, tortuous and show some caliber variations. There are only few punctate retinal hemorrhages.

Figure 287. Same eye as figure 286. Fundus periphery with numerous small retinal hemorrhages and microaneurysms.

CLINICAL NOTE: Figures 285—287 are from the same patient as figure 99, a female, aged 51. Myelomatosis was recently diagnosed. During the last two months gradually reduced vision in both eyes.
Eye examination: Visual acuity, right eye: < 6/18 with − 6.5 D sph.; left eye: 6/12 with + 3.0 D sph. Bilateral incipient cataract. Both fundi are pale. The discs show papilledema. Veins are engorged and in several places they assume the form of strings of sausages. Punctate retinal hemorrhages and microaneurysms are present, especially in the fundus peripheries.
General examination showed an anemic and fatigued patient. Hemoglobin: 8.1 g/100 ml. Sedimentation rate: 138 mm/hour. γ-globulin: 7.2 g/100 ml, containing paraprotein, but no macroglobulin. Urine showed Bence-Jones protein, and X-ray of the skull and the spine showed patchy infiltration.
The patient died nine months later.

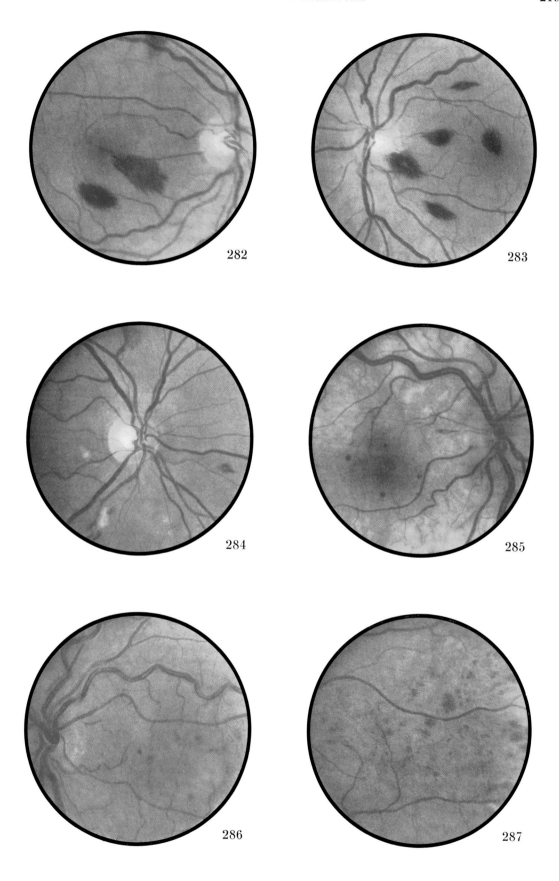

282

283

284

285

286

287

Figures 288 and 289. Same right eye. Fundus changes in macroglobulinemia. The retinal veins are engorged, tortuous and irregular in caliber. Numerous small retinal hemorrhages and some microaneurysms are diffusely scattered in the fundus. The disc is hyperemic.

Figure 290. Same eye as figures 288 and 289. Fundus periphery showing numerous small and large rounded retinal hemorrhages and some microaneurysms. The retinal vein is tortuous and slightly irregular in caliber.

CLINICAL NOTE: Figures 288—290 are from a female, aged 62. About six months ago she became ill with headache, dizziness, loss in weight and fatigue. During the following months she had a progressive loss of vision and a fortnight ago she developed convulsions. She was admitted to hospital, and macroglobulinemia was demonstrated.
Eye examination: Visual acuity, right eye: 6/18 with + 1.0 D sph.; left eye: 6/36 with + 1.5 D sph. Anterior segments are normal. Both fundi present hyperemic discs, engorged and tortuous retinal veins with marked caliber variations, and innumerable small and large rounded retinal hemorrhages, particularly in the fundus periphery. In some places the red dots resemble clusters of microaneurysms.
General examination showed an anemic patient with some enlargement of the spleen and lymph nodes. Hemoglobin: 7.2 g/100 ml. Sedimentation rate: 152 mm/hour. Serum protein: 12.8 g/100 ml. Paper-electrophoresis and immunoelectrophoresis showed lowered albumin content (3.2 g/100 ml) and marked elevation of the γ-globulin fraction (7.4 g/100 ml), especially of the macro β-globulin fraction. The white blood cells and neurological examination showed nothing abnormal.

Figure 291. Right eye (15°). Fundus changes in macroglobulinemia. Fundus periphery showing numerous small and large rounded retinal hemorrhages, and clusters of microaneurysms.

CLINICAL NOTE: Figure 291 is from the same patient as figure 98, a female, aged 41. Six years ago an unexplained high sedimentation rate was observed (144 mm/hour), and she complained of easy bruising. One year later macroglobulinemia was demonstrated. During the last year, vision has been reduced in both eyes.
Eye examination: Visual acuity, right eye: 6/36; left eye: 6/12. Unimproved by lenses. Anterior segments are normal. Both fundi present chronic papilledema, engorment of the veins —which in several places assume the form of strings of sausages—diffusely spread retinal hemorrhages and clusters of microaneurysms, especially in the fundus periphery.
General examination showed macroglobulinemia. The γ-globulin fraction was 8.7 g/100 ml and consisted of typical 20-S macroglobulin. Hemoglobin was 7.0 g/100 ml. Sedimentation rate 144 mm/hour. Blood coagulation showed a defect typical for macroglobulinemia.

Figures 292 and 293. Right and left eyes. Fundus changes in collagenosis. Both fundi present several cotton-wool exudates. The optic discs are normal. Retinal arteries are narrow, the veins are normal.

CLINICAL NOTE: Figures 292 and 293 are from a male, aged 63. Anaphylactoid purpura observed about one year ago. No visual complaints.
Eye examination: Visual acuity, both eyes: 6/6 + 2.5 D sph. Anterior segments are normal. Both fundi present hypertensive angiopathy with vascular sclerosis and several cotton-wool exudates. No retinal hemorrhages.
General examination showed anaphylactoid purpura and hypertension. Blood pressure: 180/120 mm Hg.

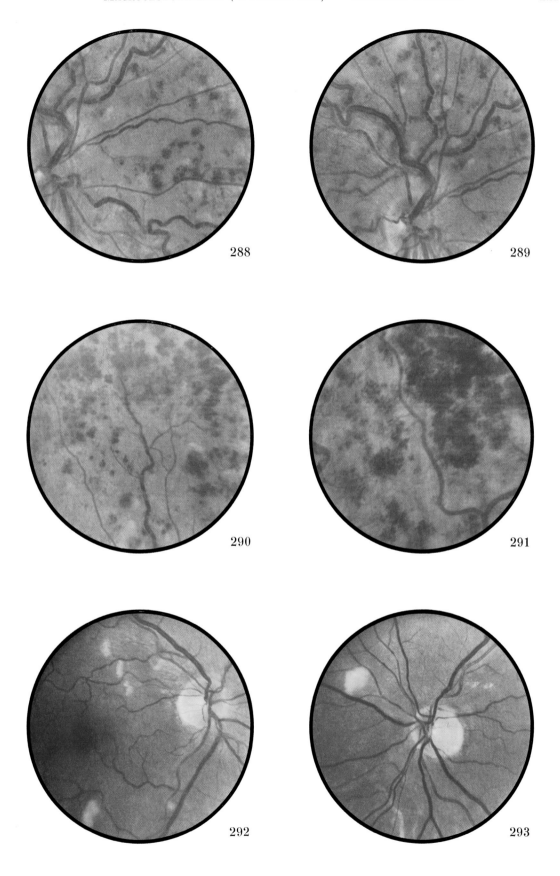

288

289

290

291

292

293

Figure 294. Composite picture. Right eye. Choroideremia. The fundus is pale, whitish with atrophy of the choroid and some choroidal pigment accumulation in the macula. The optic disc and retinal vessels are normal.

CLINICAL NOTE: Figure 294 is from a male, aged 58. Since childhood he and his brother have had defective vision and hemeralopia.
Eye examination: Visual acuity, both eyes: hand movements. Unimproved by lenses. Anterior segments are normal. Both fundi show typical choroideremia. He presents profound hemeralopia. Electroretinographic response extinguished.
General examination showed nothing abnormal.

Figure 295. Composite picture. Right eye. Choroideremia. The choroid is intact in the macular area, but elsewhere it is atrophic. Scattered clusters of pigment are seen in the fundus. The disc and retinal vessels are normal.

CLINICAL NOTE: Figure 295 is from a male, aged 20. His mother's brother has retinitis pigmentosa, otherwise no family history of fundal disease. Since infancy he has had hemeralopia, but no other visual complaints.

Eye examination: Visual acuity, both eyes: 6/6 with − 0.5 D sph. − 1.0 D cyl. axis 90°. Anterior segments are normal. Both fundi present changes typical for choroideremia. Both visual fields show concentric contraction to 20°. Profound hemeralopia. Electroretinographic response is extinguished.
General examination showed nothing abnormal.

Figures 296 and 297. Left and right eyes. Gyrate atrophy of the choroid and retina. There are confluent chorioretinal atrophies around the disc and in the fundus periphery. Scattered pigment clumping is also present. The optic disc and retinal vessels are normal.

CLINICAL NOTE: Figures 296 and 297 are from a female, aged 64. She has had reduced vision, myopia and hemeralopia since childhood. Several members of the family are weak-sighted.
Eye examination: Visual acuity, both eyes: 2/18 with − 13.0 D sph. Anterior segments are normal. Both fundi present gyrate atrophy of the choroid and retina. Profound hemeralopia. Visual fields constricted to about 10°. Electroretinographic response is extinguished.
General examination showed nothing abnormal.

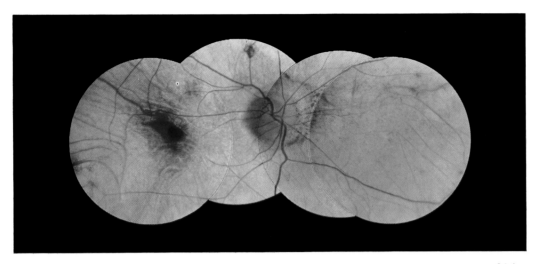

294

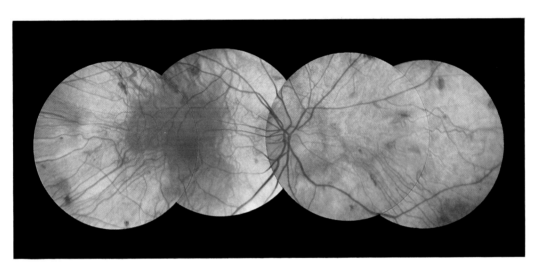

295

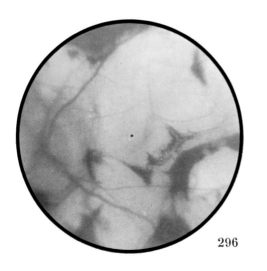

296

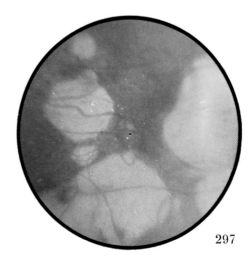

297

Figure 298. Composite picture, right eye. Retinitis pigmentosa. Typical bone corpuscle-like pigment deposits and some patchy atrophy are seen in the fundus periphery. Slight pallor of the disc. The retinal vessels are normal. Slight degenerative changes in the macula.

Figure 299. Same eye as figure 298. Fundus periphery with some retinal atrophy and pigment deposits partly ensheathing the narrow retinal vessels.

CLINICAL NOTE: Figures 298 and 299 are from a female, aged 20. No family history of ocular disease. She has been deaf and night blind since childhood. The last few years vision has been gradually reduced.
Eye examination: Visual acuity, both eyes: 6/12 with − 1.5 D sph. − 1.0 D cyl. axis 0°. Anterior segments and intraocular tension are normal. Both fundi present changes typical of retinitis pigmentosa. Both visual fields contracted to about 10°. Electroretinographic response is extinguished.
General examination showed nothing abnormal. No vacuolized lymphocytes.

Figure 300. Left eye. Retinitis pigmentosa. In the equatorial region characteristic bone corpuscle-like pigment deposits are scattered diffusely and some are ensheathing the vessels.

Figure 301. Composite picture. Right eye. From the same patient as figure 300. The optic disc is pale, atrophic, yellowish-white. The retinal vessels are narrow. Typical bone corpuscle-like pigment deposits are seen nasally. The fundus shows some patchy atrophy and the macula some degenerative changes.

CLINICAL NOTE: Figures 300 and 301 are from a male, aged 27. Several members of the family have retinitis pigmentosa, but his parents and his sister are healthy. Fifteen years ago the patient found he was night blind. Since then vision has been gradually reduced.
Eye examination: Visual acuity, right eye: 2/24; left eye: 3/24. Unimproved by lenses. Intraocular tension and anterior segments are normal. No cataract. Both fundi present changes typical of retinitis pigmentosa. Visual fields show incomplete ring scotomas. Electroretinographic response is extinguished.
General examination showed nothing abnormal. The blood showed no vacuolized lymphocytes.

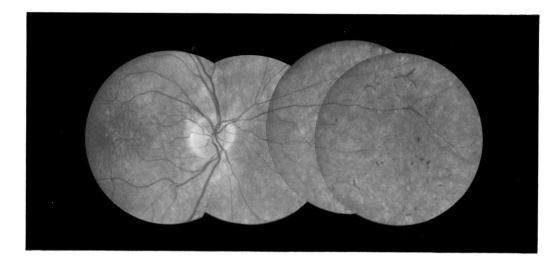

298

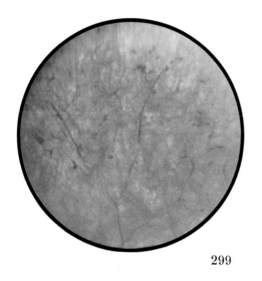

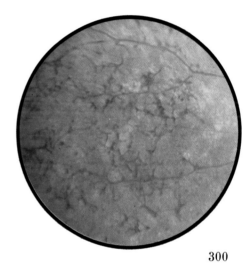

299   300

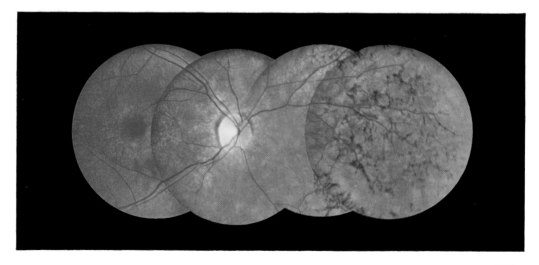

301

Figure 302. Right eye. Albipunctate dystrophy. Numerous small white dots are seen in the sparsely pigmented fundus. Choroidal vessels are seen plainly.

Figure 303. Left eye. From the same patient as figure 302. There are numerous small white dots and a single pigment deposit at the retinal vessel above.

CLINICAL NOTE: Figures 302 and 303 are from a male, aged 13. No known ocular disease in the family. He has presented night blindness since early childhood. During the last few years his central vision has decreased.
Eye examination: Visual acuity, both eyes: 6/12 with + 1.0 D cyl. axis 90°. He presents typical hemeralopia. His color vision is normal. Both visual fields are constricted to about 30°. Anterior segments are normal. Both fundi show white dots all over the fundi and there are a few corpuscular pigmentary deposits. The maculae show no obvious changes. The discs are pale and the retinal vessels are narrow. The electroretinographic response is nearly extinguished.
General examination showed nothing abnormal.

Figure 304. Right eye. Macular changes in albipunctate dystrophy. The macula shows some degenerative changes. The disc shows some atrophy and the retinal vessels are slightly narrowed. In the fundus there are some small white dots.

Figure 305. From the same eye as figure 304, showing numerous small white dots and a few pigment deposits in the fundus periphery.

CLINICAL NOTE: Figures 304 and 305 are from a female, aged 29. No known ocular disease in the family. Since childhood she has been night blind. During the last five years central vision has decreased somewhat and visual fields have shown progressive contraction.
Eye examination: Visual acuity, both eyes: 6/12 with − 0.5 D sph. + 1.0 cyl. axis 0°. She presents typical hemeralopia and color blindness. Both visual fields are contracted to about 5°. Anterior segments are normal. Both fundi present some macular degeneration. There are widespread small white dots and some small pigment clumps in the fundi. Both discs show some atrophy and retinal vessels are slightly narrowed. The electroretinographic response is nearly extinguished.
General examination showed nothing abnormal.

Figures 306 and 307. Right and left eyes. Fundus flavimaculatus, seen as yellowish, irregular flecks in the posterior pole. There is also macular degeneration with accumulation of numerous small yellowish-white dots around the fovea.

CLINICAL NOTE: Figures 306 and 307 are from a male, aged 53. His sister presents fundus flavimaculatus, but otherwise no known ocular disease in the family. During the last 15 years his central vision has gradually decreased. No general symptoms.
Eye examination: Visual acuity, both eyes: 6/60 with + 4.0 D sph. He presents no hemeralopia. Anterior segments are normal. Both fundi present macular degeneration and numerous irregular whitish flecks in the posterior pole. The discs and retinal vessels are normal. Visual fields show central scotomas, but the peripheral fields are normal. The electroretinogram is normal.
General examination showed nothing abnormal.

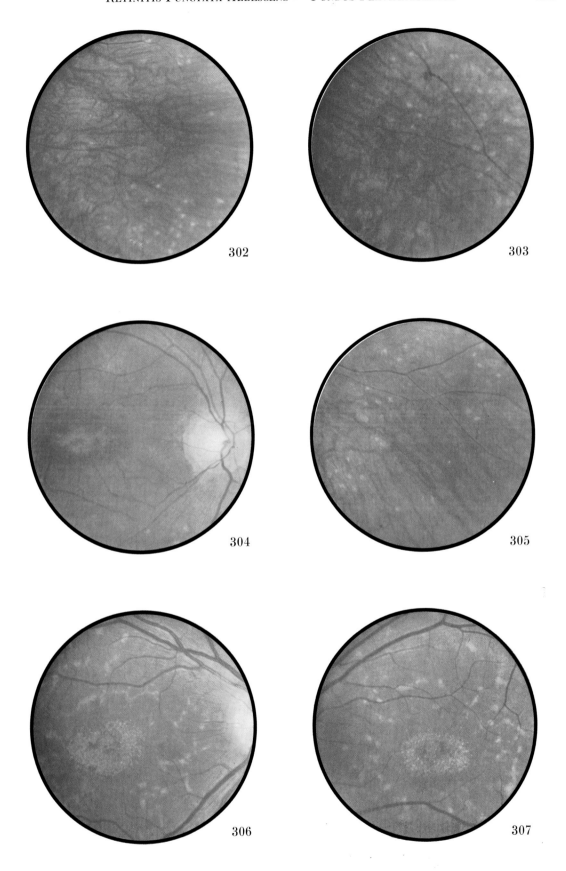

302

303

304

305

306

307

Figures 308. Left eye. Tay-Sachs' disease, advanced stage. The fovea is seen as a red spot, surrounded by an opaque, whitish zone. The disc is atrophic, and retinal arteries are narrow.

CLINICAL NOTE: Figure 308 is from a male, aged 2¾. No known neurological or metabolic diseases in the family. He was normal at birth. In the course of several months he developed progressive muscular weakness and later a spastic tetraplegia and blindness, and there has been a lack of mental development. At the age of one year, Tay-Sachs' disease was diagnosed.
Eye examination: He behaves like a blind child. Both maculae present a "cherry-red" spot. The discs show some atrophy and retinal arteries are narrow.
General examination showed a meager child with tetraplegia and severe muscle atrophy. The blood showed vacuolized lymphocytes. Serum lipids were normal.

Figure 309. Right eye. Niemann-Pick's disease. The fovea presents a "cherry-red" spot surrounded by a broad opaque whitish zone.

CLINICAL NOTE: Figure 309 is from a male, aged 3. No known neurological or metabolic diseases in the family. He developed normally during the first year of life. Since then he has shown progressive weakness and lack of mental development. Niemann-Pick's disease was diagnosed about the age of two years.
Eye examination: He follows light and objects with both eyes. Both fundi present changes similar to those in Tay-Sachs' disease, but discs and retinal vessels are normal.
General examination showed a meager child with gross enlargement of liver and spleen. Xanthomas were present in the skin. Histopathological examination of a lymph node and skin showed foam cells in the lymph node and xanthogranulomas in the skin.

Figure 310. Right eye. Spielmeyer-Vogt's disease, early stage. In the fovea there is a dark-red spot surrounded by a light-red and dark-red halo. Fundus reflexes are bright. Optic disc is pale. Retinal arteries are narrow, the veins are normal.

CLINICAL NOTE: Figure 310 is from a male, aged 7. No family history of mental or ocular disease. Since the age of six years he has shown mental retardation and gradual reduction of vision.

Eye examination: Visual acuity, both eyes: 3/24. Unimproved by lenses. Anterior segments are normal. Both fundi present some macular degeneration. Retinal arteries are narrow, the veins are normal. The discs are pale. No abnormal pigmentation. Electroretinographic response is nearly extinguished.
General examination showed a mentally retarded boy. The blood showed vacuolized lymphocytes.

Figure 311. Right eye. Spielmeyer-Vogt's disease. The optic disc is atrophic, yellowish-white. Retinal vessels are narrow and the fundus shows some patchy atrophy.

CLINICAL NOTE: Figure 311 is from a male, aged 9. No family history of mental or ocular disease. The last year he has shown progressive loss of vision and mental retardation.
Eye examination: Visual acuity, both eyes: 1/36 with + 3.0 D sph. Anterior segments are normal. Both fundi present atrophic discs, some macular degeneration and coarse pigmentation and depigmentation in the periphery. Electroretinographic response is extinguished.
General examination showed a mentally retarded boy. The blood showed vacuolized lymphocytes.

Figure 312. Left eye. Spielmeyer-Vogt's disease. The disc is pale, atrophic. The retinal arteries are very narrow and the veins slightly narrowed. The macula presents depigmentation and some clumping of pigment and is surrounded by fine radiating whitish light reflexes.

Figure 313. From the same eye as figure 312. Fundus periphery showing coarse, irregular pigmentation and depigmentation.

CLINICAL NOTE: Figures 312 and 313 are from a male, aged 6. No known neurological or ocular disease in the family. He developed normally until one year ago. Since then his vision has been gradually reduced and he has shown progressive mental deterioration.
Eye examination: Visual acuity, both eyes: 3/24. Unimproved by lenses. Anterior segments are normal. Both fundi present atrophic discs, some macular degeneration, narrowed retinal vessels and coarse pigmentation and depigmentation in the fundal peripheries. Electroretinographic response is extinguished.
General examination showed a mentally retarded boy with cerebellar ataxia. The blood showed vacuolized lymphocytes.

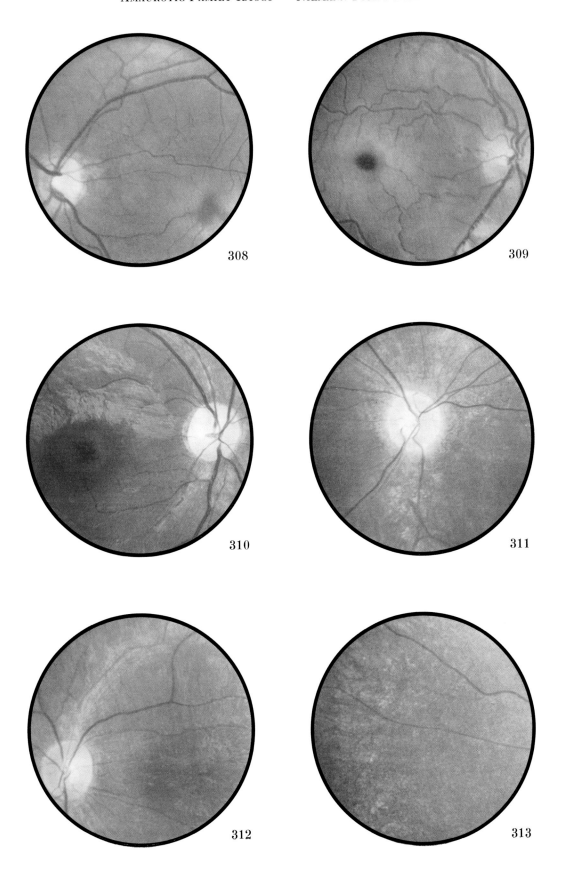

308

309

310

311

312

313

Figure 314. Right eye. Heredomacular degeneration, early stage. The macula presents slight pigment clumping and radiating light streaks. Retinal vessels and disc are normal.

CLINICAL NOTE: Figure 314 is from a male, aged 14. His two brothers and his mother's father present macular degeneration. The same condition was observed in his eyes one year ago, when his vision became slightly reduced. Since then there has been progressive reduction of central vision.
Eye examination: Visual acuity, right eye: 6/36 with − 0.5 D cyl. axis 0°; left eye: 6/12 with + 0.5 D sph. Anterior segments are normal. Both fundi present slight macular degeneration. Discs and retinal vessels are normal. Small central scotoma in both eyes. Electroretinogram is normal.
General examination showed nothing abnormal.

Figure 315. Left eye. Heredomacular degeneration, early stage. Star-shaped cracking of the macular light reflex and slight pigment migration. Disc and retinal vessels are normal.

CLINICAL NOTE: Figure 315 is from a male, aged 23. One of his three brothers has macular degeneration. Both parents have defective vision. During the last few years he has observed some reduction of central vision in both eyes.
Eye examination: Visual acuity, both eyes: 6/18. Unimproved by lenses. Anterior segments are normal. Both fundi present slight macular degeneration. Discs and retinal vessels are normal. Small central scotoma in both eyes. Electroretinogram is normal.
General examination showed nothing abnormal.

Figures 316—319. Same right eye. The development of heredomacular degeneration. The first picture presents only a small white dot in the macula.
The next picture, 18 months later, shows enlargement of the white dot, which is now surrounded by a dark-red halo.
The next pictures, ten months and 6 years later, show a further progression of the macular degeneration. Disc and retinal vessels are normal.

CLINICAL NOTE: Figures 316—319 are from a male, aged 16. His brother presents macular degeneration. His parents are healthy. Over a period of two years he has experienced a gradual reduction of central vision in both eyes. No general symptoms.
Eye examination at first admission: Visual acuity, both eyes: 6/36 with − 1.5 D sph. Anterior segments are normal. Both fundi present slight commencing macular degeneration. Optic discs and retinal vessels are normal. Visual fields show small central scotomas.
Eye examination, 18 and 28 months later: Visual acuity is unchanged, but macular changes are progressive. Electroretinogram is normal.
Eye examination, 7 years after the first examination: Visual acuity, both eyes: 6/60 with − 2.0 D sph. Anterior segments are normal. In both fundi, the macular degeneration shows further progression. Optic discs and retinal vessels are normal. Visual fields present some enlargement of the central scotomas.
General examination showed nothing abnormal. The blood showed no vacuolized lymphocytes.

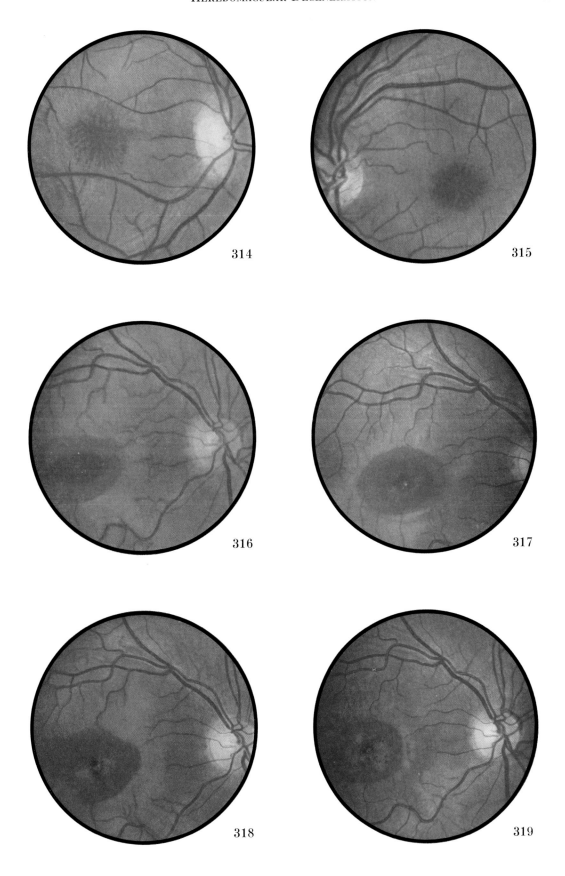

314

315

316

317

318

319

Figures 320 and 321. Right and left eyes. Heredomacular degeneration. In both macular areas there is a dark-red spot surrounded by a small atrophic zone. Discs and retinal vessels are normal.

Clinical note: Figures 320 and 321 are from a male, aged 7. No family history of macular degeneration. He has observed a gradual reduction of vision during the last six months.
Eye examination: Visual acuity, right eye: < 6/36 with − 2.5 D sph.; left eye: 6/12 with − 2.5 D sph. Anterior segments are normal. Both fundi show commencing macular degeneration. Discs and retinal vessels are normal. Both visual fields show central scotomas.
General examination showed nothing abnormal.

Figures 322 and 323. Right and left eyes. Heredomacular degeneration, advanced stage. In both macular areas there is an oval, worm-eaten, degenerative zone with pigment clumping and depigmentation. The foveal reflex is absent, but fundus reflexes are bright. The discs and retinal vessels are normal.

Figures 324 and 325. Same eyes as figures 322 and 323, five years later. The macular lesions are nearly unchanged. Fundus reflexes are now dull. In both fundi there are some irregular light patches resembling those found in fundus flavimaculatus.

Clinical note: Figures 322—325 are from a male, aged 18. His brother presents macular degeneration. His parents are healthy. Seven years ago his vision was gradually reduced in both eyes.
Eye examination: Visual acuity, both eyes: < 6/36. Unimproved by lenses. Anterior segments are normal. Both fundi present advanced macular degeneration. The discs and retinal vessels are normal. Central scotomas in both eyes. Electroretinogram is normal.
Until now, vision and fundus changes have remained nearly stationary, but lesions resembling those in fundus flavimaculatus have developed.
General examination showed nothing abnormal. The blood showed no vacuolized lymphocytes.

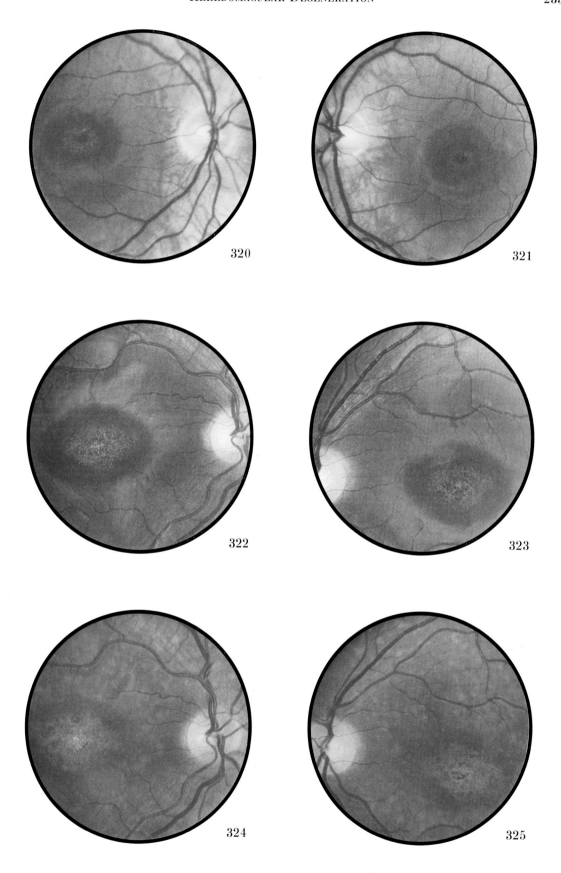

Figures 326 and 327. Right and left eyes. Toxic retinopathy (chloroquine). Both maculae show some degenerative lesions consisting of fine depigmentation and some small hard exudates. Discs and retinal vessels are normal.

CLINICAL NOTE: Figures 326 and 327 are from a female, aged 46. Disseminated lupus erythematosus was diagnosed five years ago. Since then she has received chloroquine treatment, daily dose 750 mg. Three months ago she experienced metamorphopsia and pericentral scotomas.
Eye examination: Visual acuity, both eyes: 6/9. Unimproved by lenses. Some corneal degeneration typical for chloroquine intoxication. Both fundi present some macular degeneration. There are ring-shaped pericentral scotomas for white light in both eyes and central scotomas for red light. Electroretinographic response is nearly extinguished.
General examination showed typical disseminated lupus erythematosus.

Figures 328 and 329. Right and left eyes. Toxic retinopathy (Mellaril). Both maculae show degenerative lesions with depigmentation, pigment clumping and small hemorrhages. Discs and retinal vessels are normal.

CLINICAL NOTE: Figures 328 and 329 are from a female, aged 51. Schizophrenia was diagnosed 20 years ago. The last three years she has received Mellaril (thioridazine chloridum) treatment, daily dose 200 mg. During the last year vision has been gradually reduced.
Eye examination: Visual acuity, right eye: 6/36 with + 1.0 D sph.; left eye: 6/18 with + 1.0 D sph. Anterior segments are normal. Both fundi present macular degeneration and there are central scotomas. Electroretinographic response is reduced.
General examination showed schizophrenia.

Figures 330 and 331. Right and left eyes. Toxic retinopathy (antimalarial drugs). Both macular areas show fine degenerative lesions and some edema. Retinal arteries are slightly narrowed, veins are normal. The discs are normal.

CLINICAL NOTE: Figures 330 and 331 are from a male, aged 34. Two months ago he had a malaria attack with high fever. After he had received antimalarial treatment for some days he experienced a severe reduction of vision in both eyes.
Eye examination: Visual acuity, right eye: 6/18; left eye: 6/60. Unimproved by lenses. Anterior segments are normal. Both fundi present some macular degeneration and edema. Retinal arteries are narrowed. He shows centrocecal scotoma in the right eye and central scotoma in the left eye.
General examination showed nothing abnormal. Blood pressure: 140/80 mm Hg.

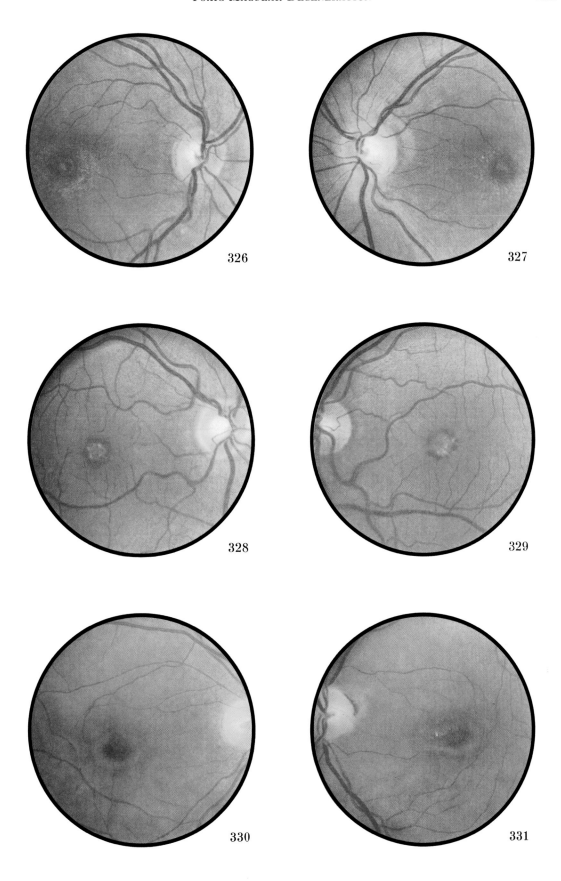

326

327

328

329

330

331

Figure 332. Right eye. Senile macular de-generation with coarse depigmentation and some pigment clumping in the macular area. Elsewhere in the fundus there are some drusen-like yellowish-white dots. Ret-inal vessels show some sclerosis and the disc is normal.

CLINICAL NOTE: Figure 332 is from a male, aged 78. He has had psoriasis for many years. The last few years he has had some heart failure and the last year some reduction of vision.
Eye examination: Visual acuity, right eye: 6/9 with + 1.0 D cyl. axis 170°; left eye: 6/9 with + 1.0 D sph. Anterior segments are normal. Both fundi present senile macular degeneration and retinal vessels show some sclerosis.
General examination showed psoriasis and some heart failure. Blood pressure: 145/70 mm Hg.

Figure 333. Right eye. Senile macular de-generation with depigmentation and fine pigment clumping. The lesion is surround-ed by numerous colloid bodies. The disc is normal.

CLINICAL NOTE: Figure 333 is from a male, aged 69. He has been healthy until two months ago, when he experienced some metamorphopsia and reduction of vision.
Eye examination: Visual acuity, right eye: < 6/6 with + 1.5 D sph.; left eye: < 6/12 with + 1.5 D sph. Anterior segments are normal. The right fundus presents senile macular de-generation, and the left fundus commencing disciform macular degeneration.
General examination showed nothing abnormal. Blood pressure: 160/100 mm Hg.

Figure 334. Right eye. Senile macular de-generation with pigment clumping in the macular area. A senile peripapillary halo is seen plainly.

CLINICAL NOTE: Figure 334 is from a male, aged 75. He has had some heart failure for about five years. Some years ago he developed a cere-bral thrombosis. The last year vision has been slightly reduced in both eyes.
Eye examination: Visual acuity, both eyes: < 6/9 with + 1.0 D sph. Incipient bilateral cataract. Both fundi show senile macular de-generation, sclerosis of the retinal vessels and senile peripapillary atrophy.
General examination showed generalized ar-teriosclerosis and some heart failure. Blood pressure: 155/70 mm Hg.

Figure 335. Left eye. Senile macular de-generation with coarse pigmentation in the macular area. There is some peripapillary atrophy and a few colloid bodies. The disc is normal.

CLINICAL NOTE: Figure 335 is from the same pa-tient as figure 340, a male, aged 75. The last few years vision has been gradually reduced in both eyes. He has just recovered from a coronary occlusion.
Eye examination: Visual acuity, right eye: 6/18; left eye: 1/60. Unimproved by lenses. In-cipient bilateral cataract. Both fundi present senile macular degeneration, some peripapil-lary atrophy and sclerosis of the retinal ves-sels. Visual fields show central scotomas.
General examination showed generalized ar-teriosclerosis, but no heart failure. Electrocar-diogram showed sequelae after a coronary oc-clusion. Blood pressure: 140/100 mm Hg.

Figure 336. Right eye. Senile macular de-generation with coarse depigmentation and slight pigment clumping in the macular area. The disc is normal.

CLINICAL NOTE: Figure 336 is from a male, aged 71. During the last ten years central vision has been seriously reduced in the right eye. No complaints from the left eye or general symp-toms.
Eye examination: Visual acuity, right eye: 6/60 with + 1.0 D sph.; left eye: 6/6 with + 1.0 D sph. Anterior segments are normal. The right fundus presents senile macular degeneration, the left macula is normal. Retinal vessels show some sclerosis. The discs are normal. Right visual field shows central scotoma, the left is normal.
General examination showed nothing abnormal. Blood pressure: 160/100 mm Hg.

Figure 337. Right eye. Senile macular de-generation surrounded by colloid bodies. The disc is normal.

CLINICAL NOTE: Figure 337 is from the same pa-tient as figure 341, a male, aged 75. During the last few years central vision has gradually di-minished in the left eye. No complaints from the right eye. No general complaints.
Eye examination: Visual acuity, right eye: 6/9; left eye: 2/60. Unimproved by lenses. Both lenses show incipient cataract. Both fundi pre-sent senile macular degeneration surrounded by colloid bodies. Retinal vessels show mod-erate sclerosis. Right visual field is normal; the left shows central scotoma.
General examination showed myocardial de-generation. Blood pressure: 160/100 mm Hg.

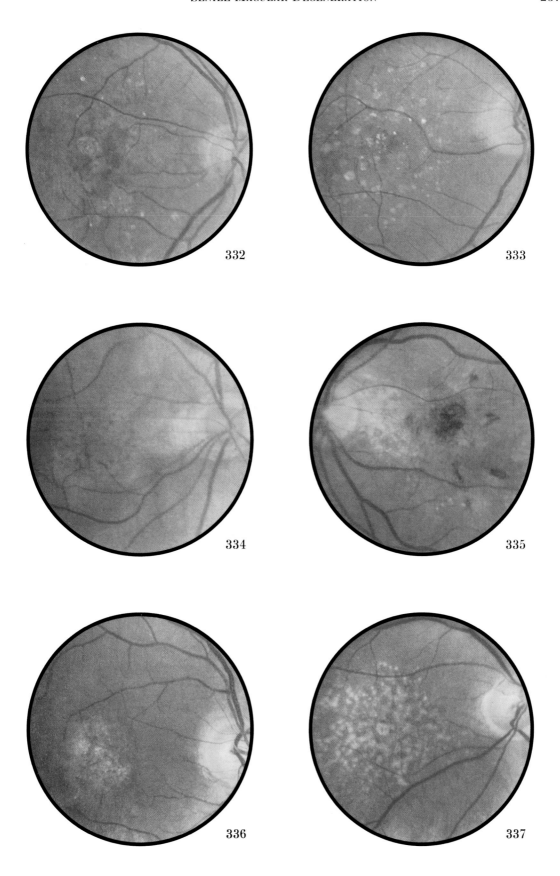

332

333

334

335

336

337

Figure 338. Right eye. Senile macular degeneration surrounded by large colloid bodies.

Clinical note: Figure 338 is from a male, aged 52. The last two years he has experienced some metamorphopsia and slight reduction of vision. No general symptoms.
Eye examination: Visual acuity, both eyes: < 6/6 with + 1.5 D sph. Anterior segments are normal. Both fundi present senile macular degeneration and many large colloid bodies. Discs and retinal vessels are normal.
General examination showed nothing abnormal.

Figure 339. Left eye. Senile macular degeneration surrounded by colloid bodies. Disc and retinal vessels are normal.

Clinical note: Figure 339 is from a female, aged 55. During the last five years vision has been gradually reduced in both eyes. No general complaints.
Eye examination: Visual acuity, both eyes: 6/18 with + 1.0 D sph. + 4.0 D cyl. axis 90°. Anterior segments are normal. Both fundi show senile macular degeneration and many colloid bodies. Discs and retinal vessels are normal.
General examination showed nothing abnormal.

Figure 340. Right eye. Senile macular degeneration surrounded by colloid bodies. There is some peripapillary atrophy. The disc is normal.

Clinical note: Figure 340 is from the same patient as figure 335, a male, aged 75. The last few years vision has been gradually reduced in both eyes. He has just recovered from a coronary occlusion.
Eye examination: Visual acuity, right eye: 6/18; left eye: 1/60. Unimproved by lenses. Incipient bilateral cataract. Both fundi present senile macular degeneration, some peripapillary atrophy and sclerosis of the retinal vessels. Visual fields show central scotomas.
General examination showed generalized arteriosclerosis, but no heart failure. Electrocardiogram showed sequelae after a coronary occlusion. Blood pressure: 140/100 mm Hg.

Figure 341. Left eye. Senile macular degeneration and colloid bodies. In the macular area there is coarse depigmentation and

some pigment clumping. The colloid bodies are situated beneath the retinal vessels.

Clinical note: Figure 341 is from the same patient as figure 337, a male, aged 75. During the last few years central vision has gradually diminished in the left eye. No complaints from the right eye. No general complaints.
Eye examination: Visual acuity, right eye: 6/9; left eye: 2/60. Unimproved by lenses. Both lenses show incipient cataract. Both fundi present senile macular degeneration surrounded by colloid bodies. Retinal vessels show moderate sclerosis. Right visual field is normal; the left shows central scotoma.
General examination showed myocardial degeneration. Blood pressure: 160/100 mm Hg.

Figure 342. Right eye. Cystoid macular degeneration. A macular cyst is seen as a well-defined, slightly elevated, round, deep-red spot. The retinal vessels show some sclerosis and the disc is normal.

Clinical note: Figure 342 is from a female, aged 75. During the last eight years central vision has been much reduced in the right eye. No complaints from the left eye. No general symptoms.
Eye examination: Visual acuity, right eye: 6/60 + 2.0 D sph.; left eye: 6/9 with + 2.0 D sph. Anterior segments are normal. The right fundus presents a macular cyst, while the left macula is normal. Retinal vessels show some sclerosis. The discs are normal. Right visual field shows central scotoma, the left is normal.
General examination showed nothing abnormal. Blood pressure: 140/70 mm Hg.

Figure 343. Right eye. Lamellar macular hole in cystoid macular degeneration.

Clinical note: Figure 343 is from a female, aged 67. During the last five months vision in the right eye has gradually decreased. No complaints from the left eye. No general symptoms.
Eye examination: Visual acuity, right eye: 6/60 with + 2.0 D sph.; left eye: 6/6 with + 2.0 D sph. Anterior segments are normal. The right fundus presents a macular hole, following the rupture of a macular cyst. The left macula is normal. Retinal vessels show some sclerosis. The discs are normal. Right visual field shows a central scotoma, the left is normal.
General examination showed nothing abnormal. Blood pressure: 170/100 mm Hg.

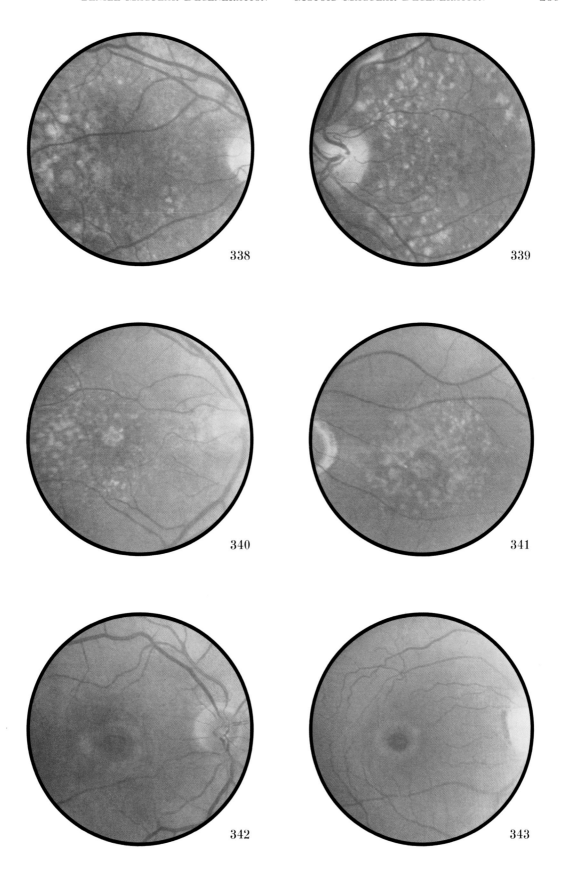

338

339

340

341

342

343

Figures 344 and 345. Right and left eyes. Central areolar choroidal atrophy, early stages. The discs and retinal vessels are normal.

CLINICAL NOTE: Figures 344 and 345 are from a female, aged 36. No family history of ocular disease. Since the age of three years she has had divergent strabismus and amblyopia of the left eye. The last year vision in the right eye has been slightly reduced. No general symptoms.
Eye examination: Visual acuity, right eye: 6/9 with − 2.5 D sph. − 1.0 D cyl. axis 20°; left eye: 6/36 with − 2.5 D sph. − 0.5 D cyl. axis 10°. She has left divergent squint of about 20°. Eye movements are normal. Anterior segments are normal. Both fundi show commencing central areolar choroidal atrophy. Discs and retinal vessels are normal. Visual field defects correspond to the fundal lesions. Electroretinographic response is normal.
General examination showed nothing abnormal.

Figure 346. Right eye. Central areolar choroidal atrophy. In the atrophic area there is some pigment clumping and choroidal vessels are seen plainly. Disc and retinal vessels are normal.

CLINICAL NOTE: Figure 346 is from a female, aged 35. No family history of ocular disease. During the last two years central vision has gradually been reduced in both eyes. No general symptoms.
Eye examination: Visual acuity, both eyes: 6/60 with − 1.0 D sph. Anterior segments are normal. Both fundi present central areolar choroidal atrophy. Discs and retinal vessels are normal. Visual fields show small central scotomas. Electroretinographic response is normal.
General examination showed nothing abnormal.

Figure 347. Right eye. Central areolar choroidal atrophy with marked sclerosis of the choroidal vessels. There is also some peripapillary atrophy.

CLINICAL NOTE: Figure 347 is from a female, aged 87. She has had psoriasis for many years. During the last five years central vision has gradually been reduced in both eyes.

Eye examination: Visual acuity, both eyes: 2/60. Unimproved by lenses. Both lenses present incipient cataract. In both fundi there is a pronounced central areolar choroidal atrophy and sclerosis of the choroidal vessels. Retinal vessels show moderate sclerosis. The discs are normal, but show some peripapillary atrophy. *General examination* showed psoriasis. Blood pressure: 160/50 mm Hg.

Figure 348. Right eye. Extensive peripapillary choroidal atrophy. Retinal vessels are narrow. The disc is atrophic.

CLINICAL NOTE: Figure 348 is from a female, aged 49. Twenty-five years ago she had polyneuritis. Since then she has had some walking incapacity and uncoordination of movements. The last ten years her vision has been reduced gradually.
Eye examination: Visual acuity, right eye: 6/60 with − 2.0 D sph.; left eye: 6/24 with − 2.0 D sph. She has bilateral ptosis. Anterior segments are normal. Both fundi present extensive peripapillary choroidal atrophy. The retinal vessels are narrow and both discs atrophic. Both visual fields show concentric contraction and defects around the blind spot, and there is a central scotoma in the right eye.
General examination showed severe ataxia. Cerebral cortex biopsy showed lipoidosis. Wassermann reaction was negative. Blood lipids: 1,040 mg/100 ml. All lipid fractions were elevated. Blood pressure: 150/110 mm Hg.

Figure 349. Right eye. Diffuse choroidal atrophy with marked pigmentation in the fundus periphery.

CLINICAL NOTE: Figure 349 is from a female, aged 57. No family history of ocular disease. During the last five years vision has been slightly reduced. No general complaints.
Eye examination: Visual acuity, both eyes: 6/9 with + 2.5 D sph. Anterior segments are normal. Both fundi present extensive choroidal atrophy and coarse pigmentation in the periphery. Retinal arteries are narrow, the veins appear normal. The optic discs are normal. Both visual fields are contracted to about 30°. The electroretinographic response is nearly extinguished.
General examination showed nothing abnormal. The Wassermann reaction was negative.

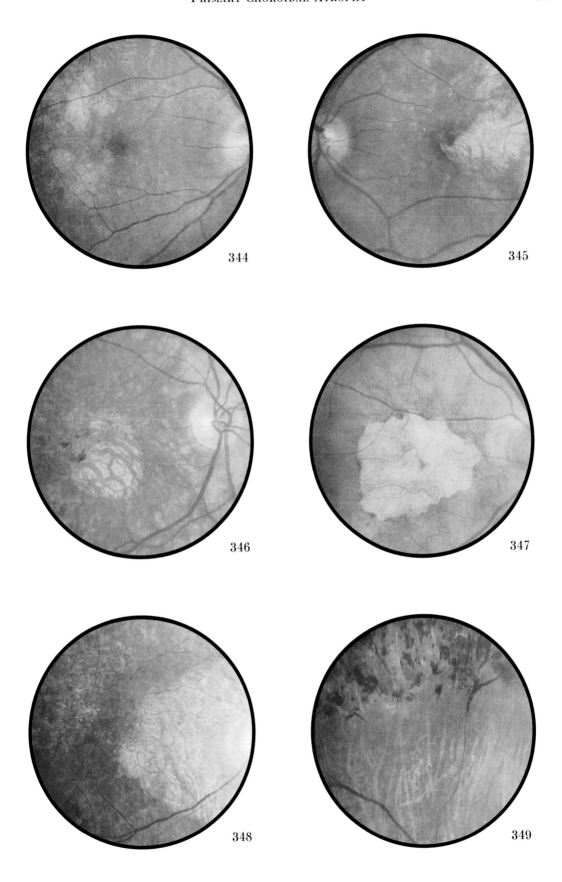

344

345

346

347

348

349

Figures 350—355. Same right eye. The pictures show the development of a juvenile disciform macular degeneration in the course of 17 months. The lesion commences with a macular subretinal hemorrhage and some edema. In the further development a new subretinal hemorrhage appears. Later on the hemorrhages are absorbed and the lesion converted into a fibrous tissue scar. Finally, some pigmentation develops at the margin of the scar. Disc and retinal vessels are normal.

Clinical note: Figures 350—355 are from a male, aged 25. No family history of ocular disease. Eighteen months ago he experienced a rapid reduction of vision and metamorphopsia in the right eye. No complaints from the left eye. No general symptoms.

Eye examination in the acute stage: Visual acuity, right eye: 6/18 with − 1.0 D sph.; left eye: 6/6 with − 1.0 D sph. The right fundus shows a macular subretinal hemorrhage surrounded by edema. The left fundus is normal.

During the following months the fundus lesion in the right eye developed further.

About six months later, the hemorrhages had been absorbed and the lesion was converted into fibrous tissue and surrounded by some hard exudates.

A year later, the fibrous tissue had been converted into a firm scar and the exudates had disappeared. Visual acuity in the right eye had now decreased to 6/60 with − 1.0 D sph. The left eye was normal and visual acuity was 6/6 with − 1.0 D sph.

General examination showed nothing abnormal.

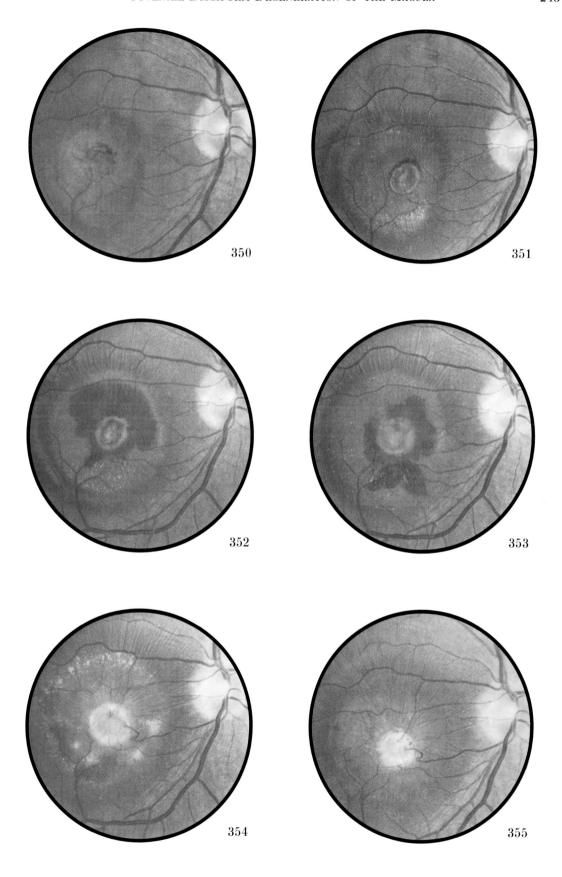

350

351

352

353

354

355

Figure 356. Left eye. Juvenile disciform macular degeneration, early stage. A slate-gray, ill-defined degenerative lesion is situated just below the fovea. The lesion is surrounded by slight edema. Retinal vessels are normal.

CLINICAL NOTE: Figure 356 is from a male, aged 32. No family history of ocular disease. The last two months he has experienced a gradual loss of central vision in the left eye. No complaints from the right eye. No general symptoms.
Eye examination: Visual acuity, right eye: 6/6 with + 1.0 D sph.; left eye: 6/60 with + 1.0 D sph. Anterior segments are normal. The right fundus is normal. The left fundus shows a commencing juvenile disciform macular degeneration. The disc and retinal vessels are normal. Visual field defect corresponds to the fundal lesion.
General examination showed nothing abnormal.

Figure 357. Right eye. Juvenile disciform macular degeneration, early stage. The grayish lesion situated just above the fovea is surrounded by subretinal hemorrhage and some edema. Disc and retinal vessels are normal.

Figure 358. Same eye as figure 357, fifteen months later. The grayish lesion is now converted into a chorioretinal scar. The scar is surrounded by some patchy fundal atrophy.

CLINICAL NOTE: Figures 357 and 358 are from a male, aged 36. No family history of ocular disease. Two years ago he experienced metamorphopsia and gradual reduction of vision in the right eye. No complaints from the left eye. No general symptoms.
Eye examination in the acute stage: Visual acuity, right eye: 6/36 with + 1.0 D sph.; left eye: 6/6 with + 1.0 D sph. Anterior segments are normal. The right fundus presents a commencing juvenile disciform macular degeneration, while the left is normal.

Eye examination, fifteen months later: Visual acuity, right eye: 6/60 with + 1.0 D sph. The fundus lesion in an atrophic scar stage. The left fundus is normal.
General examination showed nothing abnormal.

Figure 359. Left eye. Incipient juvenile disciform macular degeneration. The top of the grayish-red, ill-defined lesion in the macula projects about one diopter. The lesion is surrounded by slight choroidal atrophy. Retinal vessels are normal.

Figure 360. Same eye as figure 359, two months later. The macular lesion is still elevated, but its color has now changed to yellowish-gray and the lesion is surrounded by subretinal hemorrhage and some edema.

Figure 361. Same eye as figure 360, six years later. The macular lesion is now converted into a disciform chorioretinal scar. The fundus shows diffuse choroidal atrophy with some pigment clumping.

CLINICAL NOTE: Figures 359—361 are from a female, aged 37. Her mother, her four sisters and a brother have renal glycosuria. The brother also presents bilateral macular degeneration and disseminated chorioretinal lesions. Seven years ago she experienced a gradual reduction of central vision in both eyes.
Eye examination at the first admission: Visual acuity, right eye: 1/60; left eye: 3/60. Unimproved by lenses. Anterior segments are normal. No cataract. The right fundus presents a large disciform macular degeneration in the scar stage, and the left shows a commencing disciform macular degeneration.
Eye examination six years later: Visual acuity, right eye: 1/60; left eye: 1/36. Both fundi present disciform macular degeneration and diffuse choroidal atrophy with pigment accumulation. The discs and retinal vessels are normal.
General examination showed renal glycosuria, but no diabetes. No nephropathy or hypertension.

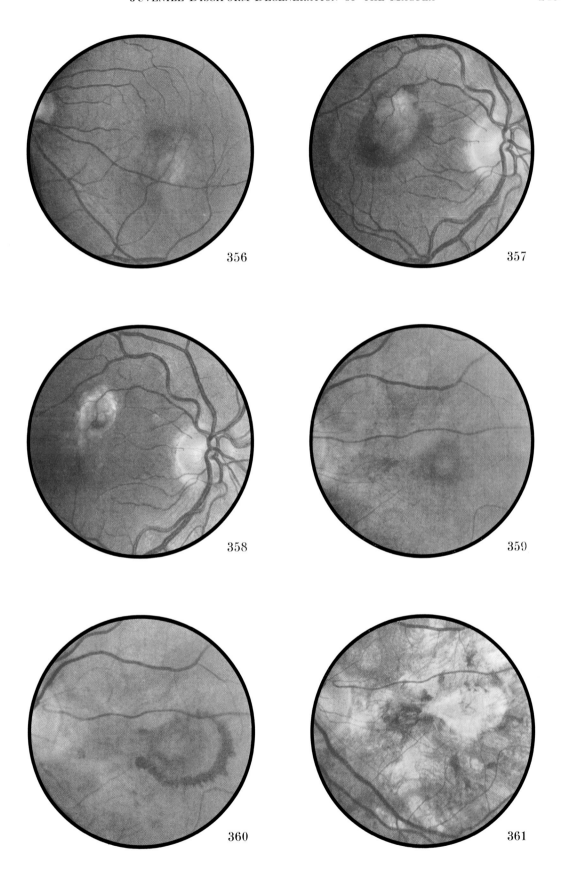

356

357

358

359

360

361

Figure 362. Right eye. Incipient senile disciform macular degeneration. The slightly elevated macular lesion is heavily pigmented centrally and bordered by a zone of diffuse slate-gray pigmentation. Disc and retinal vessels are normal.

Figure 363. Same eye as figure 362, six years later. The macular lesion has enlarged somewhat. It is now converted into a disciform atrophy, but it is still bordered by a zone of slate-gray pigmentation.

CLINICAL NOTE: Figures 362 and 363 are from a male, aged 54. No family history of ocular disease. One year ago he experienced some reduction of vision in the right eye and a subretinal hemorrhage was found in the right macular area. Since then vision has decreased further. No complaints from the left eye. No general symptoms.
Eye examination at first admission: Visual acuity, right eye: 6/12 with + 1.0 D sph.; left eye: 6/6, emmetropia. Anterior segments are normal. The right fundus shows commencing disciform macular degeneration with heavy pigmentation. The left fundus is normal.
During the following years, vision in the right eye showed a further decrease.
Eye examination, six years later: Visual acuity, right eye: 6/24 with + 1.0 D sph.; left eye: 6/6, emmetropia. The macular lesion is converted into an atrophic lesion. The lesion is still bordered by a zone of pigmentation. The left fundus is normal.
General examination showed nothing abnormal.

Figure 364. Left eye. Senile disciform macular degeneration, early stage. The lesion is ill-defined, yellowish-gray, edematous and slightly elevated. The disc and retinal vessels are normal.

Figure 365. Same eye as figure 364, six months later. The macular lesion is now converted into a disciform yellowish-white mass surrounded by glistening, whitish, circinate exudates.

CLINICAL NOTE: Figures 364 and 365 are from a male, aged 63. During the last six months,

gradually decreased central vision in the left eye. No complaints from the right eye. No general symptoms.
Eye examination at first admission: Visual acuity, right eye: 6/6 with + 3.5 D sph. + 0.5 D cyl. axis 90°; left eye: 3/36 with + 3.5 D sph. Anterior segments are normal. The right fundus presents an incipient senile macular degeneration, and the left fundus a commencing disciform macular degeneration. Retinal vessels and discs are normal.
During the following months central vision also gradually decreased in the right eye.
Eye examination, six months later: Corrected visual acuity, right eye: 6/24; left eye: 2/60. The degenerative lesions in both maculae show further progression. Visual field defects correspond to the fundal lesions.
General examination showed nothing abnormal. Blood pressure: 160/100 mm Hg.

Figure 366. Right eye. Senile disciform macular degeneration, early stage. A large subretinal hemorrhage is seen in the posterior pole of the eye. The color of the hemorrhage varies from slate-gray to nearly black. Disc and retinal vessels are normal.

Figure 367. Same eye as figure 366, four years later. The macular lesion is now converted into a large, slightly elevated yellowish-white mass of fibrous tissue. There is also some pigment clumping. Retinal vessels are narrowed.

CLINICAL NOTE: Figures 366 and 367 are from a male, aged 71. Two years ago he experienced slight reduction of vision in the right eye. A fortnight ago vision dropped suddenly in both eyes. No general complaints.
Eye examination at first admission: Visual acuity, right eye: 1/60; left eye: 1/36. Unimproved by lenses. Anterior segments are normal. Both fundi show commencing disciform macular degeneration with extensive subretinal hemorrhage in the posterior poles.
Eye examination, four years later: The visual acuity is unchanged. The macular lesions are converted into large disciform fibrous masses. Both visual fields show large central scotomas.
General examination showed nothing abnormal. Blood pressure: 160/90 mm Hg.

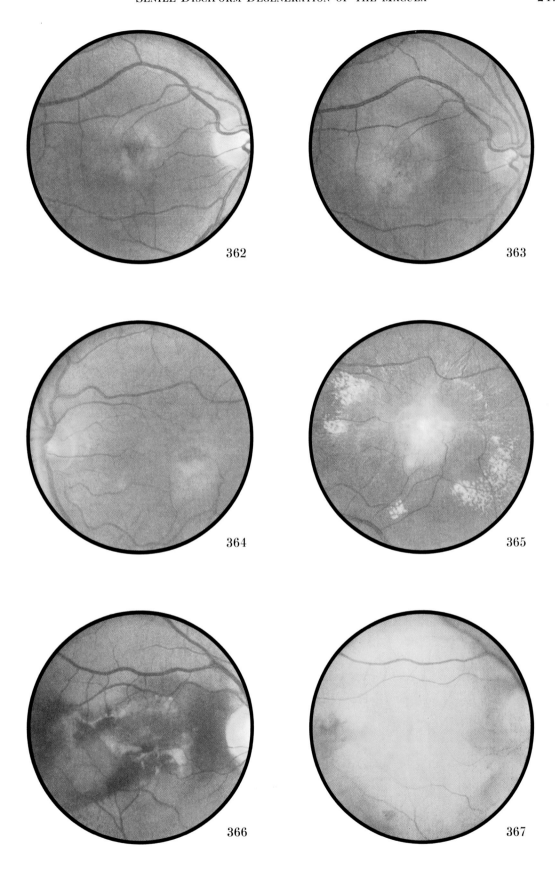

362

363

364

365

366

367

Figure 368. Left eye. Senile disciform macular degeneration, early stage. The macular area is pale and edematous. It is bordered by a subretinal hemorrhage, being red in color.

Figure 369. Same eye as figure 368, nine months later. The subretinal hemorrhage has nearly disappeared. The macula and the adjacent fundus are pale with chorioretinal atrophies and some hard exudates.

CLINICAL NOTE: Figures 368 and 369 are from a male, aged 72. During the last year vision has gradually decreased in both eyes. No general symptoms.
Eye examination, early stage: Visual acuity, right eye: 6/24 with + 5.0 D sph.; left eye: 6/18 with + 2.5 D sph. Both lenses present incipient cataract. The right fundus shows senile macular degeneration and the left a commencing disciform macular degeneration with subretinal hemorrhage.
Eye examination, nine months later: Visual acuity, right eye: 6/36 with + 5.0 D sph.; left eye: 6/36 with + 2.5 D sph. The fundus lesions have progressed in both eyes and the subretinal hemorrhage in the left eye is nearly absorbed. Retinal vessels show some sclerosis. The discs are normal. Visual fields show defects corresponding to the fundal lesions.
General examination showed nothing abnormal.

Figure 370. Left eye. Senile disciform macular degeneration, early stage. A subretinal hemorrhage, red in color, is seen in the macular area and the adjacent parts of the fundus.

Figure 371. Same eye as figure 370, eight months later. The subretinal hemorrhage has been replaced by a large yellowish-white fibrotic mass lying beneath the retinal vessels.

CLINICAL NOTE: Figures 370 and 371 are from a male, aged 70. Four months ago he observed hazy vision in the right eye, and a fortnight ago hazy vision in the left eye. No general complaints.
Eye examination, early stage: Visual acuity, right eye: 6/36 with + 2.0 D sph.; left eye: 6/60

with + 1.0 D sph. The right fundus presents an advanced disciform macular degeneration, and the left a large subretinal hemorrhage in the posterior pole. Retinal vessels show moderate sclerosis. The discs are normal.
Eye examination, eight months later: Visual acuity is nearly unchanged. Both fundi present advanced disciform macular degeneration.
General examination showed nothing abnormal. Blood pressure: 135/80 mm Hg.

Figure 372. Right eye. Circinate retinopathy, early stage. A girdle of deeply situated, sharply defined and confluent, glistening whitish exudates surround the macular area. In the macular area there are some punctate retinal hemorrhages and slight macular degeneration.

CLINICAL NOTE: Figure 372 is from a male, aged 56. The last three months he has observed reduction of vision in the right eye. No complaints from the left eye. He has been admitted for a pulmonary tumor.
Eye examination: Visual acuity, right eye: 6/60 with − 3.0 D sph.; left eye: 6/6 with − 2.0 D sph. Anterior segments are normal. The right fundus presents circinate retinopathy and slight macular degeneration. The left fundus is normal. The discs and retinal vessels are normal.
General examination: Explorative thoracotomy showed inoperable pulmonary neoplasm.

Figure 373. Left eye. Circinate retinopathy with advanced macular degeneration. A girdle of confluent, hard exudates surrounds the macular area. The macula shows a macular degeneration with pigment clumping.

CLINICAL NOTE: Figure 373 is from a male, aged 77. During the last eight years vision has gradually decreased in the left eye. During the last three months also some reduction of vision in the right eye. No general complaints.
Eye examination: Visual acuity, right eye: 6/9; left eye: hand movements. Unimproved by lenses. There is bilateral incipient cataract. The right fundus presents a commencing senile macular degeneration, the left fundus shows a disciform macular degeneration and circinate retinopathy.
General examination showed nothing abnormal. Blood pressure: 170/100 mm Hg.

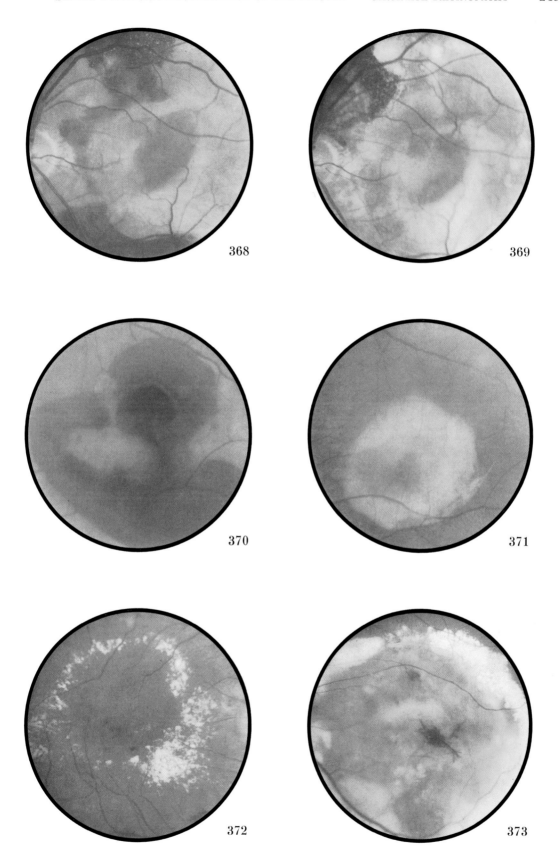

368

369

370

371

372

373

Figure 374. Right eye. Colloid bodies. There is an accumulation of small drusen in the macular area. Disc and retinal vessels are normal.

CLINICAL NOTE: Figure 374 is from a male, aged 17. No ocular or general complaints.
Eye examination: Visual acuity, both eyes: 6/6, emmetropia. Anterior segments are normal. Both fundi present drusen in the macular area. Discs and retinal vessels are normal.
General examination showed nothing abnormal.

Figure 375. Right eye. Large colloid bodies in the macular area. Disc and retinal vessels are normal.

CLINICAL NOTE: Figure 375 is from a female, aged 55. Diabetes was diagnosed nine years ago. Insulin treatment since then. No ocular complaints.
Eye examination: Visual acuity, both eyes: < 6/6 with + 1.0 D cyl. axis 90°. Anterior segments are normal. Both fundi show numerous large colloid bodies in the macular area. No signs of diabetic retinopathy. Discs and retinal vessels are normal.
General examination showed diabetes without nephropathy. Blood pressure: 120/80 mm Hg.

Figure 376. Right eye. Colloid bodies. The fundus is speckled by yellowish-white pinpoint dots and larger spots situated beneath the normal retinal vessels.

CLINICAL NOTE: Figure 376 is from a female, aged 39. She has always been healthy. No family history of ocular disease. No ocular or general complaints.
Eye examination: Visual acuity, right eye: 6/6 with + 0.5 D sph. + 1.0 D cyl. axis 90°; left eye: 6/6 with + 1.0 D sph. Anterior segments are normal. Both fundi show innumerable colloid bodies. Retinal vessels and discs are normal.
General examination showed nothing abnormal.

Figure 377. Left eye. Central serous retinopathy seen as a slightly prominent, well-defined oval area of indistinctness, bordered by a light reflex. Some small whitish dots are seen within the affected area. Retinal vessels are normal. There is a small crater-like hole in the optic disc.

CLINICAL NOTE: Figure 377 is from a female, aged 30. Four weeks ago she observed some hazy vision in the left eye. This haze was followed at first by a positive and later by a negative central scotoma. No complaints from the right eye. No general symptoms.
Eye examination: Visual acuity, right eye: 6/6, emmetropia; left eye: 1/60, unimproved by lenses. Anterior segments and the right fundus are normal. The left fundus presents a central serous retinopathy and a small hole in the optic disc.
In the course of some months the serous retinopathy subsided and vision gradually increased to normal.
General examination showed nothing abnormal.

Figure 378. Composite picture. Right eye. Central serous retinopathy, seen as a slightly prominent area of indistinctness in the macular area, bordered by a light reflex. Numerous whitish dots are seen in the affected area.

CLINICAL NOTE: Figure 378 is from a female, aged 37. She has had myopia since the age of 14 years. The last two years she has had recurrent attacks of central serous retinopathy in the right eye. No complaints from the left eye. No general symptoms.
Eye examination: Visual acuity, right eye: 6/12 with − 3.5 D sph.; left eye: 6/6 with − 1.0 D sph. Anterior segments and the left fundus are normal. The right fundus presents central serous retinopathy. Retinal vessels are normal. Both discs present myopic conus.
General examination showed nothing abnormal.

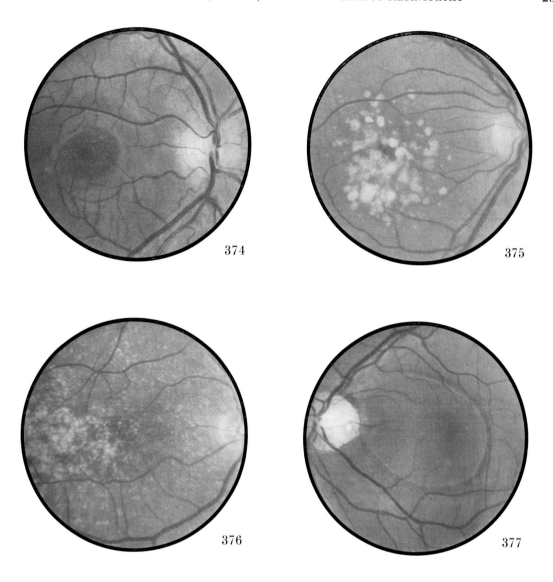

374

375

376

377

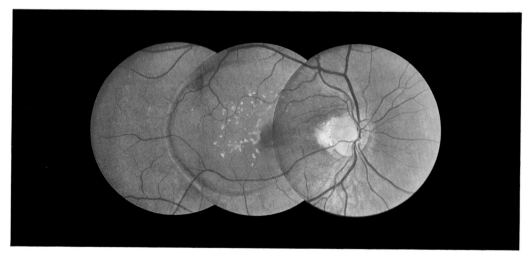

378

Figure 379. Right eye. Coats' syndrome. Large, confluent and slightly prominent, but deeply situated whitish exudates are seen in the fundus. The retinal vessels lie superficial to the exudates. A dense vitreous haze partly obscures the fundus.

CLINICAL NOTE: Figure 379 is from a male, aged 9. On routine examination vision in the right eye was found to be severely reduced. No subjective ocular or general complaints.
Eye examination: Visual acuity, right eye: 6/60, unimproved by lenses; left eye: 6/6 with + 1.0 D sph. Anterior segments and the left fundus are normal. The right vitreous presents a dense haze and the fundus shows large, confluent, deeply situated exudates. No hemorrhages or visible vascular aneurysms.
General examination showed nothing abnormal. No signs of tuberculosis, toxoplasmosis or syphilis.

Figure 380. Right eye. Coats' syndrome. Area with sheathing of retinal vessels and some miliary arterial aneurysms seen through a vitreous haze.

Figure 381. Same eye as figure 380. The fundus presents numerous miliary arterial aneurysms and confluent, deeply situated exudates.

CLINICAL NOTE: Figures 380 and 381 are from a male, aged 28. On routine examination Coats' syndrome was diagnosed in the right eye two years ago. Since then the fundus lesions have shown a steady progression and vision has been gradually reduced. No general symptoms.
Eye examination: Visual acuity, right eye: 6/24, unimproved by lenses; left eye: 6/6, emmetropia. Anterior segments and left fundus are normal. The right vitreous shows some haze and the fundus presents confluent, deeply situated exudates, sheathing of the retinal vessels and miliary arterial aneurysms.
Three years later, the fundus lesion was complicated by a large retinal detachment.
General examination showed nothing abnormal.

Figure 382. Right eye. Coats' syndrome. There is a confluent, deeply situated yellowish-white exudate, on top of which there

are numerous microaneurysms and punctate retinal hemorrhages.

CLINICAL NOTE: Figure 382 is from a male, aged 51. During the last few years vision has gradually been reduced in the right eye. No complaints from the left eye. No general symptoms.
Eye examination: Visual acuity, right eye: hand movements; left eye: 6/6, emmetropia. Anterior segments and left fundus are normal. The right fundus shows extensive lesions typical for Coats' syndrome.
General examination showed nothing abnormal.

Figure 383. Left eye. Coats' syndrome. The fundus shows confluent, deeply situated exudates, several miliary arterial aneurysms and a small angiomatous tumor.

CLINICAL NOTE: Figure 383 is from a female, aged 11. Two months ago she experienced a severe reduction of vision in the left eye. No complaints from the right eye. No general symptoms.
Eye examination: Visual acuity, right eye: 6/6, emmetropia; left eye: 3/60, unimproved by lenses. Anterior segments and right fundus are normal. The left fundus shows extensive deeply situated exudates, numerous miliary arterial aneurysms and several small angiomatous tumors.
General examination showed no evidence of intracranial angiomas, but moderate cerebral atrophy and an abnormal electroencephalogram.

Figure 384. Left eye. Coats' syndrome. Leber's multiple miliary aneurysms. There are miliary arterial aneurysms, but only a few small exudates.

CLINICAL NOTE: Figure 384 is from a male, aged 20. Diabetes diagnosed two years ago. Since then insulin treatment. No ocular complaints.
Eye examination: Visual acuity, both eyes: 6/6, emmetropia. Anterior segments and right fundus are normal. The left fundus presents numerous miliary arterial aneurysms, but only a few small patches of exudate. No diabetic retinopathy.
A year later the fundus lesions were unchanged.
General examination showed diabetes without nephropathy or hypertension.

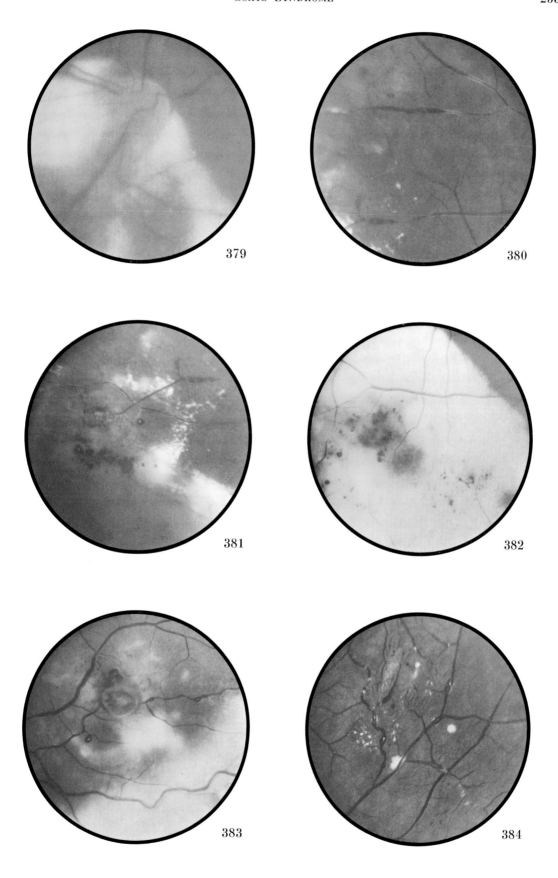

379

380

381

382

383

384

Figure 385. Right eye. Angioid streaks, seen as irregular red-brown and grayish bands around the disc. The disc and retinal vessels are normal.

CLINICAL NOTE: Figure 385 is from a male, aged 35. His sister has pseudoxanthoma elasticum and angioid streaks. He has always felt healthy and has had no ocular complaints.
Eye examination: Visual acuity, both eyes: 6/6, emmetropia. Anterior segments are normal. Both fundi present some angioid streaks.
General examination showed pseudoxanthoma elasticum and hypertension. Blood pressure: 200/110 mm Hg.

Figure 386. Right eye. Angioid streaks seen very plainly as irregular red-brown wavy anastomosing bands situated beneath the retinal vessels.

CLINICAL NOTE: Figure 386 is from the same patient as figure 388, a male, aged 24. He has always been healthy, and has no ocular or general complaints.
Eye examination: Visual acuity, both eyes: 6/6 with − 1.0 D sph. Anterior segments are normal. Both fundi present angioid streaks and peau d'orange configuration in the perimacular areas and the fundus peripheries.
General examination showed pseudoxanthoma elasticum.

Figure 387. Composite picture. Left eye. There are numerous angioid streaks nasally. Only a few angioid streaks traverse the macular area. In the perimacular area the fundus has assumed a peau d'orange configuration.

CLINICAL NOTE: Figure 387 is from a male, aged 25. His brother presents pseudoxanthoma elasticum and angioid streaks. He has had symptoms of gastroduodenal ulcer for several years. About one year ago he observed light streaks in the skin of the neck. He has been myopic since the age of 14. No visual complaints.

Eye examination: Visual acuity, both eyes: 6/6 with − 1.5 D sph. Anterior segments are normal. Both fundi present numerous angioid streaks and perimacular peau d'orange configuration.
General examination showed pseudoxanthoma elasticum. X-ray examinations showed gastroduodenal ulcer and arteriosclerosis of the vessels of the legs.

Figure 388. Left eye. Angioid streaks accompanied by irregular, wavy, deeply situated whitish lines of fibrous tissue. In the fundus periphery there is some mottling, assuming a peau d'orange-like configuration.

CLINICAL NOTE: Figure 388 is from the same patient as figure 386, a male, aged 24. For further clinical information, see clinical note to figure 386.

Figure 389. Right eye. Angioid streaks in the fundus periphery together with yellowish-white glistening dots, known as "salmon"-spots.

CLINICAL NOTE: Figure 389 is from the same patient as figures 392—394, a male, aged 46. Following a slight trauma to the right eye nine years ago vision was severely reduced in the right eye. Following a blunt injury to the left eye one year ago vision was also reduced severely in that eye. During the last few years he has developed some heart failure and intermittent claudication.
Eye examination: Visual acuity, right eye: 3/60 with + 1.0 D sph.; left eye: 6/60 with + 1.0 D sph. Anterior segments are normal. Both fundi present angioid streaks and macular involvement with scar tissue formation.
General examination showed pseudoxanthoma elasticum, some heart failure and intermittent claudication. Blood pressure: 140/85 mm Hg.

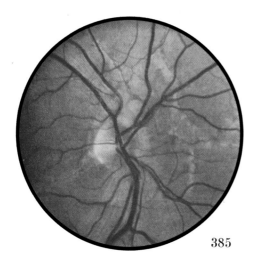

385

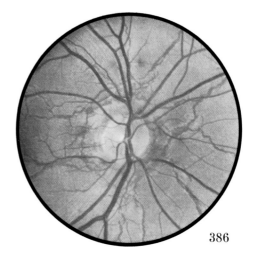

386

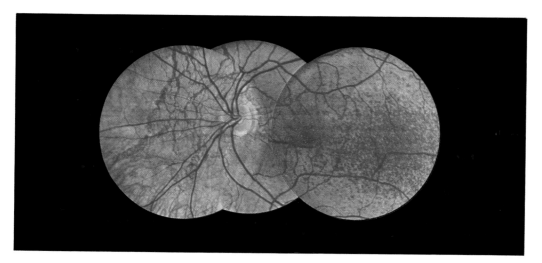

387

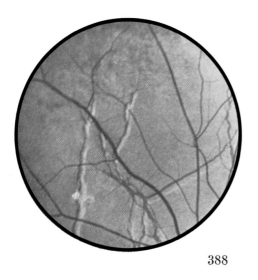

388

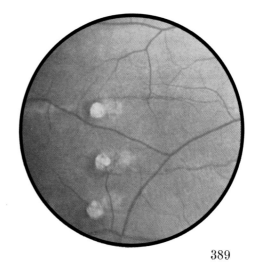

389

256   Angioid Streaks

Figure 390. Left eye. Macular subretinal hemorrhage and angioid streaks.

Figure 391. Same eye as figure 390, nine months later. The subretinal hemorrhage has been absorbed and has been replaced by a pigmented, atrophic scar. The scar is surrounded by some small hemorrhages.

Clinical note: Figures 390 and 391 are from a male, aged 45. A cousin has pseudoxanthoma elasticum and angioid streaks. He had a duodenal ulcer ten years ago. Four years ago, he experienced metamorphopsia in the right eye. After some time, this metamorphopsia was followed by an abrupt loss of vision. Some months ago he observed a reduction of vision in the left eye.
Eye examination at first admission: Visual acuity, right eye: 1/60; left eye: 6/18. Unimproved by lenses. Anterior segments are normal. Both fundi present angioid streaks. In the right macula there is a large chorioretinal scar. In the left macula there is a subretinal hemorrhage.
Eye examination, nine months later: Visual acuity, right eye: 1/60; left eye: 3/36. The lesions in the right fundus are unchanged. In the left macula the subretinal hemorrhage has been replaced by a pigmented, atrophic scar.
General examination showed pseudoxanthoma elasticum.

Figure 392. Left eye. Chorioretinal macular scar, early stage, and angioid streaks. The macular lesion is bordered by some hemorrhage.

Figure 393. Same eye as figure 392, two years later. The macular lesion is now converted into firm fibrous tissue with some pigmentation.

Figure 394. Right eye. From the same patient as figures 392—393. Extensive chorioretinal macular scarring in angioid streaks.

Clinical note: Figures 392—394 are from the same patient as figure 389, a male, aged 46. Following a slight trauma to the right eye nine years ago vision was severely reduced in the right eye. Following a blunt injury to the left eye one year ago vision was also reduced severely in that eye. During the last few years he has developed some heart failure and intermittent claudication.
Eye examination: Visual acuity, right eye: 3/60 with + 1.0 D sph.; left eye: 6/60 with +1.0 D sph. Anterior segments are normal. Both fundi present angioid streaks and macular involvement with scar tissue formation.
General examination showed pseudoxanthoma elasticum, some heart failure and intermittent claudication. Blood pressure: 140/85 mm Hg.

Figure 395. Right eye. Extensive, heavy chorioretinal atrophy in angioid streaks.

Clinical note: Figure 395 is from a female, aged 60. During the last ten years she has had several periods with symptoms of duodenal ulcer. Pseudoxanthoma elasticum was observed about 20 years ago. Since then vision has gradually decreased in both eyes.
Eye examination: Visual acuity, right eye: hand movements; left eye: 6/36. Unimproved by lenses. Anterior segments are normal. Both fundi present extensive chorioretinal atrophy with exposure of sclerosed choroidal vessels. Angioid streaks are not present.
General examination showed pseudoxanthoma elasticum and duodenal ulcer.

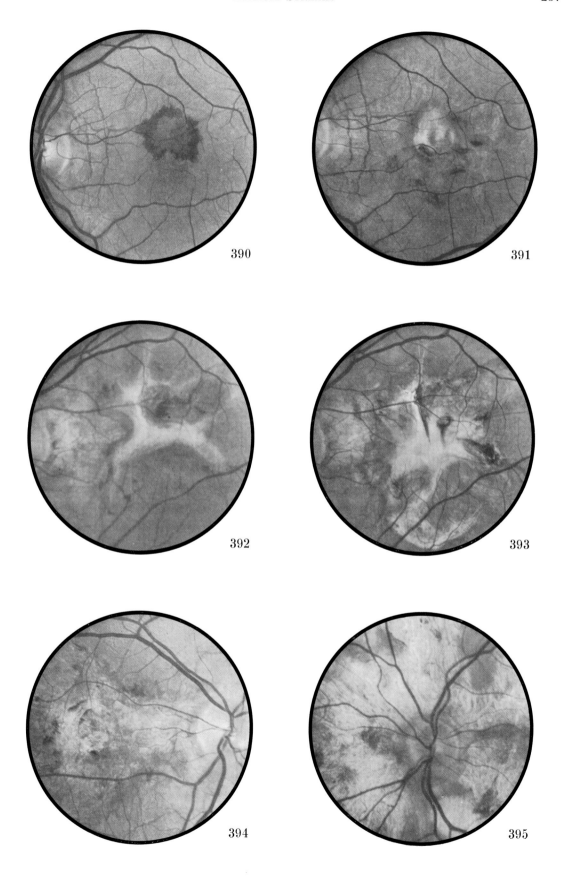

390

391

392

393

394

395

Figure 396. Left eye. Fundus changes in Eales' disease. Periphlebitis is seen as fluffy whitish exudates accompanying and partly obscuring the retinal veins.

CLINICAL NOTE: Figure 396 is from a male, aged 21. The last year he has had recurrent vitreous hemorrhages in both eyes. After the first attacks the vitreous cleared perfectly within a short time. After the last attack, however, dense opacities and blood remained in the right vitreous. No general complaints.
Eye examination: Visual acuity, right eye: 1/36, unimproved by lenses; left eye: 6/6, emmetropia. Anterior segments are normal. A dense vitreous haze obscures the right fundus. The left fundus shows massive periphlebitic changes and numerous small chorioretinal scars.
General examination, including blood studies, showed nothing abnormal. No signs of tuberculosis, toxoplasmosis or syphilis.

Figure 397. Right eye. Fundus changes in Eales' disease. Above, retinal veins are partly obscured by sheathing. There is also a single small tuft of new-formed vessels.

CLINICAL NOTE: Figure 397 is from a male, aged 36. During the last year he has had several vitreous hemorrhages in the left eye. No complaints from the right eye. No general symptoms.
Eye examination: Visual acuity, right eye: 6/6, emmetropia; left eye: light perception. Anterior segments are normal. The right fundus shows perivasculitis and small tufts of new-formed vessels in the fundus periphery. Left fundus is obscured by vitreous hemorrhage.
General examination, including blood studies, showed nothing abnormal.

Figure 398. Right eye. Fundus changes in Eales' disease. In the fundus periphery, there is an elongated preretinal vascular proliferation and above this there is a fine veil of fibrous tissue.

Figure 399. Left eye. From the same patient as figure 398. Fundus periphery showing sheathing of retinal vessels and a small preretinal mass of fibrous tissue.

CLINICAL NOTE: Figures 398 and 399 are from a male, aged 55. As a child he had left strabismus. Since then, the left eye has been ambly-

opic. The last eight years he has had recurrent vitreous hemorrhages in both eyes. For about five years the left fundus has been obscured by vitreous hemorrhage, but after that time the vitreous has cleared up gradually.
Eye examination: Visual acuity, right eye: 6/24; left eye: 6/9. Unimproved by lenses. Anterior segments are normal. Both vitreous bodies show opacities, and fundi present extensive perivasculitis and some new-vessel proliferation and connective tissue formation in the periphery.
General examination, including blood studies, showed nothing abnormal.

Figure 400. Right eye. Fundus changes in multiple sclerosis. The retinal veins are more or less obscured by fluffy whitish exudates, which ensheath the veins for some distance.

CLINICAL NOTE: Figure 400 is from a female, aged 33. During the last year she has had two attacks of retrobulbar neuritis in the right eye and she presents signs of multiple sclerosis.
Eye examination: Visual acuity, both eyes: 6/6, emmetropia. Anterior segments are normal. Both fundi present periphlebitic changes. The optic discs are normal. Visual fields are normal.
General examination, including neurological examination, showed signs of multiple sclerosis.

Figure 401. Right eye. Fundus changes in multiple sclerosis. The vein is accompanied by whitish exudates which partly ensheath the vessel. The arteries are normal.

CLINICAL NOTE: Figure 401 is from a male, aged 42. Twenty-seven years ago he had transient diplopia. Twenty years ago he developed transient signs of multiple sclerosis. Three years ago the neurological symptoms recurred, and they have progressed steadily since then. No ocular complaints.
Eye examination: Visual acuity, both eyes: 6/6, emmetropia. Eye movements are normal. No diplopia. Anterior segments are normal. Both fundi present periphlebitic changes. The discs are normal.
General examination, including neurological examination, showed signs of multiple sclerosis.

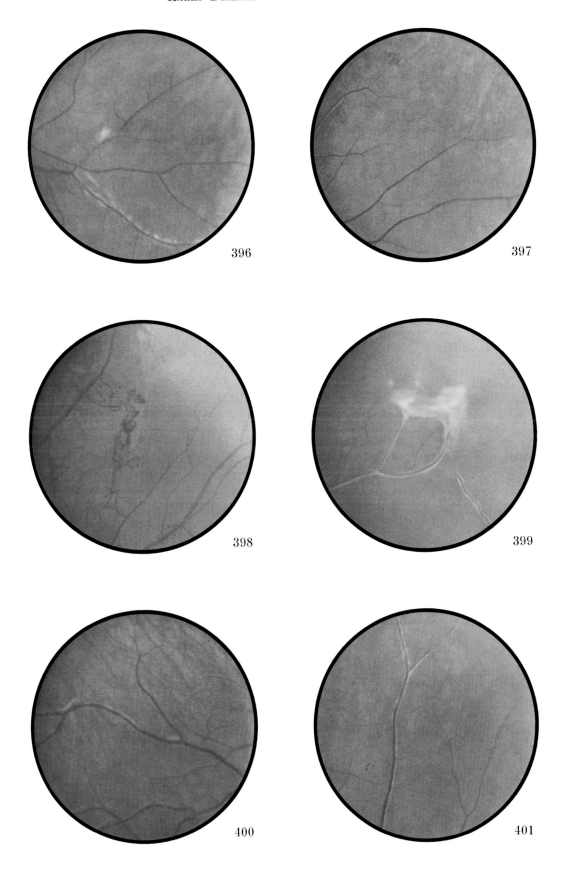

396

397

398

399

400

401

Figure 402. Left eye. Uveitis and choroiditis with macular edema.

Clinical note: Figure 402 is from the same patient as figures 414—415, a male, aged 14. Since early childhood central choroiditis and amblyopia have been observed in the right eye. Six days ago he observed hazy vision in the left eye. No general complaints.
Eye examination, acute stage: Visual acuity, right eye: 6/60, unimproved by lenses; left eye: 6/24 with + 2.0 D sph. Right divergent strabismus of about 10°. Eye movements are normal. Right anterior segment is normal. The right fundus presents a chorioretinal scar in the macula. The left anterior chamber shows some aqueous flare and precipitates. The fundus is partly obscured by vitreous haze and opacities. In the fundus there is a juxtapapillary choroiditis and massive retinal edema. Right visual field shows central scotoma, and the left a centrocecal scotoma.
General examination showed toxoplasmosis.

Figure 403. Right eye. Periphlebitis in uveitis. The retinal vein is partly hidden by fluffy whitish exudates.

Clinical note: Figure 403 is from a female, aged 43. During the last three years she has had several attacks of iridocyclitis in both eyes. After the last attack she has developed low-grade chronic posterior uveitis. No general complaints.
Eye examination: Visual acuity, both eyes: 6/6, emmetropia. Anterior segments show no sequelae after the iridocyclitis. Both vitreous bodies show some opacities and slight haze. In both fundi there is some periphlebitis.
She received steroid therapy for some months.
Eye examination, six months later: The vitreous opacities and the vitreous haze have disappeared and the retinal veins have become normal.
General examination showed nothing abnormal.

Figures 404 and 405. Right and left eyes. Sequelae after uveitis. Both maculae present hard exudates following an inflammatory retinal edema.

Clinical note: Figures 404 and 405 are from a male, aged 46. Two months ago he developed bilateral iridocyclitis. Following systemic steroid therapy, the reaction in the anterior segments disappeared quickly, while vitreous haze and retinal edema persisted for about six weeks. No general complaints.
Eye examination: Visual acuity, right eye: 6/18; left eye: 6/36. Unimproved by lenses. Anterior segments show only slight sequelae after the iridocyclitis. Both maculae present hard exudates. Discs and retinal vessels are normal.
General examination showed nothing abnormal. Blood pressure: 130/85 mm Hg.

Figure 406. Right eye. Preretinal vitreous opacities in sarcoidosis, seen as small opaque, whitish masses, partly obscuring the retina.

Clinical note: Figure 406 is from a male, aged 50. Eleven years ago sarcoidosis was diagnosed. No visual complaints until two weeks ago, when he observed hazy vision in the left eye.
Eye examination: Visual acuity, right eye: 6/6 with − 0.5 D cyl. axis 0°; left eye: 6/18 with — 0.5 D cyl. axis 0°. Right anterior segment is normal, the left shows precipitates of the cornea and aqueous flare. In both eyes there are dense preretinal vitreous opacities. Both fundi present periphlebitis. The optic discs are normal. There is slight edema in the left macular area.
General examination showed sarcoidosis.

Figure 407. Left eye. Synchysis scintillans. Innumerable small, round, yellowish-white glistening opacities are seen in the vitreous. The disc and retinal vessels are seen faintly.

Clinical note: Figure 407 is from a female, aged 48. Diabetes demonstrated 18 years ago. Insulin treatment since then. Simple diabetic retinopathy was observed one year ago. The last few months she has experienced hazy vision in the left eye. No complaints from the right eye.
Eye examination: Visual acuity, right eye: 6/6, emmetropia; left eye: 6/18, unimproved by lenses. Anterior segments are normal. The right vitreous is normal, the left shows synchysis scintillans. Both fundi present simple diabetic retinopathy.
General examination showed diabetes without nephropathy. Blood pressure: 130/70 mm Hg. Serum cholesterol: 210 mg/100 ml.

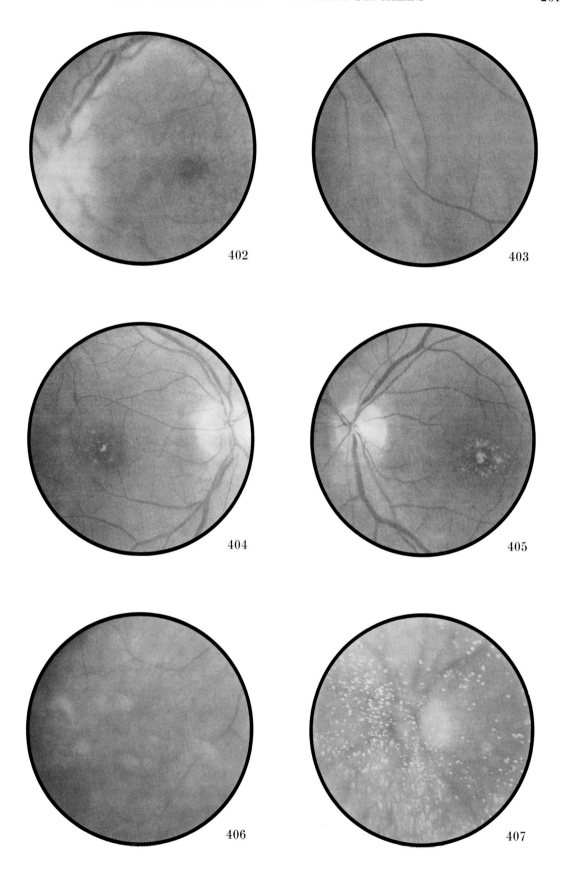

Figure 408. Left eye. Acute retinal peri-arteritis with ensheathing of retinal arteries and fluffy exudates.

Figure 409. Same eye as figure 408, one year later. The fluffy exudates and most of the retinal arterial sheathing have disappeared, but the retinal arteries still show slight caliber variations.

CLINICAL NOTE: Figures 408 and 409 are from a male, aged 68. About one year ago he observed some blurring of vision in the left eye. No complaints from the right eye. No general symptoms.
Eye examination, acute stage: Visual acuity, right eye: 6/6, emmetropia; left eye: 6/9 with − 0.5 D sph. Anterior segments are normal. The right fundus is normal. The left fundus presents heavy periarteritis and some cotton-wool exudates.
Eye examination, one year later: The arterial sheathing has nearly disappeared, but retinal arteries show variations in caliber.
General examination showed nothing abnormal. Blood pressure: 140/80 mm Hg.

Figure 410. Left eye. Posterior uveitis and retinal periarteritis, acute stage. Around the disc there are several ill-defined whitish, fluffy infiltrates. The retinal arteries show heavy sheathing, and there is some vitreous haze.

Figure 411. Same eye as figure 410, three years later. Nasally, there is now a large chorioretinal atrophy with some pigmentation.

Figure 412. Left eye. Posterior uveitis and retinal periarteritis, acute stage. There is a whitish infiltrate at the disc and retinal arteries show heavy sheathing.

Figure 413. Same eye as figure 412, three years later (15°). The retinal arteries still show some sheathing.

CLINICAL NOTE: Figures 410—413 are from a female, aged 39. About three years ago she developed retrobulbar pain and hazy vision in the left eye. No complaints from the right eye. No general symptoms.
Eye examination, acute stage: Visual acuity, both eyes: 6/6, emmetropia. Anterior segments and the right fundus are normal. The left eye presents vitreous haze, acute choroiditis and retinal periarteritis.
Eye examination, three years later: The left fundus shows a chorioretinal scar and some sheathing of the retinal vessels. The right eye is normal. Vision unchanged.
General examination showed nothing abnormal.

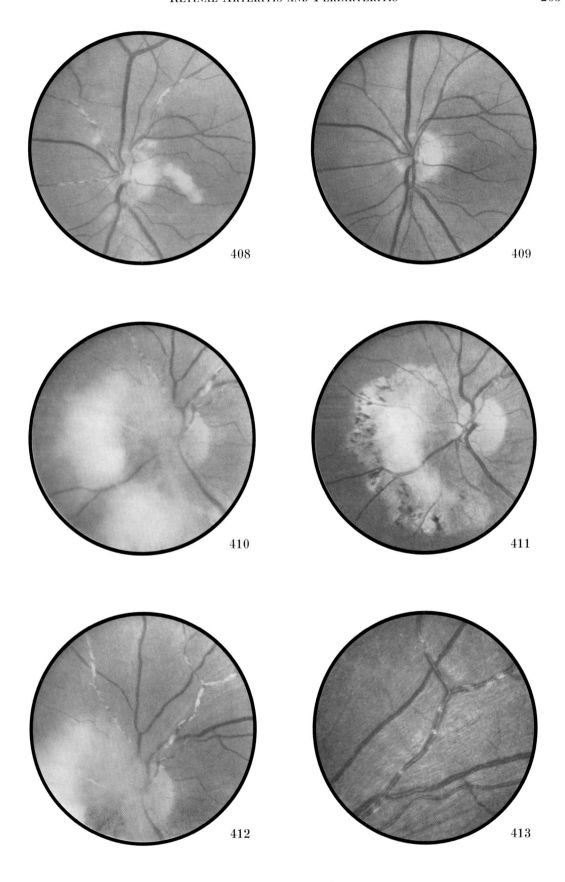

408

409

410

411

412

413

*Figure 414. Left eye. Juxtapapillary cho-
roiditis, acute stage. The optic disc and the
peripapillary area are obscured by some
vitreous haze, massive yellowish-white retinal edema and a fluffy exudate.*

*Figure 415. Same eye as figure 414, six
years later. Juxtapapillary choroiditis, scar
stage.*

CLINICAL NOTE: Figures 414 and 415 are from
the same eye as figure 402, a male, aged 14.
Since early childhood central choroiditis and
amblyopia have been observed in the right eye.
Six days ago he observed hazy vision in the
left eye. No general complaints.
Eye examination, acute stage: Visual acuity,
right eye: 6/60, unimproved by lenses; left eye:
6/24 with + 2.0 D sph. Right divergent strabismus of about 10°. Eye movements are normal.
Right anterior segment is normal. The right
fundus presents a chorioretinal scar in the macula. The left anterior chamber shows some
aqueous flare and precipitates. The fundus is
partly obscured by vitreous haze and opacities.
In the fundus there is a juxtapapillary choroiditis and massive retinal edema. Right visual field shows central scotoma, and the left a
centrocecal scotoma.
General examination in the acute stage showed
a positive toxoplasmosis reaction.
Eye examination, six years later: The left fundus shows a juxtapapillary chorioretinal scar.

*Figure 416. Left eye. Central choroiditis,
acute stage. In the macular area there is an
ill-defined whitish patch of exudate, some
edema and a chorioretinal scar.*

*Figure 417. Same eye as figure 416, two
years later. The fundus shows central choroiditis in scar stage.*

CLINICAL NOTE: Figures 416 and 417 are from
a female, aged 10. During the last week she has
complained of hazy vision in the left eye. No
complaints from the right eye. No general
symptoms.
Eye examination: Visual acuity, right eye: 6/6,
emmetropia; left eye: 1/60, unimproved by
lenses. Anterior segments and right fundus are

normal. The left fundus presents an acute central choroiditis and a chorioretinal scar. Left
visual field shows a central scotoma.
Eye examination, two years later: Central choroiditis in scar stage.
General examination, including blood studies,
showed nothing abnormal.

*Figure 418. Right eye. Central choroiditis,
acute stage. In the macular area there is a
deeply situated, ill-defined yellowish-white
patch of exudate, some edema and two chorioretinal scars.*

*Figure 419. Same eye as figure 418, one
month later. Choroiditis in the healing
stage. The fundal edema has subsided, and
the exudate has decreased in size. The lesion is partly transformed into a chorioretinal scar.*

CLINICAL NOTE: Figures 418 and 419 are from a
female, aged 19. She has been BCG-vaccinated
three times. Just after the last vaccination,
about four years ago, she had a period with
fever, but at that time she had no ocular complaints. She is now six months pregnant. A
fortnight ago she observed hazy vision in the
right eye. No complaints from the left eye. No
general symptoms.
Eye examination in the acute stage: Visual acuity, right eye: hand movements; left eye: 6/6
with − 2.5 D sph. The right anterior chamber
shows some aqueous flare, but no precipitates
or nodules in the iris. Left anterior segment is
normal. The right vitreous shows many opacities, and the fundus presents acute central
choroiditis and chorioretinal scars. The left
vitreous is normal, but in the fundus there are
some chorioretinal scars above the disc. Visual
fields show scotomas corresponding to the fundal lesions.
Eye examination after systemic steroid therapy
for one month: The anterior segments are normal. There are still some opacities in the right
vitreous. The choroiditis is in the healing
stage. Five months later the fundus lesion was
converted into a chorioretinal scar.
General examination showed nothing abnormal. No signs of tuberculosis, toxoplasmosis or
syphilis.

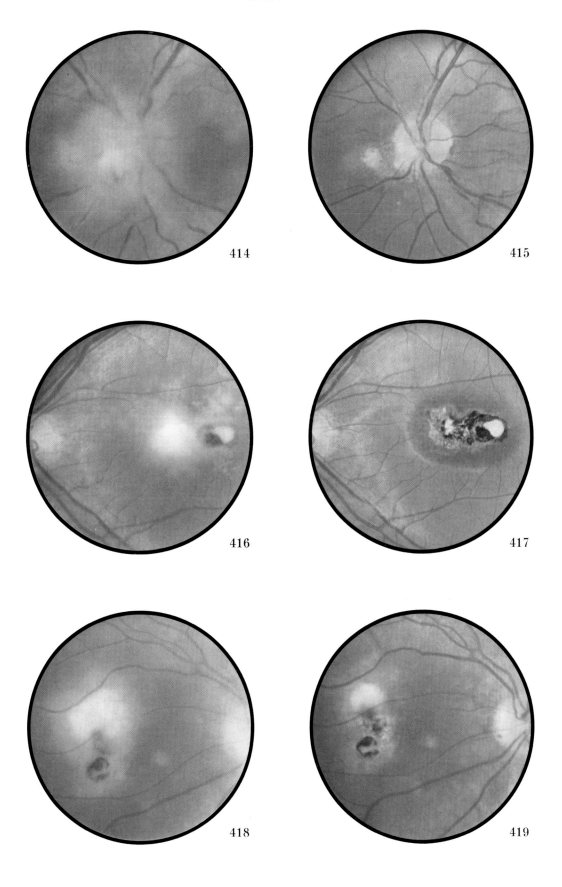

414

415

416

417

418

419

Figure 420. Right eye. Central choroiditis, scar stage. A whitish chorioretinal scar with dense pigmentation centrally is seen in the macular area.

CLINICAL NOTE: Figure 420 is from a female, aged 19. On routine examination three years ago, an old central choroiditis was observed in the right eye. No general symptoms.
Eye examination: Visual acuity, right eye: 6/60, unimproved by lenses; left eye: 6/6, emmetropia. Anterior segments are normal. In the right fundus there is a central chorioretinal scar. Left fundus is normal.
General examination showed nothing abnormal.

Figure 421. Right eye. Central choroiditis, scar stage. The lesion consists of an atrophic scar, which is partly obscured by a large pigment accumulation. A rounded pigment patch is also seen below the upper temporal vessels.

CLINICAL NOTE: Figure 421 is from a female, aged 23. Since the age of 12 years vision has been slightly reduced in her right eye and seriously reduced in her left eye. No complaints of general illness.
Eye examination: Visual acuity, right eye: 6/9; left eye: 3/36. Unimproved by lenses. Anterior segments are normal. The right vitreous is normal, the left contains dense opacities, which partly obscure the fundus. Both fundi present chorioretinal scars in the macular area.
General examination showed nothing abnormal. No signs of tuberculosis, toxoplasmosis or syphilis.

Figure 422. Right eye. Circumscribed choroiditis, scar stage. There is an atrophic chorioretinal lesion bordered by pigmentation. In the central part of the lesion, there is a fluffy exudate.

CLINICAL NOTE: Figure 422 is from a female, aged 22. Fifteen years ago she developed left divergent squint, and a central chorioretinal scar was found in the left eye. Five years ago she had acute iridocyclitis and choroiditis in the right eye. The Sabin-Feldman reaction was positive, and she reacted well to specific therapy. A week ago, she suddenly observed hazy vision in the right eye.
Eye examination: Visual acuity, right eye: < 6/6; left eye: 6/36. Unimproved by lenses. Left divergent squint of about 10°. Anterior segments are normal. The right vitreous shows some haze, the left is normal. The right fundus shows a chorioretinal scar with a fluffy exudate centrally. The left fundus presents a macular chorioretinal scar.

General examination showed a slightly positive toxoplasmosis reaction.

Figure 423. Right eye. Circumscribed choroiditis, scar stage. There are two whitish chorioretinal scars, bordered by some pigment.

CLINICAL NOTE: Figure 423 is from a female, aged 16. At the age of seven years she had tuberculous meningitis, which was followed by bilateral choroiditis. After the acute stage, vision regained its normal acuity. No general symptoms.
Eye examination: Visual acuity, both eyes: 6/6, emmetropia. Anterior segments are normal. Both fundi present several chorioretinal scars.
General examination showed no sequelae after tuberculous meningitis.

Figure 424. Left eye. Old central choroiditis with massive pigmentation.

CLINICAL NOTE: Figure 424 is from a female, aged 21. Bilateral choroiditis was observed at the age of six years. During the last month she has experienced hazy vision in the right eye. No general symptoms.
Eye examination: Visual acuity, right eye: 6/36; left eye: 1/36. Unimproved by lenses. Anterior segments are normal. The right vitreous body presents a dense haze, which partly obscures the fundus, the left is normal. In the right fundus there are large fluffy exudates and retinal edema. The left fundus presents a chorioretinal scar in the macula.
General examination showed nothing abnormal. The Sabin-Feldman dye test was positive in 1:1,250 and complement fixation test positive in 1:16.

Figure 425. Right eye. Central choroiditis, scar stage. The macular lesion consists of a grayish center surrounded by two rings of pigment, which are connected by pigment like spokes in a wheel.

CLINICAL NOTE: Figure 425 is from a male, aged 10. His mother was well during pregnancy, and he was normal at birth. Since infancy chorioretinal scars have been observed in both eyes.
Eye examination: Visual acuity, right eye: 1/36; left eye: < 6/6 with − 1.0 D sph. Anterior segments are normal. The right fundus shows a large chorioretinal scar in the macular area, and the left fundus presents chorioretinal scars outside the macula.
General examination showed nothing abnormal. The Sabin-Feldman dye test was slightly positive in 1:10.

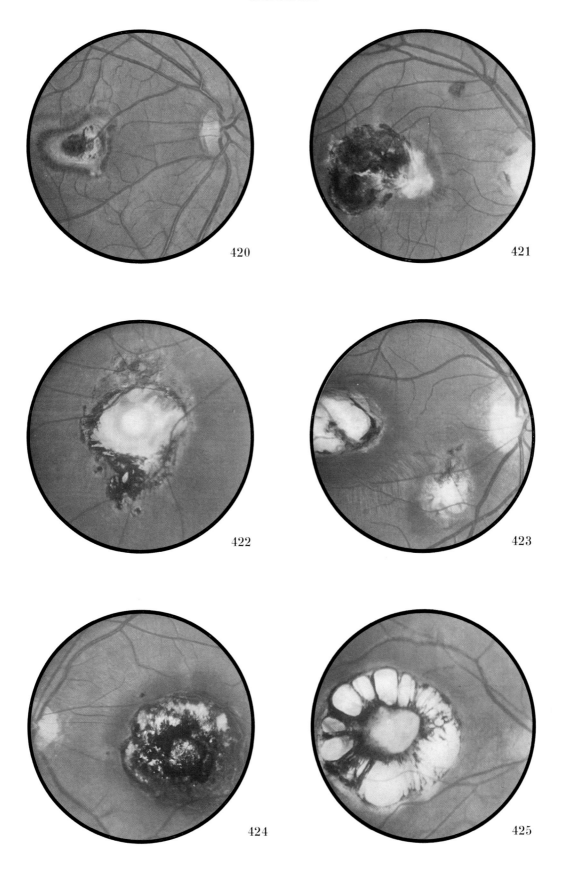

420

421

422

423

424

425

Figure 426. Right eye. Disseminated cho-roiditis, scar stage. There are pale, ill-de-fined patches of choroidal atrophy and some patchy pigment clumping.

CLINICAL NOTE: Figure 426 is from a male, aged 59. Twenty-four years ago he had undulant fever and bilateral uveitis. Since then vision has been reduced. Seven years ago he had a perforating injury of the left eye. After some time the eye was enucleated.
Eye examination: Visual acuity, right eye: 3/36, unimproved by lenses; left eye: anophthalmos. Right anterior chamber is normal. There is incipient cataract. The fundus presents an old disseminated choroiditis.
General examination showed nothing abnormal.

Figures 427 and 428. Same left eye. Dis-seminated choroiditis, scar stage. The fun-dus presents multiple atrophic chorioreti-nal scars with pigment accumulation and exposure of the choroidal vessels.

Figure 429. Same eye as figures 427 and 428. The optic disc is surrounded by ex-tensive chorioretinal atrophy and some pig-ment accumulation.

CLINICAL NOTE: Figures 427—429 are from a male, aged 56. A serious reduction of vision in the right eye was observed by chance about 20 years ago, and an old disseminated cho-roiditis was demonstrated. Ten years ago he had choroiditis in the left eye. Since then vision has been slightly reduced in this eye.
Eye examination: Visual acuity, right eye: 1/60, unimproved by lenses; left eye: < 6/9 with − 1.0 D sph. Anterior segments are normal. Both fundi present disseminated chorioretinal scars. The discs and retinal vessels are normal. Visual fields show numerous scotomas.
General examination showed nothing abnormal. No signs of tuberculosis, toxoplasmosis or syphilis.

Figure 430. Composite picture, right eye. Disseminated choroiditis, scar stage. The fundus shows extensive chorioretinal atro-phy with pigment clumping and exposure of the whitish sclera.

CLINICAL NOTE: Figure 430 is from a male, aged 34. Eight years ago he had acute bilateral cho-roiditis. Three years ago he had a new attack. During both attacks he received systemic cor-tisone treatment with some result.
Eye examination: Visual acuity, right eye: 1/24, unimproved by lenses; left eye: 6/18 with − 1.0 D sph. Anterior segments are normal. Both fundi present old disseminated choroidi-tis. The discs and retinal vessels are normal. Visual fields show numerous scotomas.
General examination showed nothing abnor-mal. No signs of tuberculosis, toxoplasmosis or syphilis.

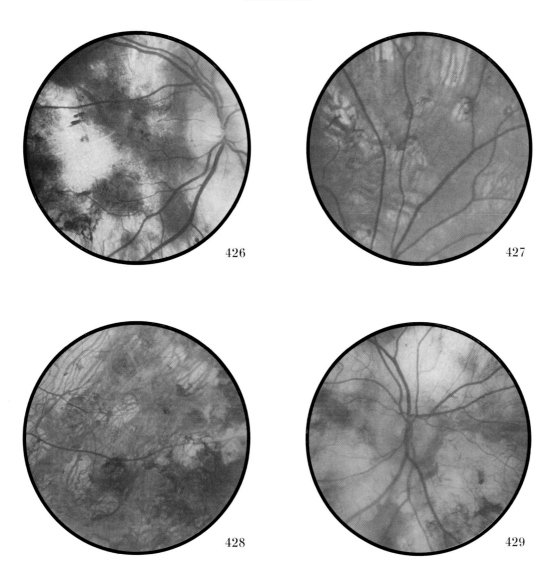

426

427

428

429

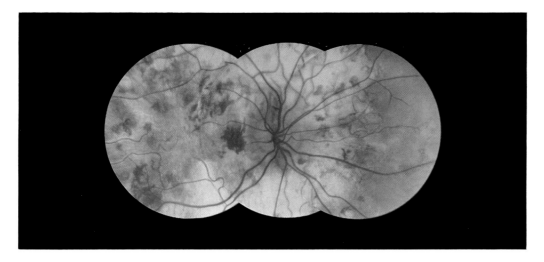

430

Figure 431. Left eye. Diffuse choroiditis, scar stage. The fundus shows numerous small patchy atrophies and some pigment clumping. Below, there is a small distinct chorioretinal scar.

CLINICAL NOTE: Figure 431 is from a male, aged 9. His mother had rubella when she was two months pregnant. He has developed normally, but his vision has always been defective.
Eye examination: Visual acuity, both eyes: 6/12. Unimproved by lenses. Anterior segments are normal. No cataract. Both fundi present old diffuse choroiditis.
General examination showed nothing abnormal.

Figure 432. Left eye. Diffuse choroiditis, scar stage. The fundus has assumed a salt-and-pepper appearance with numerous pinpoint pigmentations and atrophies.

CLINICAL NOTE: Figure 432 is from a female, aged 10. Her mother had rubella when she was two months pregnant. At birth her right eye was microphthalmic and later she developed cataract in that eye. She has had irregular nystagmus since the age of one year. Five years ago she was operated on for persistent ductus arteriosus and pulmonary valvular stenosis with good result. The cataract was needled two years ago.
Eye examination: Visual acuity, right eye: hand movements; left eye: 6/12 with − 0.5 D cyl. axis 35°. Right eye is microphthalmic and shows some membranaceous cataract. There is slight irregular nystagmus. The left fundus shows diffuse salt-and-pepper choroiditis.
General examination showed sequelae after the heart operation.

Figure 433. Right eye (15°). Diffuse choroiditis, scar stage. There are numerous small chorioretinal scars with atrophy and pigment clumping.

CLINICAL NOTE: Figure 433 is from a female, aged 57. Some years ago she experienced some blurring of vision in the right eye, but in the course of some months vision became normal again. Since then she has had no visual or general complaints.
Eye examination: Visual acuity, both eyes: 6/6 with − 1.0 D sph. Anterior segments and the left fundus are normal. The right fundus pre-sents an old diffuse choroiditis, leaving the macula free. The electroretinogram is normal.
General examination showed nothing abnormal.

Figure 434. Left eye. Diffuse choroiditis with some pigment clumping, scar stage.

CLINICAL NOTE: Figure 434 is from a female, aged 59. One year ago diabetes was diagnosed. Since then treated with oral antidiabetic drugs. During the last year vision in her left eye has decreased rapidly. No complaints from the right eye.
Eye examination: Visual acuity, right eye: 6/6 with + 1.0 D sph.; left eye: light perception. Anterior segments are normal. The right fundus shows slight senile macular degeneration and the left fundus presents an old diffuse choroiditis.
General examination showed diabetes without nephropathy or hypertension.

Figure 435. Right eye. Diffuse choroiditis, scar stage. The fundus shows diffuse chorioretinal atrophy with pallor of the fundus, pigment clumping, sclerosis of the choroidal vessels and marked narrowing of the retinal vessels. The disc is dirty-pink, atrophic and slightly cupped.

Figure 436. Same eye as figure 435. The nasal periphery shows heavy choroidal sclerosis and marked pigment accumulation.

CLINICAL NOTE: Figures 435 and 436 are from a female, aged 63. At the age of 29 years she had an infection of the genital organs. Five years later she observed a gradual reduction of vision in both eyes, but it was not until another five years had elapsed, when she first consulted a doctor, that syphilis, syphilitic choroiditis and optic atrophy were diagnosed. Antisyphilitic treatment was given for many years, but the fundus changes and vision remained unaltered. During the last few years vision has decreased to light perception.
Eye examination: Visual acuity, both eyes: light perception. Both lenses show immature nuclear and cortical cataract. Both fundi present severe chorioretinal atrophy with pigment clumping. The discs are atrophic.
General examination showed a woman in the tertiary stage of syphilis. The Wassermann reaction was ±. Blood pressure: 150/100 mm Hg.

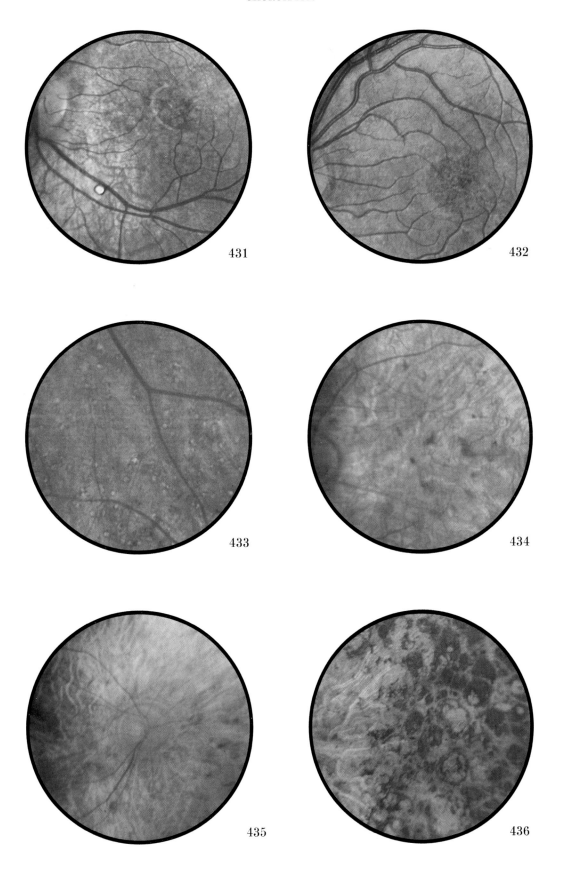

431

432

433

434

435

436

Figure 437. Right eye. Retinochoroiditis juxtapapillaris, acute stage. At the disc and below there are fluffy whitish exudates, and retinal vessels show some sheathing.

Figure 438. Same eye as figure 437, four years later. The exudates are converted into whitish scars. Below, the scar is surrounded by some pigment. The lower retinal artery still shows some sheathing.

CLINICAL NOTE: Figures 437 and 438 are from a female, aged 36. Four years ago she experienced some blurring of vision in the right eye and juxtapapillary retinochoroiditis was observed. No complaints from the left eye. No general symptoms.
Eye examination, acute stage: Visual acuity, right eye: < 6/6 with + 0.5 D sph.; left eye: 6/6 with + 0.5 D sph. Right anterior chamber shows slight aqueous flare and some precipitates, the left is normal. The right fundus presents an acute retinochoroiditis and there is a sector-formed scotoma extending from the blind spot. The left fundus is normal.
Eye examination, four years later: Visual acuity, both eyes: 6/6 with + 0.5 D sph. The juxtapapillary retinochoroiditis is in the scar stage and visual field defect is unaltered.
General examination showed nothing abnormal.

Figure 439. Left eye. Retinochoroiditis juxtapapillaris, acute stage. There is some vitreous haze. At the nasal side of the disc there is a fluffy whitish exudate.

Figure 440. Same eye as figure 439, three years later. There is still slight vitreous haze above, but the exudate has been converted into chorioretinal scars.

CLINICAL NOTE: Figures 439 and 440 are from a male, aged 42. Three years ago he experienced some blurring of vision in the left eye and juxtapapillary retinochoroiditis was observed. No complaints from the right eye. No general symptoms.
Eye examination, acute stage: Visual acuity, right eye: 6/6, emmetropia; left eye: < 6/6, em-

metropia. Right anterior segment is normal, the left shows some corneal precipitates. The right fundus is normal, the left presents an acute juxtapapillary retinochoroiditis and there is a sector-formed scotoma extending from the blind spot.
Eye examination, three years later: Visual acuity, both eyes: 6/6, emmetropia. Anterior segments are normal. The juxtapapillary retinochoroiditis is in the scar stage and visual field defect is unaltered.
General examination showed nothing abnormal.

Figure 441. Left eye. Retinochoroiditis juxtapapillaris, acute and scar stage. There is some vitreous haze. Just above the disc there is a fluffy exudate, and nasally there are some retinal hemorrhages. Above the fluffy exudate there is a chorioretinal scar.

CLINICAL NOTE: Figure 441 is from a male, aged 24. During the last week he has experienced some hazy vision in both eyes. No general symptoms.
Eye examination: Visual acuity, right eye: 6/18; left eye: 6/12. Unimproved by lenses. Anterior segments are normal. Both vitreous bodies show some haze and opacities. Both fundi present juxtapapillary retinochoroiditis and there are sector-formed visual field defects extending from the blind spots.
General examination showed nothing abnormal.

Figure 442. Right eye. Retinochoroiditis juxtapapillaris, scar stage. There is a large chorioretinal scar in the lower nasal quadrant. The disc and retinal vessels are normal.

CLINICAL NOTE: Figure 442 is from a male, aged 66. Many years ago he had several attacks of hazy vision in the right eye. Since then he has had no ocular complaints.
Eye examination: Visual acuity, both eyes: 6/6 with + 2.0 D sph. Anterior segments are normal. The right fundus presents a large juxtapapillary chorioretinal scar, the left is normal. Right visual field shows sector-formed scotoma extending from the blind spot.
General examination showed nothing abnormal.

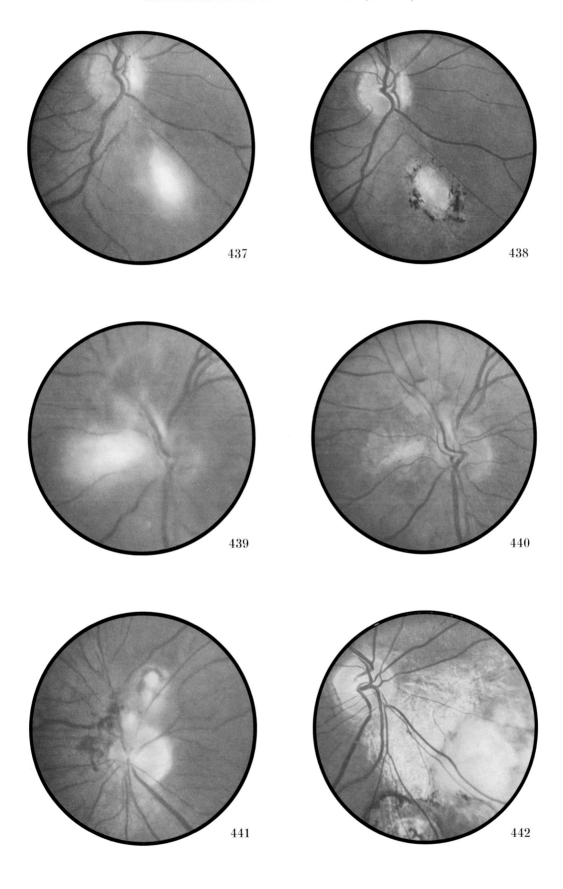

437

438

439

440

441

442

Figure 443. Right eye. Retinoschisis. The superficial layers of the retina are slightly elevated and between these layers and the profound layers there is a fine network of whitish connective tissue and some small cystic spaces.

CLINICAL NOTE: Figure 443 is from a male, aged 59. During the last year he has experienced a shadow in the lower part of the right visual field. No complaints from the left eye.
Eye examination: Visual acuity, both eyes: 6/6, emmetropia. Anterior segments are normal. The right fundus presents retinoschisis in the upper part of the fundus, while the lower part is normal. The left fundus is normal. Visual field defect corresponds to the fundus lesion.
General examination showed nothing abnormal.

Figure 444. Left eye. Retinoschisis, seen as fine, branching, whitish, intraretinal demarcation lines. Below, the retina is slightly elevated.

CLINICAL NOTE: Figure 444 is from a female, aged 23. Six months ago she experienced hazy vision in the left eye. No complaints from the right eye.
Eye examination: Visual acuity, right eye: 6/6, emmetropia; left eye: 6/36 with − 1.0 D sph. Anterior segments are normal. The right fundus is normal, the left presents retinoschisis and a retinal cyst in the lower temporal quadrant and a retinal detachment extending from 2 to 6 o'clock. There is a visual field defect corresponding to the fundus lesion.
General examination showed nothing abnormal.

Figures 445 and 446. Same right eye. Retinoschisis, seen as fine, branching, whitish intraretinal lines and diffuse whitish veils.

CLINICAL NOTE: Figures 445 and 446 are from a female, aged 22. She has been myopic since the age of 15. About six months ago she experienced reduced vision in the right eye. No complaints from the left eye.
Eye examination: Visual acuity, right eye: 6/60 with − 2.5 D sph.; left eye: 6/6 with − 2.5 D sph. Anterior segments are normal. The right fundus presents retinoschisis in the lower quadrants and the macula is involved. The left fundus is normal. Visual field defect corresponds to the fundal lesion.
General examination showed nothing abnormal.

Figures 447 and 448. Same right eye. Retinoschisis and retinal cyst. There are several whitish intraretinal lines, and below, there is a grayish-pink elevated area, a retinal cyst.

CLINICAL NOTE: Figures 447 and 448 are from a male, aged 27. During some months he has observed some hazy vision in the right eye. No complaints from the left eye.
Eye examination: Visual acuity, right eye: 6/12 with − 2.75 D sph.; left eye: 6/6 with − 2.5 D sph. Anterior segments are normal. The right fundus presents retinoschisis and a retinal cyst in the lower nasal quadrant. The left fundus is normal. Visual field defect corresponds to the fundal lesion.
General examination showed nothing abnormal.

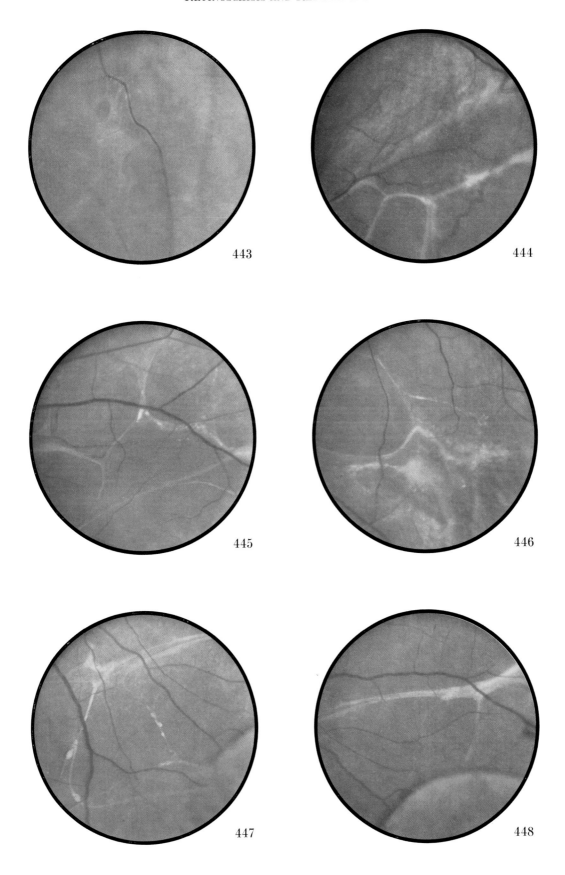

443

444

445

446

447

448

Figure 449. Left eye. Ruptured retinal cyst. The cyst has ruptured through the oval hole. The surface of the ruptured cyst is uneven as indicated by the curled retinal vessel.

CLINICAL NOTE: Figure 449 is from a male, aged 46. He had been healthy until a week ago, when he felt as if a curtain were drawn in front of his left eye. No complaints from the right eye. No known ocular trauma.
Eye examination: Visual acuity, right eye: 6/6 with + 1.0 D sph.; left eye: 2/36, unimproved by lenses. Anterior segments are normal. The right fundus presents retinoschisis in the lower temporal quadrant. The left fundus presents retinoschisis and a retinal cyst with a hole in the lower temporal quadrant, and there is a retinal detachment extending from 2 to 8 o'clock. Visual field defects correspond to the fundal lesions.
General examination showed nothing abnormal.

Figure 450. Left eye. A retinal cyst surrounded by retinal detachment.

CLINICAL NOTE: Figure 450 is from a female, aged 38. During the last month she has experienced some hazy vision in the left eye, and the last week she has observed a shadow in the visual field. No complaints from the right eye. No known ocular trauma.
Eye examination: Visual acuity, right eye: 6/6 with + 1.0 D sph.; left eye: 6/9 with + 1.0 D sph. Anterior segments and the right fundus are normal. The left fundus presents a retinal cyst surrounded by retinal detachment in the upper nasal quadrant. Visual field defect corresponds to the detachment.
General examination showed nothing abnormal.

Figures 451 and 452. Same right eye. Choroidal detachment. The detached area is slightly elevated. The surface shows fine striation and the color is grayish-red in contrast to the normal fundus color. Retinal vessels appear normal.

CLINICAL NOTE: Figures 451 and 452 are from a male, aged 58. Two years ago intracapsular cataract extraction was performed in the left eye. One month ago the same operation was performed in the right eye. A week ago, he observed hazy vision in the right eye.
Eye examination: Visual acuity, right eye: 6/18 with + 11.0 D sph.; left eye: < 6/6 with + 11.0 D sph. Anterior segments show aphakia. The right fundus presents a nearly ring-shaped choroidal detachment, but no retinal detachment. Visual field defect corresponds to the fundal lesion. The left fundus is normal.
General examination showed nothing abnormal.

Figure 453. Right eye (15°). Pigment migration in long-standing choroidal detachment.

CLINICAL NOTE: Figure 453 is from a male, aged 39. Three years ago he presented a choroidal detachment in the left eye. A year later he developed a total retinal detachment. On suspicion of tumor the eye was removed. Histopathological examination revealed no tumor but choroidal and retinal detachment. A month ago he experienced some hazy vision in the right eye, and a choroidal detachment was observed.
Eye examination: Visual acuity, right eye: < 6/9, unimproved by lenses; left eye: anophthalmos. Apart from some aqueous flare the anterior segment is normal. The fundus presents a ring-shaped choroidal detachment. In the lower quadrants it extends nearly to the disc.
General examination showed nothing abnormal.

Figure 454. Right eye. Localized vitreous detachment. The hyaloid membrane is opaque, corresponding to the detachment.

CLINICAL NOTE: Figure 454 is from a male, aged 45. Some days ago he experienced photopsia and hazy vision in the right eye. No complaints from the left eye.
Eye examination: Visual acuity, right eye: 6/9, unimproved by lenses; left eye: 6/6, emmetropia. Anterior segments and the left fundus are normal. The right fundus presents a localized opaque vitreous detachment in the posterior pole. A relative scotoma corresponds to the lesion.
General examination showed nothing abnormal.

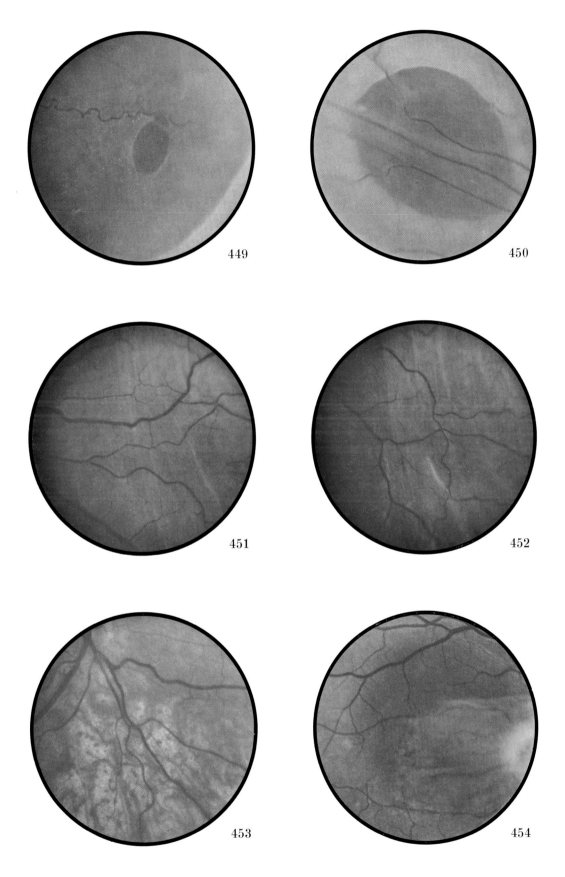

449

450

451

452

453

454

Figure 455. Left eye. Retinal detachment. In the macular area there is a shallow retinal detachment, recognized by fine, wavy, whitish lines.

CLINICAL NOTE: Figure 455 is from a male, aged 53. Four brothers and sisters, and a daughter have had retinal detachment. A week ago he felt as if a curtain were drawn in front of his left eye. No complaints from the right eye. No known ocular trauma.
Eye examination: Visual acuity, right eye: 6/6 with + 1.0 D sph.; left eye: 3/60 with + 1.0 D sph. Anterior segments and the right fundus are normal. The left fundus presents a retinal detachment extending from 1 to 6 o'clock. Two large horseshoe-shaped tears are seen in the upper temporal quadrant. Visual field defect corresponds to the detachment.
General examination showed nothing abnormal.

Figure 456. Right eye. Retinal detachment. In the macular area there is a shallow retinal detachment, recognized by fine, wavy, whitish lines. The detachment shows a vertical demarcation against the normal fundus.

CLINICAL NOTE: Figure 456 is from a male, aged 18. Two months ago he observed a reduction of vision in the right eye. No complaints from the left eye. No known ocular trauma.
Eye examination: Visual acuity, right eye: hand movements; left eye: 6/6, emmetropia. Anterior segments and the left fundus are normal. The right fundus presents a retinal detachment extending from 6 to 11 o'clock. In the involved area there are whitish demarcation lines, indicating retinoschisis. In the lower temporal quadrant there is a large retinal disinsertion at the ora. Visual field defect corresponds to the detachment.
General examination showed nothing abnormal.

Figure 457. Right eye. Retinal detachment with an apparent macular hole, a pseudo-hole.

CLINICAL NOTE: Figure 457 is from a male, aged 65. He has been healthy until one week ago, when he experienced a gradual loss of vision in the right eye. No complaints from the left eye. No known ocular trauma.
Eye examination: Visual acuity, right eye: hand movements; left eye: 6/6 with + 1.5 D sph. Anterior segments and the left fundus are

normal. The right fundus presents a retinal detachment extending from 4 to 11 o'clock. Three tears are seen in the upper temporal quadrant and there is a macular pseudo-hole. Visual field defect corresponds to the detachment.
General examination showed nothing abnormal.

Figure 458. Right eye. Retinal detachment. The detachment is shallow below and prominent above.

CLINICAL NOTE: Figure 458 is from the same patient as figures 461 and 465, a female, aged 59. She has had myopia since school-age. Four weeks ago she observed hazy vision in the right eye. Since then she has had many flickers of light in the right visual field and there has been a gradual loss of vision. No known ocular trauma.
Eye examination: Visual acuity, right eye: light perception; left eye: 6/9 with − 3.5 D sph. − 1.0 D cyl. axis 15°. Anterior segments are normal. The right fundus presents a total retinal detachment, prominent above and shallow below. A retinal tear is seen at 10 o'clock. The left fundus is normal.
General examination showed nothing abnormal.

Figures 459 and 460. Same left eye. Retinal detachment. The detachment is shallow, projecting forward about two to three diopters. The detachment is recognized by discrete wavy whitish lines and some bending of the retinal vessels.

CLINICAL NOTE: Figures 459 and 460 are from a male, aged 29. Six months ago and again three months ago he had vitreous hemorrhage in the left eye. The hemorrhages were absorbed quickly. An angiomatous tumor was observed in the temporal fundal periphery. A week ago he observed an abrupt reduction of vision in the left eye. No complaints from the right eye. No known ocular trauma.
Eye examination: Visual acuity, right eye: 6/6, emmetropia; left eye: 3/60, unimproved by lenses. Anterior segments are normal. The right fundus presents nasally a fan-shaped meshwork of new-formed preretinal vessels, but no retinal detachment. The left fundus shows temporally a yellowish-white angiomatous tumor surrounded by a shallow retinal detachment extending from 2 to 9 o'clock. Visual field defects correspond to the fundal lesions.
General examination, including neurological examination and angiography, showed no signs of cerebellar cysts.

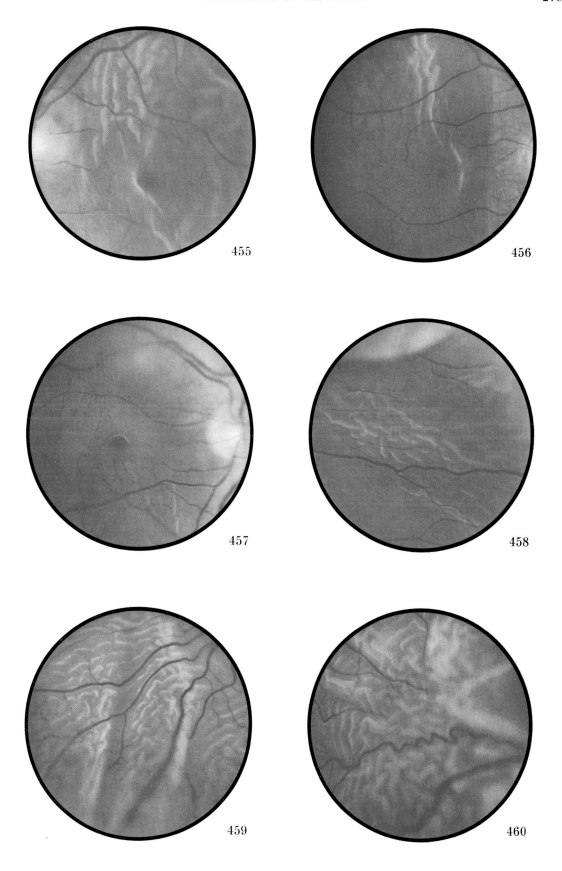

Figure 461. Right eye. Retinal detachment. The detachment is prominent, projecting forward about ten diopters and the detached retina is seen as a yellowish-pink uneven membrane. The retinal vessels show some bending and appear darker than normal.

CLINICAL NOTE: Figure 461 is from the same patient as figures 458 and 465, a female, aged 59. She has had myopia since school-age. Four weeks ago she observed hazy vision in the right eye. Since then she has had many flickers of light in the right visual field and there has been a gradual loss of vision. No known ocular trauma.
Eye examination: Visual acuity, right eye: light perception; left eye: 6/9 with − 3.5 D sph. − 1.0 D cyl. axis 15°. Anterior segments are normal. The right fundus presents a total retinal detachment, prominent above and shallow below. A retinal tear is seen at 10 o'clock. The left fundus is normal.
General examination showed nothing abnormal.

Figure 462. Right eye. Retinal detachment in the lower part of the fundus. The detached retina projects forward about five to six diopters.

CLINICAL NOTE: Figure 462 is from a male, aged 38. The last month he has experienced some shadows in the right visual field. No complaints from the left eye. No known ocular trauma.
Eye examination: Visual acuity, right eye: < 6/6 with − 0.5 D sph. − 1.0 D cyl. axis 90°; left eye: 6/6 with − 0.75 D sph. Anterior segments and the left fundus are normal. The right fundus presents a retinal detachment extending from 5 to 8 o'clock, leaving the macula free. Visual field defect corresponds to the detachment.
General examination showed nothing abnormal.

Figure 463. Left eye. Sickle-shaped hole in the macula without retinal detachment.

CLINICAL NOTE: Figure 463 is from a male, aged 48. Six weeks ago he observed some hazy vision in the left eye. No complaints from the right eye. No known ocular trauma.
Eye examination: Visual acuity, right eye: 6/6, emmetropia; left eye: 6/12 with + 2.0 D sph. Anterior segments and the right fundus are normal. In the left fundus there is a sickle-shaped hole in the macula without retinal detachment. Visual field shows a small paracentral scotoma.
General examination showed nothing abnormal.

Figure 464. Left eye. Retinal tear without retinal detachment. The horseshoe-shaped tear has an operculum projecting slightly forward.

CLINICAL NOTE: Figure 464 is from a male, aged 33. Chronic granulocytic leukemia was observed one year ago. He has no visual complaints.
Eye examination: Visual acuity, both eyes: 6/6, emmetropia. Anterior segments are normal. Both fundi present several flame-shaped retinal hemorrhages with a fluffy whitish center. In the left fundus, at 2 o'clock, there is a retinal tear without retinal detachment. No visual field defect.
General examination showed chronic granulocytic leukemia in remission.

Figure 465. Right eye. Retinal detachment with tear. The oval red hole has an operculum at both ends and is surrounded by a shallow retinal detachment temporally and a prominent detachment nasally.

CLINICAL NOTE: Figure 465 is from the same patient as figures 458 and 461, a female, aged 59. For further clinical information, see clinical note to figures 458 and 461.

Figure 466. Right eye. Retinal detachment with tear. The detached retina is grayish-red. The oval tear is sharply outlined and a whitish operculum is attached to the central end of the tear.

CLINICAL NOTE: Figure 466 is from the same patient as figure 45, a male, aged 50. He and his five siblings have had progressive myopia since childhood. A fortnight ago, he felt as if a curtain were drawn in front of his right eye. No complaints from the left eye. No known ocular trauma.
Eye examination: Visual acuity, right eye: hand movements with − 12.0 D sph.; left eye: 6/9 with − 8.5 D sph. Anterior segments are normal. Some opacities are present in the right vitreous. Both fundi show myopic conus and some diffuse myopic atrophy. In the right fundus there is a retinal detachment extending from 9 to 12 o'clock and an oval retinal tear at 11 o'clock. Visual field defect corresponds to the detachment.
General examination showed nothing abnormal.

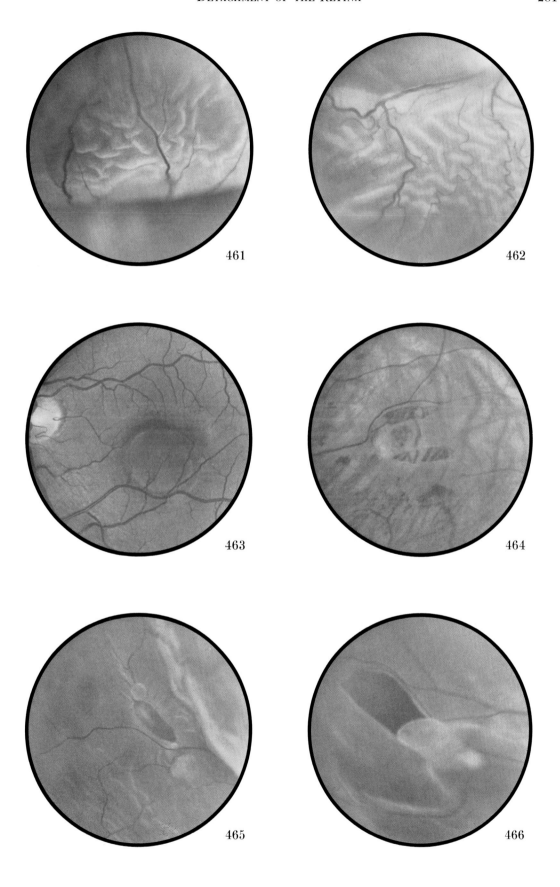

461

462

463

464

465

466

Figure 467. Left eye. Retinal detachment with tear. There is a large horseshoe-shaped retinal tear with operculum.

CLINICAL NOTE: Figure 467 is from a female, aged 53. She has had simple myopia since the age of 15. Two months ago she had some muscae volitantes in the left eye and a month later she experienced flickers of light in the same eye. Shortly afterwards she had a loss of vision in the left eye. No known ocular trauma.
Eye examination: Visual acuity, right eye: 6/6 with − 1.0 D sph.; left eye: hand movements. Anterior segments and the right fundus are normal. The left fundus presents a retinal detachment extending from 1 to 6 o'clock. There are two horseshoe-shaped retinal tears about 3 o'clock. Visual field defect corresponds to the detachment.
General examination showed nothing abnormal.

Figure 468. Left eye. Retinal detachment and tear. Above the disc there is a retinal tear with a whitish operculum.

CLINICAL NOTE: Figure 468 is from a male, aged 41. Six years ago he observed some reduction of vision in the left eye. Eye examination showed some vitreous opacities and a preretinal connective tissue band above the disc. Three weeks ago he experienced a sudden reduction of vision in the left eye. No known ocular trauma.
Eye examination: Visual acuity, right eye: 6/6, emmetropia; left eye: 6/36, unimproved by lenses. Anterior segments and the right fundus are normal. The left fundus presents a retinal detachment extending from 10 to 3 o'clock and with a tear above the disc. Visual field defect corresponds to the detachment.
General examination showed nothing abnormal.

Figure 469. Right eye. Retinal detachment and tear. In the upper temporal quadrant there is a giant tear. The choroid is seen faintly through the hole.

CLINICAL NOTE: Figure 469 is from a male, aged 58. He has had progressive myopia since childhood. Two months ago he felt as if a curtain were drawn in front of his right eye. No known ocular trauma.
Eye examination: Visual acuity, right eye: 6/18 with − 12.5 D sph. − 2.0 D cyl. axis 10°; left eye: < 6/9 with − 9.5 D sph. − 1.0 D cyl. axis 25°. Anterior segments are normal. The right fundus presents a retinal detachment extending from 10 to 6 o'clock. There are giant tears at 11 and 2 o'clock. Visual field defect corresponds to the detachment. The left fundus shows typical myopic changes.
General examination showed nothing abnormal.

Figure 470. Right eye. Retinal detachment with tear. In the lower part of the fundus there is a giant horseshoe-shaped retinal tear. The choroid is seen faintly through the hole.

CLINICAL NOTE: Figure 470 is from a male, aged 63. His right eye has been myopic for many years. A week ago he felt as if a curtain were drawn in front of his right eye. No known ocular trauma.
Eye examination: Visual acuity, right eye: 6/36 with − 3.0 D sph.; left eye: 6/9 with + 0.5 D sph. Both lenses show incipient cataract. In the right fundus there is a retinal detachment extending from 4 to 9 o'clock and there is a giant horseshoe-shaped tear at 6 o'clock. Left fundus is normal. Visual field defect corresponds to the detachment.
General examination showed nothing abnormal.

Figure 471. Right eye. Retinal detachment with tears. There is a retinal detachment and two small oval tears. The tears are surrounded by whitish connective tissue projecting far into the vitreous.

CLINICAL NOTE: Figure 471 is from a female, aged 10. After a trauma one year ago vision in her right eye has been reduced severely.
Eye examination: Visual acuity, right eye: 6/36, unimproved by lenses; left eye: 6/6, emmetropia. Anterior segments and the left fundus are normal. The right fundus presents retinoschisis and a retinal cyst in the lower temporal quadrant. There is a retinal detachment in both nasal quadrants and two tears at 1 o'clock. The tears are surrounded by connective tissue projecting far into the vitreous. Visual field defect corresponds to the fundal lesions.
General examination showed nothing abnormal.

Figure 472. Left eye. Exudative retinal detachment in uveitis.

CLINICAL NOTE: Figure 472 is from a male, aged 63. He has had chronic polyarthritis for many years. Two weeks ago he experienced blurred vision in the left eye. No complaints from the right eye.
Eye examination: Visual acuity, right eye: 6/6, emmetropia; left eye: 6/24, unimproved by lenses. Right anterior segment and fundus are normal. The left eye shows chemosis, iritis with synechiae and vitreous opacities. In the left fundus there is an exudative, nearly ring-shaped retinal detachment. No retinal tears. Visual field defect corresponds to the detachment.
General examination showed nothing abnormal.

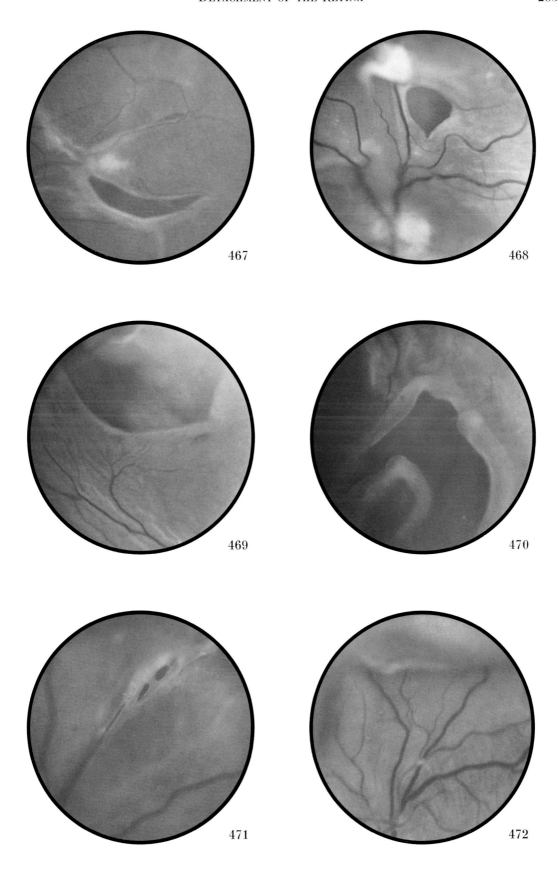

467

468

469

470

471

472

Figure 473. Left eye. Grouped pigmentation of the retina, seen as sharply defined rounded dark-brown patches, grouped like footprints of an animal.

CLINICAL NOTE: Figure 473 is from a female, aged 35. Grouped pigmentation has been present in both fundi for many years. Some months ago a tumor without relation to the grouped pigmentation was found in the right fundus. The eye was enucleated and histopathological examination showed malignant choroidal melanoma. No complaints from the left eye. No general symptoms.
Eye examination: Visual acuity, right eye: anophthalmos; left eye: 6/6, emmetropia. Anterior segment is normal. Grouped pigmentation is seen in the fundus.
General examination showed nothing abnormal.

Figure 474. Left eye. Grouped pigmentation of the retina. The dark pigment is grouped like footprints of an animal.

CLINICAL NOTE: Figure 474 is from the same patient as figure 42, a female, aged 11. No family history of myopia. She has had myopia since the age of eight years.
Eye examination: Visual acuity, right eye: 6/6 with − 2.25 D sph.; left eye: 6/6 with − 3.75 D sph. Anterior segments are normal. Both fundi are lightly pigmented except in and around the macular area. Scattered grouped pigmentation is present in both eyes.
General examination showed nothing abnormal.

Figure 475. Left eye. Choroidal nevus, seen as a flat, oval, dark grayish-green patch of uniform density.

CLINICAL NOTE: Figure 475 is from a female, aged 24. She has had myopia since childhood. No visual complaints.
Eye examination: Visual acuity, both eyes: 6/6 with − 2.5 D sph. Both lenses are luxated upwards and show slight cataract. Intraocular tension and visual fields are normal. In the left

fundus there is a choroidal nevus, but otherwise fundi are normal.
General examination showed nothing abnormal.

Figure 476. Right eye. Choroidal nevus, seen as a flat, oval, grayish-green patch of uniform density. The retinal vessels lying in front of the nevus appear darker than normal.

CLINICAL NOTE: Figure 476 is from a female, aged 38. A choroidal nevus was observed by chance four years ago. Several control examinations have shown it to be stationary. No ocular or general complaints.
Eye examination: Visual acuity, both eyes: 6/6, emmetropia. Visual fields and anterior segments are normal. In the right fundus there is a choroidal nevus, but otherwise fundi are normal.
General examination showed nothing abnormal.

Figure 477. Left eye. Choroidal nevus, seen as a flat, grayish-black area between the disc and the fovea.

CLINICAL NOTE: Figure 477 is from a female, aged 32. She has had myopia since childhood. No visual or general complaints.
Eye examination: Visual acuity, both eyes: 6/6 with − 3.5 D sph. − 0.5 D cyl. axis 90°. Anterior segments are normal. In the left fundus there is a choroidal nevus, but otherwise fundi are normal.
General examination showed nothing abnormal.

Figure 478. Right eye. Choroidal nevus, seen as a flat, rounded, nearly black pigmentation lying beneath the retinal vessels.

CLINICAL NOTE: Figure 478 is from a female, aged 38. No ocular or general complaints.
Eye examination: Visual acuity, both eyes: 6/6, emmetropia. Anterior segments are normal. In the right fundus there is a choroidal nevus, but otherwise fundi are normal.
General examination showed nothing abnormal.

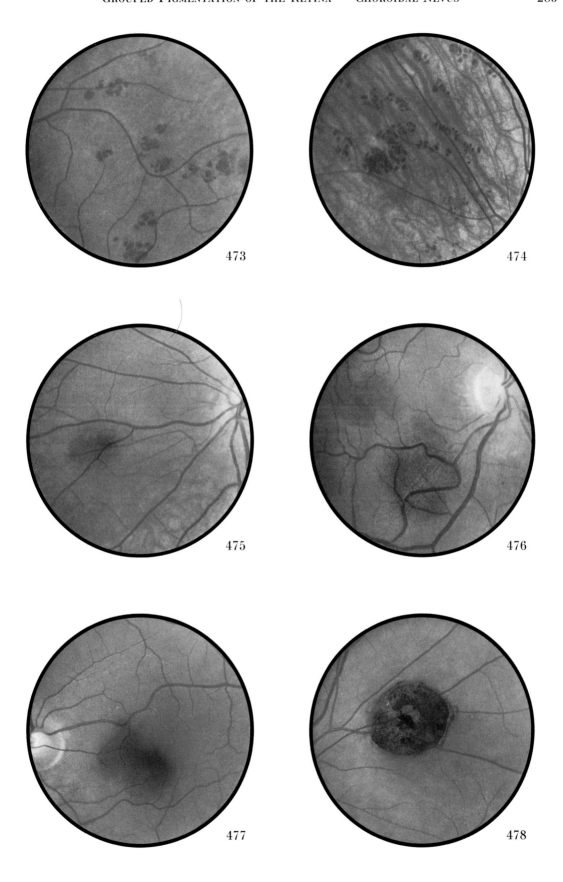

473

474

475

476

477

478

Figure 479. Right eye. Malignant choroidal melanoma. In the macular area there is a large, slightly prominent, mottled, grayish-green choroidal tumor.

CLINICAL NOTE: Figure 479 is from a female, aged 60. During the last six months vision in the right eye has gradually decreased. No complaints from the left eye. No general symptoms. *Eye examination:* Visual acuity, right eye: 3/60 with + 2.5 D sph.; left eye: 6/9 with + 1.5 D sph. Anterior segments and the left fundus are normal. The right fundus presents a large, flat choroidal tumor in the macular area. Transillumination shows a massive shadow corresponding to the site of the tumor. Visual field defect corresponds to the tumor. The eye was enucleated and histopathological examination showed malignant choroidal melanoma of spindle-cell type. *General examination* showed nothing abnormal.

Figure 480. Left eye. Malignant choroidal melanoma. In the posterior pole there is a large, slightly prominent, mottled, grayish-green choroidal tumor.

CLINICAL NOTE: Figure 480 is from a male, aged 59. During the last six months vision in his left eye has gradually decreased. No complaints from the right eye. No general symptoms. *Eye examination:* Visual acuity, right eye: 6/6, emmetropia; left eye: 6/36 with + 3.0 D sph. Anterior segments and right fundus are normal. The left fundus presents a large, flat choroidal tumor in the posterior pole. Transillumination shows a massive shadow corresponding to the site of the tumor. Visual field defect corresponds to the tumor. The eye was enucleated and histopathological examination showed malignant choroidal melanoma of spindle-cell type. *General examination* showed nothing abnormal.

Figure 481. Right eye. Malignant choroidal melanoma. There is a large, slightly prominent mottled, yellowish-gray choroidal tumor.

CLINICAL NOTE: Figure 481 is from a male, aged 50. One year ago he observed a shadow in the right visual field, but vision was not impaired. No general symptoms. *Eye examination:* Visual acuity, both eyes: 6/6 with + 1.5 D sph. Anterior segments and the left fundus are normal. The right fundus presents a choroidal tumor in the perimacular area. Transillumination shows a shadow at the site of the tumor and visual field defect corresponds to the tumor. The eye was enucleated and histopathological examination showed malignant choroidal melanoma of mixed type. *General examination* showed nothing abnormal.

Figure 482. Right eye. Malignant choroidal melanoma. There is a transition from the normal fundus below to the slightly prominent, mottled, yellowish-green tumor above.

CLINICAL NOTE: Figure 482 is from a female, aged 59. During the last six months she has observed a shadow in the right visual field and some reduction of vision. No complaints from the left eye. No general symptoms. *Eye examination:* Visual acuity, right eye: 6/9 with + 2.5 D sph.; left eye: 6/6 with + 2.5 D sph. Anterior segments and left fundus are normal. The right fundus presents a choroidal tumor in the upper temporal quadrant. Transillumination shows a shadow corresponding to the site of the tumor and visual defect corresponds to the tumor. The eye was enucleated and histopathological examination showed malignant choroidal melanoma of fascicular type. *General examination* showed nothing abnormal.

Figure 483. Right eye. Malignant choroidal melanoma. The choroidal tumor is slightly prominent and has a mottled yellowish color.

CLINICAL NOTE: See clinical note to figure 486.

Figure 484. Right eye. Malignant choroidal melanoma. The slightly prominent choroidal tumor is yellowish and contains some scattered pigment.

CLINICAL NOTE: Figure 484 is from a male, aged 60. During the last year he has observed a shadow in the right visual field. No visual complaints. No general symptoms. *Eye examination:* Visual acuity, both eyes: 6/6 with + 4.0 D sph. Anterior segments and the left fundus are normal. The right fundus presents a choroidal tumor above the disc. Transillumination shows a slight shadow, and visual field defect corresponds to the tumor. The eye was enucleated and histopathological examination showed malignant choroidal melanoma of mixed type. *General examination* showed nothing abnormal.

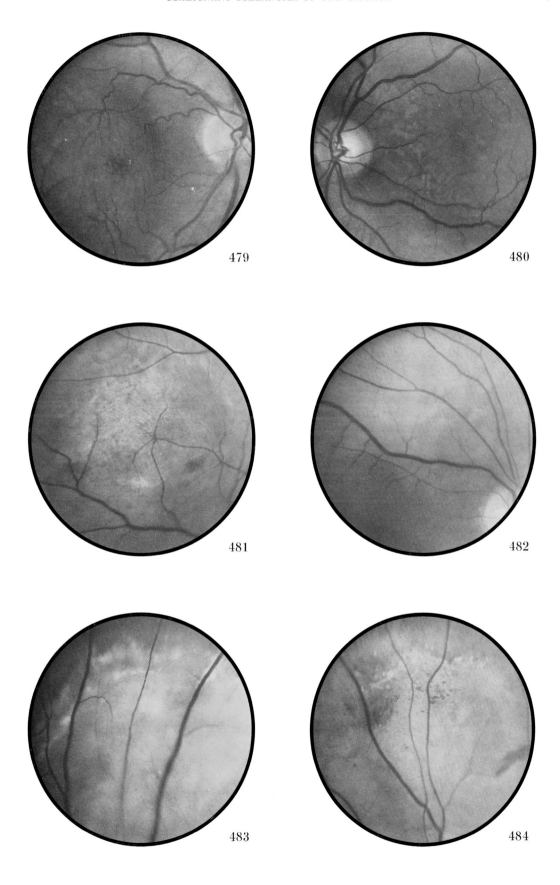

479

480

481

482

483

484

Figure 485. Left eye (15°). Preretinal pigment migration from a malignant choroidal melanoma.

CLINICAL NOTE: Figure 485 is from a male, aged 60. Two months ago he observed slight blurring of vision in the left eye and soon afterwards a shadow in the visual field. No symptoms of general illness.
Eye examination: Visual acuity, both eyes: 6/9 with + 1.0 D sph. Anterior segments and the right fundus are normal. The left fundus presents a large choroidal tumor in the lower nasal quadrant and diffuse pigment dispersion preretinally. Transillumination shows a dark shadow and visual field defect corresponds to the tumor. The eye was enucleated and histopathological examination showed malignant choroidal melanoma of mixed type.
General examination showed nothing abnormal.

Figure 486. Right eye. Malignant choroidal melanoma obscures the optic disc. Prepapillary the tumor contains many vessels. Above, choroidal tumor vessels are not visible.

CLINICAL NOTE: Figure 486 is from the same patient as figure 483, a male, aged 55. Three months ago he experienced a shadow in the right visual field. No visual complaints. No general symptoms.
Eye examination: Visual acuity, both eyes: 6/6, emmetropia. Anterior segments and the left fundus are normal. The right fundus presents a choroidal tumor extending from the disc to the upper part of the fundus. Transillumination shows a slight shadow, and visual field defect corresponds to the tumor. The eye was enucleated and histopathological examination showed malignant choroidal melanoma of spindle-cell type.
General examination showed nothing abnormal.

Figure 487. Right eye. Malignant choroidal melanoma seen as a large, prominent, yellowish mass in the lower part of the fundus. The disc is obscured by the tumor.

CLINICAL NOTE: Figure 487 is from a male, aged 43. One week ago he observed hazy vision and a visual field defect in the right eye. No general symptoms.
Eye examination: Visual acuity, right eye: 6/9 with + 0.5 D sph.; left eye: 6/6, emmetropia. Anterior segments and the left fundus are normal. The right fundus presents a choroidal tumor in the lower part of the fundus. The disc is obscured by the tumor. Transillumination shows a shadow and visual field defect corresponds to the tumor. The eye was enucleated and histopathological examination showed malignant choroidal melanoma of mixed type.
General examination showed nothing abnormal.

Figure 488. Left eye. Malignant choroidal melanoma and some retinal detachment seen as a large, prominent whitish mass in the perimacular area.

CLINICAL NOTE: Figure 488 is from a male, aged 65. Three weeks ago he observed a shadow in the left visual field. No visual complaints. No general symptoms.
Eye examination: Visual acuity, both eyes: 6/6 with + 0.5 D sph. Anterior segments and the right fundus are normal. The left fundus presents a large whitish choroidal tumor in the perimacular area together with some retinal detachment. Transillumination shows a shadow and visual field defect corresponds to the tumor. The eye was enucleated and histopathological examination showed malignant choroidal melanoma of spindle-cell type.
General examination showed nothing abnormal.

Figure 489. Left eye. Malignant choroidal melanoma seen as a prominent, yellowish-green, irregularly pigmented, rounded mass.

CLINICAL NOTE: Figure 489 is from a male, aged 52. During the last few months he has observed some blurring of vision and a gradually increasing shadow in the left visual field. No general complaints.
Eye examination: Visual acuity, right eye: 6/6, emmetropia; left eye: < 6/18 with + 1.0 D sph. Anterior segments and the right fundus are normal. The left fundus shows a large, prominent choroidal tumor temporally. Transillumination shows massive shadow and visual field defect corresponds to the tumor. The eye was enucleated and histopathological examination showed malignant choroidal melanoma of mixed type.
General examination showed nothing abnormal.

Figure 490. Left eye. Benign medulloepithelioma seen as a large, prominent, grayish-green mass.

CLINICAL NOTE: Figure 490 is from a female, aged 45. During the last four years a slowly enlarging tumor has been observed in the left fundus, and vision has gradually decreased. No general symptoms.
Eye examination: Visual acuity, right eye: 6/6 with + 0.5 D sph.; left eye: 6/18 with + 1.0 D sph. Anterior segments and the right fundus are normal. In the left fundus there is a large, prominent tumor in the lower temporal quadrant surrounded by some retinal detachment. Transillumination shows a dark shadow and visual field defect corresponds to the fundus lesion. The eye was enucleated and histopathological examination showed benign medulloepithelioma.
General examination showed nothing abnormal.

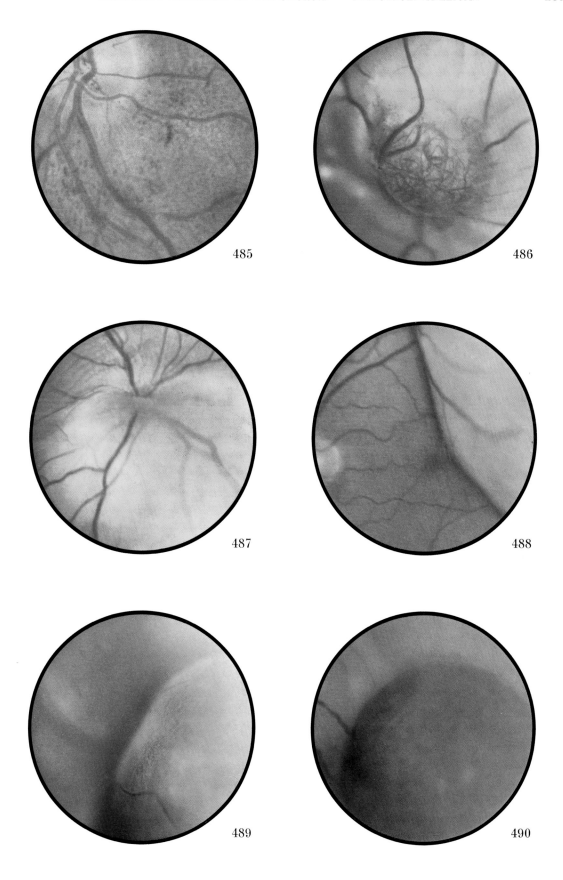

485

486

487

488

489

490

Figure 491. Left eye. Metastatic choroidal carcinoma, seen as a soft-edged, rounded, slightly raised, opaque yellowish area about the size of three disc diameters.

Clinical note: Figure 491 is from a female, aged 38. Six months ago she was operated on for mammary adenocarcinoma with extension to the axillary lymph nodes. A fortnight ago she had transient blurring of vision in the left eye.
Eye examination: Visual acuity, both eyes: 6/6, emmetropia. Anterior segments and the right fundus are normal. The left fundus shows two large choroidal metastases at the temporal side of the disc. Visual field shows a relative scotoma corresponding to the fundal lesions.
General examination showed a woman in good condition following the removal of a mammary cancer.
Shortly afterwards, however, her general condition deteriorated and a few months later she died from metastases.

Figure 492. Right eye. Metastatic choroidal carcinoma seen as a slightly prominent, soft-edged, opaque yellowish area in the macula.

Clinical note: Figure 492 is from a female, aged 44. Two months ago she was operated on for mammary scirrhous carcinoma. About ten days ago she observed blurring of vision in both eyes.
Eye examination: Visual acuity, both eyes: 6/18 with + 1.0 D sph. Anterior segments are normal. Both fundi present choroidal metastases in the macular area, and relative scotomas correspond to the fundal lesions.
General examination showed a woman with widespread metastases following a mammary cancer.
One month later she died from her metastases.

Figure 493. Left eye. Retinal ridging from an orbital tumor, seen as numerous oblique retinal ripples. The disc and retinal vessels are normal.

Clinical note: Figure 493 is from a female, aged 54. During the last year she has had progressive proptosis of the left eye and diplopia without reduction of vision. No general symptoms.
Eye examination: Visual acuity, both eyes: 6/6 with + 2.5 D sph. The left eye is displaced forwards and downwards. Eye movements are normal. Anterior segments and the right fundus are normal. The left fundus presents extensive retinal ridging. Disc and retinal vessels are normal.

General examination aroused suspicion of meningioma. Craniotomy revealed a large meningioma in the left sphenoid ridge with extension into the orbit.

Figure 494. Right eye. Retinal ridging from an orbital tumor, seen as numerous parallel retinal ripples. The disc is atrophic. The retinal vessels are normal.

Clinical note: Figure 494 is from a male, aged 44. Four years ago and again two years ago he was operated on for a meningioma arising from the olfactory groove. During the last year he has had progressive proptosis and loss of vision in the right eye.
Eye examination: Visual acuity, right eye: light perception; left eye: 6/6 with − 1.5 D sph. The right eye is displaced forwards and downwards. Eye movements are normal. Anterior segments and the left fundus are normal. The right fundus presents retinal ridging in the macular area and optic atrophy.
General examination aroused suspicion of tumor in the ethmoidal sinuses with extension to the right orbit. The tumor, a spinocellular carcinoma, was removed.

Figure 495. Retinoblastoma, seen as an yellowish-pink mass through the right pupil.

Clinical note: Figure 495 is from a female, aged 2. No known cases of retinoblastoma in the family. The last six months the parents have observed a yellowish-pink reflex from her right pupil.
Eye examination: Anterior segments and the left fundus are normal. The right fundus presents a large tumor filling nearly the whole vitreous cavity. The eye was enucleated and histopathological examination showed retinoblastoma of rosette type with invasion of the optic nerve and the choroid.
General examination showed nothing abnormal.

Figure 496. Left eye. Retinoblastoma, seen as several ill-defined, slightly raised whitish tumors in the retina.

Clinical note: Figure 496 is from a male, aged 2. No known cases of retinoblastoma in the family. A month ago the parents observed a whitish reflex from his left pupil.
Eye examination: Anterior segments and the right fundus are normal. The left fundus presents extensive retinal tumor growth. The eye was enucleated and histopathological examination showed retinoblastoma of rosette type without invasion of the optic nerve or choroid.
General examination showed nothing abnormal.

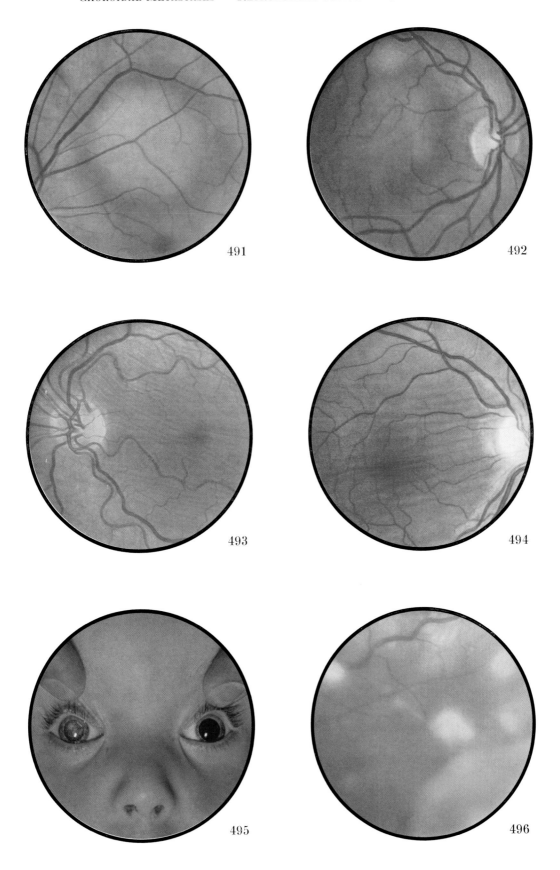

491

492

493

494

495

496

Figure 497. Right eye. Retinoblastoma, seen as a prominent grayish-red tumor at the nasal side of the disc. Some whitish calcareous concrements are seen on top of the tumor. The tumor is surrounded by chorioretinal scars following light coagulation and radiation therapy one month ago.

Figure 498. Same eye as figure 497, four months later. The tumor is in regression. There are still some calcareous concrements on top of the tumor.

Figure 499. Composite picture. Same eye as figure 498, four months later. The tumor has completely disappeared and there is a large area of chorioretinal atrophy. The calcareous nodules are still present at the nasal side of the disc, but they are difficult to distinguish in the atrophic area.

Clinical note: Figures 497—499 are from a male, aged 3. No known cases of retinoblastoma in the family. About a year ago the parents observed a whitish reflex from his left pupil. On admission to hospital eight months ago a retinoblastoma was found in both eyes. In the right fundus there was a solitary tumor at the nasal side of the disc. The left fundus presented extensive tumor growth. The left eye was enucleated and histopathological examination showed retinoblastoma of rosette type with commencing invasion of the choroid. No invasion of the optic nerve.

The right eye received one series of radiation therapy, and repeated light coagulation at intervals over a period of four months.

Eight months after the first treatment the retinoblastoma had completely disappeared.

General examination showed nothing abnormal.

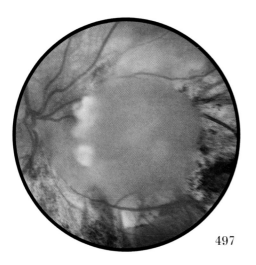

497

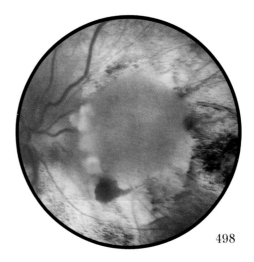

498

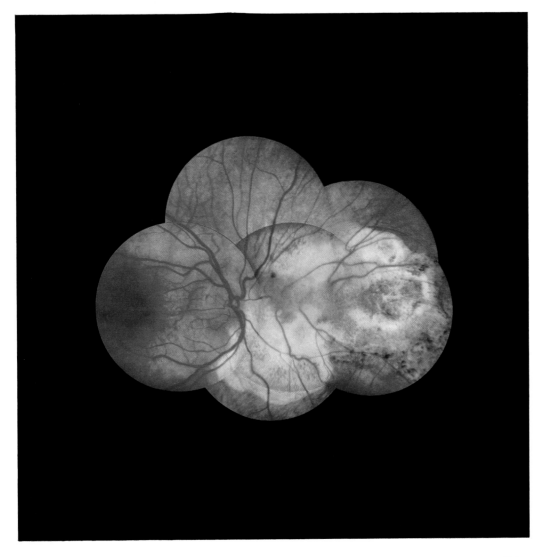

499

Figure 500. Left eye. Traumatic macular edema seen as a grayish, ill-defined area with radiating whitish light reflexes surrounding the red-brown fovea.

CLINICAL NOTE: Figure 500 is from a male, aged 9. Six days ago he received a blunt injury to his left eye with a stick. Just after the injury he presented a hyphema, but vision was normal. During the following days, however, he complained of blurred vision in the left eye.
Eye examination: Visual acuity, right eye: 6/6, emmetropia; left eye: 6/12, unimproved by lenses. Hyphema has subsided. Anterior segments and the right fundus are normal. The left fundus presents traumatic macular edema, and a choroidal rupture in the periphery. The disc and retinal vessels are normal.
General examination showed nothing abnormal.

Figure 501. Right eye. Traumatic macular edema, in subsidence. A slight grayish zone and fine radiating whitish light reflexes surround the red-brown fovea.

CLINICAL NOTE: Figure 501 is from a male, aged 17. A fortnight ago he received a small perforating lesion of the right sclera and cornea with a knife. The wound was sutured, but during the following days he complained of blurred vision in the right eye, and a traumatic fundal edema was observed.
Eye examination: Visual acuity, right eye: 6/24, unimproved by lenses; left eye: 6/6, emmetropia. The corneoscleral wound is healed. Anterior chambers, the lenses and the left fundus are normal. The right fundus presents traumatic macular edema in subsidence. The disc and retinal vessels are normal.
General examination showed nothing abnormal.

Figure 502. Right eye. Traumatic macular lesion. In the fovea there is some pigmentation and depigmentation and the fovea is surrounded by abnormal light reflexes. Below there is some patchy pigmentation of the fundus.

CLINICAL NOTE: Figure 502 is from the same patient as figure 504, a male, aged 19. Ten days ago he received a blunt injury to the right eye from a single shot fired from a shotgun. Since then vision has been blurred in the right eye.

Eye examination: Visual acuity, right eye: 6/60 with − 2.0 D sph.; left eye: 6/6 with − 1.0 D sph. Anterior segments are normal, but the right vitreous shows opacities and erythrocytes. The right fundus shows traumatic macular degeneration, retinal hemorrhages and patchy pigmentation. The disc and retinal vessels are normal. The left fundus is normal.
General examination showed nothing abnormal.

Figure 503. Right eye. Traumatic preretinal and retinal hemorrhages.

CLINICAL NOTE: Figure 503 is from a male, aged 26. Ten days ago he was hit by a football in his right eye. He was admitted for hyphema and blurred vision.
Eye examination: Visual acuity, right eye: 6/9 with − 0.5 D cyl. axis 0°; left eye: 6/6 with − 0.75 D cyl. axis 0°. The hyphema has subsided. Anterior segments and left fundus are normal. The right fundus still presents preretinal and retinal hemorrhages. The macula, retinal vessels and the disc are normal.
General examination showed nothing abnormal.

Figure 504. Right eye. Sequelae after traumatic retinal hemorrhages, seen as atrophic fundal areas with some pigmentation.

CLINICAL NOTE: Figure 504 is from the same patient as figure 502, a male, aged 19. For further clinical information, see clinical note to figure 502.

Figure 505. Right eye. Traumatic macular hole, seen as a sharply outlined red-brown area with whitish dots and surrounded by slight retinal folding.

CLINICAL NOTE: Figure 505 is from a male, aged 24. Five years ago he received a blunt injury to the right eye from a single shot fired from a shotgun. Since then central vision has been reduced in the right eye.
Eye examination: Visual acuity, right eye: 1/36, unimproved by lenses; left eye: 6/6, emmetropia. Anterior segments and the left fundus are normal. The right fundus shows a traumatic macular hole. Disc and retinal vessels are normal. Visual field defect corresponds to the fundal lesion.
General examination showed nothing abnormal.

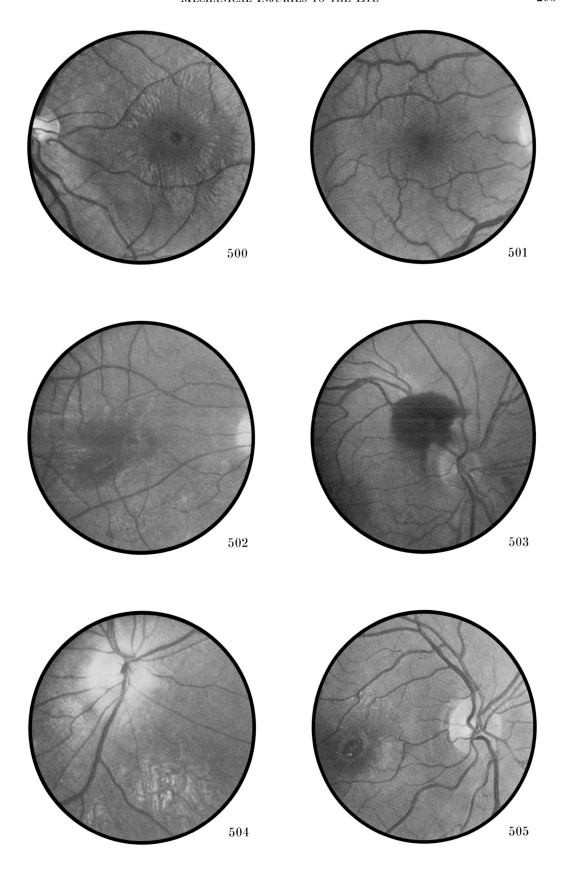

500

501

502

503

504

505

Figures 506 and 507. Same left eye. Fresh choroidal ruptures, seen as a whitish crescent surrounding the lower part of the disc and a whitish line outside the macula. There are some retinal hemorrhages in relation to the ruptures. The retina shows some wrinkling in the macular area.

CLINICAL NOTE: Figures 506 and 507 are from a female, aged 31. A week ago she received a blunt injury to the left eye from a piece of wood. Since then vision has been slightly blurred in the left eye.
Eye examination: Visual acuity, right eye: 6/6 with + 1.0 D sph. + 0.5 D cyl. axis 40°; left eye: 6/9 with − 1.0 D sph. − 0.5 D cyl. axis 10°. Anterior segments and the right fundus are normal. The left fundus shows fresh choroidal ruptures and retinal hemorrhages. Visual field defects correspond to the fundal lesions.
General examination showed nothing abnormal.

Figure 508. Right eye. Fresh choroidal rupture, seen as an irregular yellowish-white area outside the macular area, surrounded and partly obscured by deeply situated large flat hemorrhages.

CLINICAL NOTE: Figure 508 is from the same patient as figure 516, a male, aged 16. Eighteen days ago he received a blunt injury to the right eye from a single shot fired from a shotgun. On admission he presented hyphema, iridodialysis and vitreous hemorrhage. When the hyphema had subsided and the vitreous cleared somewhat, a choroidal rupture was observed.
Eye examination eighteen days after the injury: Visual acuity, right eye: 2/60, unimproved by lenses; left eye: 6/6, emmetropia. No hyphema. In the right eye there is iridodialysis between 7 and 9 o'clock, the lens is subluxated downwards and the vitreous hazy from blood. The disc shows papilledema and in the perimacular area there are a choroidal rupture and fundal hemorrhages. The left anterior segment and fundus are normal.
General examination showed nothing abnormal.

Figure 509. Right eye. Fresh choroidal ruptures, seen as yellowish lines. There is also retinal edema, and retinal and subretinal hemorrhages.

CLINICAL NOTE: Figure 509 is from the same patient as figure 7, a female, aged 13. A fortnight ago she received a blunt injury to the right eye from a single shot fired from a shotgun. Since then central vision in the right eye has been severely reduced.
Eye examination: Visual acuity, right eye: 3/36, unimproved by lenses; left eye: 6/6, emmetropia. Anterior segments are normal. In the right fundus there are fresh choroidal ruptures surrounded by retinal edema, and by retinal and subretinal hemorrhages. Visual field defect corresponds to the fundal lesion. The left fundus is normal.
General examination showed nothing abnormal.

Figure 510. Right eye. Old choroidal rupture, seen as a whitish crescent of exposed sclera, at some distance from the optic disc.

CLINICAL NOTE: Figure 510 is from a female, aged 23. Many years ago she received a blunt injury to the right eye, followed by transient blurred vision. Since then she has had no visual disturbances.
Eye examination: Visual acuity, both eyes: 6/6, emmetropia. The right pupil is large and reacts less to light than the left. Anterior chambers, the lenses and the left fundus are normal. The right fundus presents an old choroidal rupture. Disc and retinal vessels are normal. Visual field shows a relative defect corresponding to the fundal lesion.
General examination showed nothing abnormal.

Figure 511. Right eye. Old choroidal ruptures with some pigmentation in the macular area.

CLINICAL NOTE: Figure 511 is from a male, aged 19. Three years ago he received from a horse a blunt injury to his right eye. Since then vision in the right eye has been severely reduced.
Eye examination: Visual acuity, right eye: 6/60, unimproved by lenses; left eye: 6/6, emmetropia. Anterior segments and the left fundus are normal. The right macular area presents old choroidal ruptures. The disc and retinal vessels are normal. Visual field defects correspond to the fundal lesions.
General examination showed nothing abnormal.

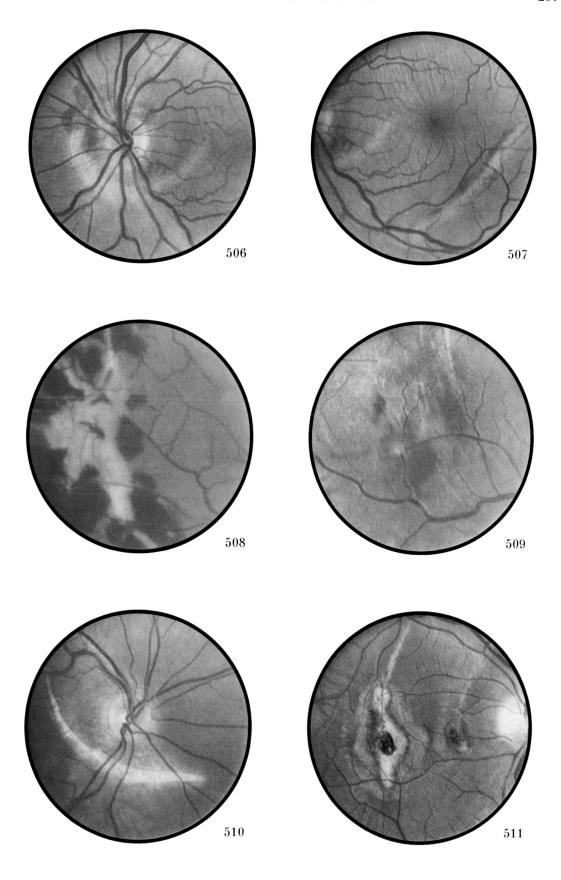

506

507

508

509

510

511

Figure 512. Left eye. Metallic foreign body in the fundus. There are small retinal hemorrhages and some of the retinal vessels are pale and bloodless.

CLINICAL NOTE: Figure 512 is from a male, aged 21. A few hours ago a metallic splinter from a hammer perforated his left sclera.
Eye examination: Visual acuity, both eyes: 6/6 with + 0.75 D sph. The anterior chambers, the lenses and the right fundus are normal. The left eye presents a sceral wound at 9 o'clock about 4 mm behind the limbus and there is a metallic foreign body in the fundus. The foreign body was extracted by a magnet.
General examination showed nothing abnormal.

Figure 513. Left eye. Metallic foreign body lying preretinally. It is partly obscured by hemorrhage.

CLINICAL NOTE: Figure 513 is from a male, aged 40. A few hours ago a metallic splinter from a hammer perforated his left sclera.
Eye examination: Visual acuity, both eyes: 6/6, emmetropia. Anterior chambers, the lenses and the right fundus are normal. The left eye presents a scleral wound at 2 o'clock just behind the limbus. There is some blood in the vitreous, and preretinally there is a metallic foreign body. The foreign body was extracted by a magnet.
General examination showed nothing abnormal.

Figure 514. Right eye. Remnants of a fibrin cap, which had obscured a metallic foreign body. There is also some depigmentation of the fundus.

Figure 515. Same eye as figure 514, a fortnight later. The fibrin has been absorbed, but the fundus shows some degeneration with depigmentation and pigment clumping.

CLINICAL NOTE: Figures 514 and 515 are from a male, aged 27. Two days ago a splinter from a hammer hit his right eye. The following day vision became hazy in his right eye.
Eye examination two days after the injury: Visual acuity, right eye: 6/9, unimproved by lenses; left eye: 6/6 with + 0.5 D sph. The right eye presents a corneal wound and a small perforation of the iris but no damage of the lens.

In the fundus there is a metallic foreign body obscured by a fibrin cap. The left anterior segment and fundus are normal. The foreign body was extracted by a magnet.
Eye examination a fortnight later: Visual acuity unaltered. The corneal wound is healed and the fundus shows some degenerative changes in the area where the foreign body had been lodged.
General examination showed nothing abnormal.

Figure 516. Right eye. Papilledema ex vacuo. The optic disc is swollen and the retinal veins engorged.

CLINICAL NOTE: Figure 516 is from the same patient as figure 508, a male, aged 16. Eighteen days ago he received a blunt injury to the right eye from a single shot fired from a shotgun. On admission he presented hyphema, iridodialysis and vitreous hemorrhage. When the hyphema had subsided and the vitreous cleared somewhat, a choroidal rupture was observed.
Eye examination eighteen days after the injury: Visual acuity, right eye: 2/60, unimproved by lenses; left eye: 6/6 emmetropia. No hyphema. In the right eye there is iridodialysis between 7 and 9 o'clock, the lens is subluxated downwards and the vitreous hazy from blood. The disc shows papilledema. In the perimacular area there are a choroidal rupture and fundal hemorrhages. The left anterior segment and fundus are normal.
General examination showed nothing abnormal.

Figure 517. Left eye. Perforating lesion in the fundus. A metallic foreign body has crushed a retinal vessel and produced an ischemic fundal area surrounded by subretinal hemorrhage. A preretinal hemorrhage is seen below.

CLINICAL NOTE: Figure 517 is from a male, aged 39. A few hours ago a metallic splinter from a hammer perforated his left cornea.
Eye examination a few hours after the injury: Visual acuity, right eye: 6/6, emmetropia; left eye: < 6/6, unimproved by lenses. The right anterior segment and fundus are normal. The left eye presents a corneal wound, a small perforation of the lens, some vitreous hemorrhage and a perforating lesion in the fundus just below the macula. The metallic foreign body was extracted by a magnet.
General examination showed nothing abnormal.

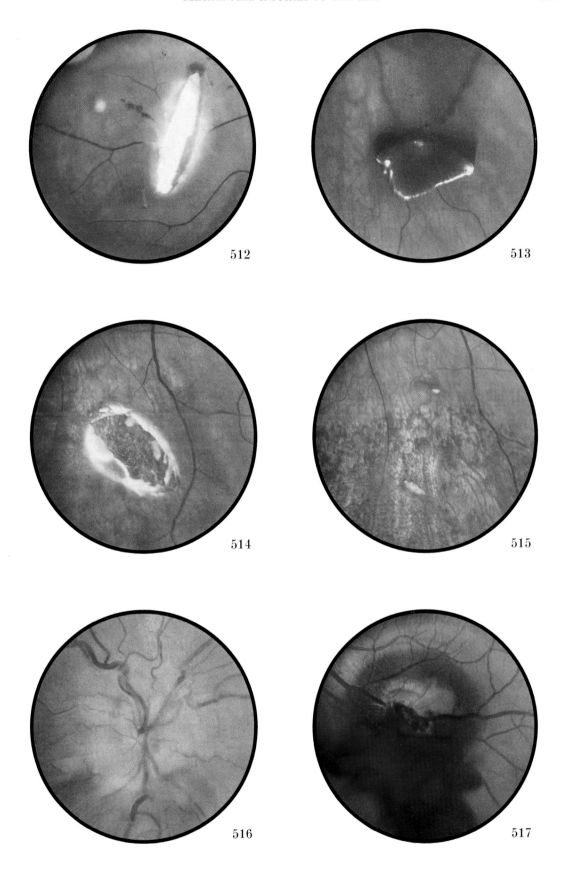

512

513

514

515

516

517

Figure 518. Right eye. Perforating lesion in the fundus partly obscured by hemorrhages.

Figure 519. Same eye as figure 518, four years later. There is an atrophic chorioretinal scar partly obscured by dense vitreous opacities.

CLINICAL NOTE: Figures 518 and 519 are from a male, aged 27. Four years ago he received a scleral perforation in the right eye from a large metallic splinter.
Eye examination just after the injury: Visual acuity, both eyes: 6/6 with + 1.0 D sph. Anterior segments and the left fundus are normal. The right eye presents a scleral wound about 6 o'clock and a metallic splinter is removed from the wound. In the fundus there is a perforating lesion and some hemorrhage.
Eye examination, four years later: Visual acuity unaltered. In the right fundus there is a chorioretinal scar partly obscured by dense vitreous opacities.
General examination showed nothing abnormal.

Figure 520. Left eye. Purtscher's retinopathy. The fundus shows cotton-wool exudates and streaky hemorrhages at the temporal side of the disc.

CLINICAL NOTE: Figure 520 is from a male, aged 60. A fortnight ago he received a thorax compression in a traffic accident. Some days later he observed hazy vision in the left eye.
Eye examination: Visual acuity, right eye: 6/6 with + 1.25 D sph.; left eye: 1/60, unimproved by lenses. Anterior segments and the right fundus are normal. The left fundus presents a traumatic retinopathy with fluffy exudates and retinal hemorrhages.
General examination showed rib fractures and pleural exudate.
Four months later vision was normal and the fundus lesion had subsided.

Figure 521. Left eye. Fundus lesions from strangulation, seen as preretinal, retinal and subretinal hemorrhages. The whitish

lesion in the macula is a macular degeneration, and independent of the strangulation lesion.

CLINICAL NOTE: Figure 521 is from a male, aged 43. Ten days ago he was found unconscious after a strangulation. He had presented macular degeneration for many years.
Eye examination: Visual acuity, both eyes: 2/60, unimproved by lenses. Anterior segments are normal. Both fundi present preretinal, retinal and subretinal hemorrhages and a macular degeneration consisting of whitish, confluent elements.
General examination still showed marks at the neck from the strangulation.

Figure 522. Left eye. Sun eclipse injury, seen as an elongated chorioretinal scar.

CLINICAL NOTE: Figure 522 is from a male, aged 41. As a child he looked with the left eye through a slightly opened door at the sun during a sun eclipse. Ever since he has had a scotoma in the left eye. He has had hypertension for many years.
Eye examination: Visual acuity, both eyes: 6/6 with + 0.5 D sph. Anterior segments are normal. Both fundi present hypertensive angiopathy. The left fundus presents a long, oblique chorioretinal scar nasally. Visual field defect corresponds to the fundal lesion.
General examination showed hypertension and uremia. Blood pressure: 160/100 mm Hg. Serum creatinine: 6.0 mg/100 ml.

Figure 523. Right eye. Sun eclipse injury, seen as a large macular chorioretinal scar with heavy pigmentation.

CLINICAL NOTE: Figure 523 is from a female, aged 75. As a child she looked with the right eye, which was unprotected, at the sun during a sun eclipse. Ever since she has had a large central scotoma in her right eye.
Eye examination: Visual acuity, right eye: hand movements; left eye: 6/6 with − 0.5 D cyl. axis 140°. Anterior segments and the left fundus are normal. The right fundus presents a large pigmented macular chorioretinal scar.
General examination showed nothing abnormal.

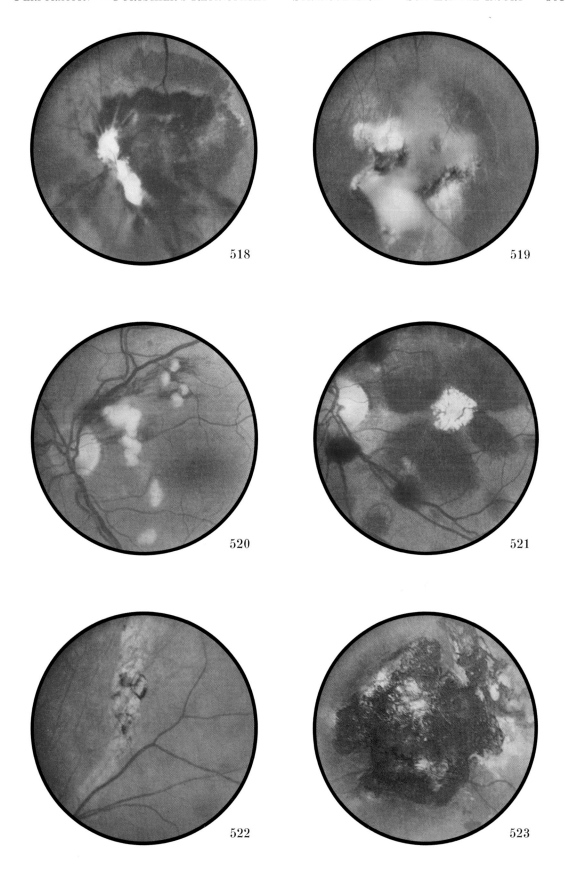

List of Patients

The abbreviation RH refers to Copenhagen University Hospital (Rigshospitalet), KH refers to Copenhagen Municipal Hospital (Kommunehospitalet), NSH refers to the Steno Memorial Hospital (Niels Steensens Hospital), KASGe refers to Copenhagen County Hospital (Københavns Amts-sygehus i Gentofte), and HWL refers to the author's own practice.

Figure no.	Name	Born	Hospital	Figure no.	Name	Born	Hospital
1	I. L.	6/12–28	HWL	44	J. P. L.	14/6–02	RH
2	C. B.	12/1–47	RH	45	E. H.	26/2–11	RH
3	D. R.	29/5–15	RH	46	M. J.	2/6–14	RH
4	G. R.	15/3–33	HWL	47	A. R. J.	13/12–85	RH
5	U. T.	2/4–32	HWL	48	K. W. A.	7/9–38	HWL
6	S. V.	31/12–12	HWL	49	K. W. A.	7/9–38	HWL
7	J. B.	8/5–50	RH	50	K. W. A.	7/9–38	HWL
8	M. O.	13/1–43	RH	51	E. C.	22/7–07	KH
9	M. O.	13/1–43	RH	52	L. K.	17/6–39	RH
10	D. L.	15/1–57	RH	53	J. P. P.	23/12–48	RH
11	D. L.	15/1–57	RH	54	C. B.	12/1–47	RH
12	L. J.	6/8–42	RH	55	B. H.	6/6–21	HWL
13	L. J.	6/8–42	RH	56	P. T.	16/2–21	RH
14	B. L.	11/4–44	RH	57	G. R.	15/3–33	HWL
15	R. H.	27/11–30	RH	58	E. C.	22/4–17	RH
16	J. J.	30/12–27	KASGe	59	J. A.	25/5–46	RH
17	R. P.	9/11–16	RH	60	B. J.	5/5–23	RH
18	E. J.	29/7–48	RH	61	M. M.	1/12–44	HWL
19	E. J.	29/7–48	RH	62	C. E.	7/7–41	KH
20	K. G.	19/5–58	RH	63	E. L.	10/10–08	HWL
21	K. G.	19/5–58	RH	64	C. B.	12/1–47	RH
22	N. M.	8/4–41	RH	65	E. H.	18/1–84	KH
23	I. N.	14/4–44	RH	66	K. H.	9/12–64	RH
24	A. J.	31/5–31	RH	67	J. M.	1/12–45	RH
25	K. M. A.	28/4–39	RH	68	H. L.	21/5–47	HWL
26	M. M.	7/3–49	RH	69	G. R.	13/6–20	RH
27	L. A. T.	1/12–31	RH	70	D. A.	5/3–11	RH
28	C. L.	30/3–33	RH	71	E. M.	15/5–96	RH
29	A. H.	26/8–30	RH	72	V. S. J.	1/8–96	KH
30	R. S.	30/7–24	RH	73	H. A.	16/1–97	HWL
31	P. J.	19/6–59	RH	74	E. N.	22/12–15	KH
32	U. A.	12/10–57	RH	75	O. N.	18/3–12	KH
33	U. A.	12/10–57	RH	76	G. K.	11/3–11	RH
34	S. T.	27/1–61	RH	77	H. A.	16/1–97	HWL
35	S. T.	27/1–61	RH	78	B. A.	25/3–56	HWL
36	S. T.	27/1–61	RH	79	I. P.	15/1–46	HWL
37	M. E.	5/1–68	RH	80	H. J.	9/4–55	HWL
38	M. E.	5/1–68	RH	81	U. M.	4/6–55	HWL
39	M. E.	5/1–68	RH	82	A. C.	27/4–95	RH
40	L. J.	18/10–66	RH	83	J. C.	19/2–52	HWL
41	J. N.	5/1–67	RH	84	K. M.	11/2–46	RH
42	S. C.	25/11–54	HWL	85	K. M.	11/2–46	RH
43	J. P. L.	14/6–02	RH	86	E. P.	3/10–17	RH

Figure no.	Name	Born	Hospital	Figure no.	Name	Born	Hospital
87	E. P.	3/10–17	RH	145	K. M.	11/2–46	RH
88	H. J.	9/4–55	HWL	146	K. M.	11/2–46	RH
89	P. H.	6/1–05	RH	147	K. M.	11/2–46	RH
90	C. C.	13/11–16	RH	148	K. M.	11/2–46	RH
91	C. C.	13/11–16	RH	149	K. M.	11/2–46	RH
92	C. C.	24/3–91	RH	150	K. M.	11/2–46	RH
93	S. K. H.	7/4–62	RH	151	K. M.	11/2–46	RH
94	A. N.	2/9–26	RH	152	K. M.	11/2–46	RH
95	A. N.	2/9–26	RH	153	K. M.	11/2–46	RH
96	P. N.	17/4–45	RH	154	K. M.	11/2–46	RH
97	L. S.	21/4–57	RH	155	K. M.	11/2–46	RH
98	M. O.	15/11–18	NSH	156	K. M.	11/2–46	RH
99	E. K.	21/7–12	KASGe	157	K. M.	11/2–46	RH
100	I. L.	13/10–23	KH	158	E. S.	13/7–20	RH
101	G. O.	28/10–15	RH	159	E. S.	13/7–20	RH
102	J. J.	14/9–12	RH	160	B. R.	27/1–52	RH
103	J. J.	14/9–12	RH	161	F. M.	31/8–50	RH
104	O. P.	2/3–53	RH	162	Å. H.	7/11–02	KH
105	O. P.	2/3–53	RH	163	J. P.	26/3–93	KH
106	K. S.	18/7–43	RH	164	A. B.	22/4–95	RH
107	V. H.	12/11–43	KH	165	A. B.	22/4–95	RH
108	S. A.	3/2–02	RH	166	E. B.	20/3–04	NSH
109	H. S.	13/7–09	RH	167	E. B.	20/3–04	NSH
110	J. J.	8/12–17	RH	168	V. S.	2/4–44	RH
111	B. J.	25/11–61	RH	169	J. H.	23/3–29	RH
112	A. H.	19/12–07	HWL	170	L. P.	19/8–52	RH
113	A. H.	19/12–07	HWL	171	L. P.	19/8–52	RH
114	H. B.	6/6–21	RH	172	E. N.	17/10–41	RH
115	H. B.	6/6–21	RH	173	E. N.	17/10–41	RH
116	M. T.	3/1–09	RH	174	H. A.	6/6–15	RH
117	U. J.	14/3–13	RH	175	R. K.	1/10–12	RH
118	P. J.	1/7–48	RH	176	R. K.	1/10–12	RH
119	E. P.	31/10–17	RH	177	A. P.	25/12–08	RH
120	F. M.	31/8–50	RH	178	I. B.	12/2–38	RH
121	O. F.	23/6–41	RH	179	C. N.	15/1–18	RH
122	G. H.	3/11–17	RH	180	C. N.	15/1–18	RH
123	M. B.	11/4–04	KH	181	C. N.	15/1–18	RH
124	K. B.	31/5–12	RH	182	I. B.	12/2–38	RH
125	A. P.	1/12–20	RH	183	E. P.	3/5–23	RH
126	I. C.	31/10–03	RH	184	E. P.	3/5–23	RH
127	R. R.	18/1–30	RH	185	D. S.	9/1–15	RH
128	G. J.	23/12–22	HWL	186	P. N.	17/4–45	RH
129	J. H.	9/10–40	KH	187	P. N.	17/4–45	RH
130	E. M.	9/3–04	RH	188	V. S.	14/10–18	RH
131	B. R.	27/1–52	RH	189	V. S.	14/10–18	RH
132	K. F.	19/7–21	RH	190	J. O.	7/3–46	RH
133	H. H.	4/3–30	HWL	191	I. M.	10/3–42	RH
134	T. J.	26/6–21	RH	192	L. P.	19/8–62	RH
135	A. C.	18/1–23	RH	193	L. P.	19/8–62	RH
136	J. A.	17/11–43	RH	194	L. P.	19/8–62	RH
137	R. J.	15/12–57	RH	195	L. P.	19/8–62	RH
138	T. F.	14/12–19	RH	196	L. P.	19/8–62	RH
139	O. J.	30/4–86	KASGe	197	L. P.	19/8–62	RH
140	E. F.	15/9–10	RH	198	J. C.	1/12–44	RH
141	B. J.	21/6–49	RH	199	J. C.	1/12–44	RH
142	B. J.	21/6–49	RH	200	M. N.	31/1–08	RH
143	H. S.	30/9–43	RH	201	M. N.	31/1–08	RH
144	K. M.	11/2–46	RH	202	O. T.	13/12–02	HWL

Figure no.	Name	Born	Hospital	Figure no.	Name	Born	Hospital
203	O. T.	13/12–02	HWL	261	T. P.	10/7–21	RH
204	T. J.	1/6–49	HWL	262	E. A.	22/4–25	NSH
205	B. P.	6/10–35	HWL	263	E. A.	22/4–25	NSH
206	B. P.	6/10–35	HWL	264	L. J.	29/5–45	NSH
207	B. P.	6/10–35	HWL	265	C. H.	20/5–13	NSH
208	M. N.	18/8–01	HWL	266	E. S.	17/8–21	NSH
209	I. P.	19/3–22	RH	267	S. J.	24/3–36	NSH
210	E. G.	27/3–86	RH	268	H. S.	24/6–27	NSH
211	G. J.	23/12–22	HWL	269	B. O.	20/12–28	KASGe
212	R. F.	16/9–41	RH	270	I. N.	11/2–23	NSH
213	R. F.	16/9–41	RH	271	H. S.	3/3–32	NSH
214	E. R.	17/1–08	RH	272	H. S.	3/3–32	NSH
215	E. R.	17/1–08	RH	273	B. O.	20/12–28	KASGe
216	O. S.	28/5–05	RH	274	B. O.	20/12–28	KASGe
217	J. P.	25/10–03	NSH	275	B. O.	20/12–28	KASGe
218	N. L.	15/7–97	RH	276	K. A.	26/5–23	HWL
219	H. J.	5/7–04	KH	277	K. A.	26/5–23	HWL
220	E. K.	22/2–17	RH	278	A. O.	19/7–00	RH
221	E. K.	22/2–17	RH	279	A. O.	19/7–00	RH
222	E. J.	18/5–25	RH	280	L. J.	19/1–05	KH
223	E. J.	18/5–25	RH	281	L. J.	19/1–05	KH
224	K. I.	18/7–38	RH	282	K. M.	10/1–06	RH
225	K. R.	23/6–91	RH	283	K. M.	10/1–06	RH
226	K. R.	23/6–91	RH	284	L. B.	29/4–12	KASGe
227	K. R.	23/6–91	RH	285	E. K.	21/7–12	KASGe
228	H. N.	28/7–86	KH	286	E. K.	21/7–12	KASGe
229	H. N.	28/7–86	KH	287	E. K.	21/7–12	KASGe
230	A. N.	18/5–07	HWL	288	A. L.	18/11–01	KASGe
231	V. R.	16/1–09	RH	289	A. L.	18/11–01	KASGe
232	E. L.	10/10–08	HWL	290	A. L.	18/11–01	KASGe
233	E. L.	10/10–08	HWL	291	M. O.	5/11–18	NSH
234	V. F.	1/3–02	NSH	292	A. B.	9/12–00	KH
235	R. K.	23/4–07	RH	293	A. B.	9/12–00	KH
236	P. J.	29/8–01	RH	294	H. W.	11/1–07	RH
237	P. J.	29/8–01	RH	295	T. E.	31/1–48	RH
238	P. J.	29/8–01	RH	296	M. K.	1/9–04	RH
239	T. A.	22/3–23	RH	297	M. K.	1/9–04	RH
240	H. B.	6/6–21	RH	298	L. O.	17/1–47	RH
241	J. F.	29/3–43	RH	299	L. O.	17/1–47	RH
242	J. F.	29/3–43	RH	300	A. E.	11/3–35	RH
243	J. F.	29/3–43	RH	301	A. E.	11/3–35	RH
244	I. J.	2/6–03	KH	302	E. A.	6/1–50	RH
245	S. S.	28/12–20	RH	303	E. A.	6/1–50	RH
246	V. T.	19/11–36	NSH	304	T. A.	16/9–39	RH
247	V. T.	19/11–36	NSH	305	T. A.	16/9–39	RH
248	J. C.	27/5–40	NSH	306	S. N.	19/7–11	RH
249	S. C.	24/8–93	NSH	307	S. N.	19/7–11	RH
250	L. J.	29/5–45	NSH	308	K. R.	25/1–60	KH
251	A. N.	11/5–44	RH	309	P. L.	26/9–59	KH
252	H. L.	14/12–33	NSH	310	T. H.	22/12–58	HWL
253	E. S.	13/4–30	NSH	311	B. M.	29/4–54	RH
254	S. J.	24/3–36	NSH	312	B. P.	16/5–55	RH
255	P. P.	21/4–16	NSH	313	B. P.	16/5–55	RH
256	K. H.	6/4–32	NSH	314	O. M.	2/7–51	HWL
257	M. H.	10/11–29	NSH	315	K. O.	27/1–39	RH
258	T. P.	10/7–21	RH	316	O. S.	16/1–47	RH
259	R. M.	22/5–01	NSH	317	O. S.	16/1–47	RH
260	A. S.	29/6–13	NSH	318	O. S.	16/1–47	RH

Figure no.	Name	Born	Hospital	Figure no.	Name	Born	Hospital
319	O. S.	16/1–47	RH	377	H. S.	22/8–30	RH
320	J. E.	11/9–59	HWL	378	E. A.	4/7–39	RH
321	J. E.	11/9–59	HWL	379	E. N.	20/3–52	RH
322	J. S.	12/6–50	RH	380	M. H.	29/10–36	RH
323	J. S.	12/6–50	RH	381	M. H.	29/10–36	RH
324	J. S.	12/6–50	RH	382	P. R.	27/4–15	RH
325	J. S.	12/6–50	RH	383	G. R.	8/4–55	RH
326	E. I.	20/8–18	RH	384	J. R.	19/3–47	HWL
327	E. I.	20/8–18	RH	385	L. N.	18/6–30	RH
328	G. M.	24/8–13	RH	386	L. B.	19/11–38	KH
329	G. M.	24/8–13	RH	387	K. P.	25/2–39	RH
330	P. J.	29/11–34	HWL	388	L. B.	19/11–38	KH
331	P. J.	29/11–34	HWL	389	B. M.	5/10–18	RH
332	C. H.	20/8–84	RH	390	E. L.	15/10–20	RH
333	E. L.	5/6–99	HWL	391	E. L.	15/10–20	RH
334	S. H.	29/7–87	KH	392	B. M.	5/10–18	RH
335	T. H.	4/9–93	RH	393	B. M.	5/10–18	RH
336	R. S.	20/12–91	KH	394	B. M.	5/10–18	RH
337	L. N.	17/12–87	KH	395	H. N.	5/5–02	HWL
338	H. B.	23/11–10	KH	396	P. L.	8/9–40	RH
339	D. S.	23/1–12	RH	397	J. T.	28/7–31	RH
340	T. H.	4/9–93	RH	398	I. G.	4/9–12	HWL
341	L. N.	17/12–87	KH	399	I. G.	4/9–12	HWL
342	M. N.	31/10–83	KH	400	A. J.	15/1–39	RH
343	K. J.	15/6–97	RH	401	K. H.	15/3–19	RH
344	R. W.	14/8–31	RH	402	E. P.	22/1–48	KH
345	R. W.	14/8–31	RH	403	E. K.	14/8–24	RH
346	G. A.	18/8–32	RH	404	B. N.	13/2–20	RH
347	M. A.	7/8–75	RH	405	B. N.	13/2–20	RH
348	E. K.	1/8–13	KH	406	Å. P.	20/6–18	KASGe
349	H. S.	17/10–06	RH	407	I. P.	5/3–10	NSH
350	P. C.	15/11–42	RH	408	G. N.	30/8–00	RH
351	P. C.	15/11–42	RH	409	G. N.	30/8–00	RH
352	P. C.	15/11–42	RH	410	G. J.	2/2–29	RH
353	P. C.	15/11–42	RH	411	G. J.	2/2–29	RH
354	P. C.	15/11–42	RH	412	G. J.	2/2–29	RH
355	P. C.	15/11–42	RH	413	G. J.	2/2–29	RH
356	A. N.	1/5–29	RH	414	E. P.	22/1–48	KH
357	K. R.	6/8–29	RH	415	E. P.	22/1–48	KH
358	K. R.	6/8–29	RH	416	P. L.	24/2–56	RH
359	E. N.	8/8–23	RH	417	P. L.	24/2–56	RH
360	E. N.	8/8–23	RH	418	J. H.	13/5–43	RH
361	E. N.	8/8–23	RH	419	J. H.	13/5–43	RH
362	J. C.	10/11–08	KH	420	L. L.	21/3–45	RH
363	J. C.	10/11–08	KH	421	T. P.	23/3–37	RH
364	M. J.	25/11–96	RH	422	G. B.	31/5–44	RH
365	M. J.	25/11–96	RH	423	J. L.	10/8–46	KH
366	C. F.	1/2–97	RH	424	K. J.	2/9–44	RH
367	C. F.	1/2–97	RH	425	B. S.	29/10–50	RH
368	H. L.	26/6–90	RH	426	B. P.	22/12–05	RH
369	H. L.	26/6–90	RH	427	V. L.	24/7–05	RH
370	J. N.	2/6–90	RH	428	V. L.	24/7–05	RH
371	J. N.	2/6–90	RH	429	V. L.	24/7–05	RH
372	T. R.	27/6–11	RH	430	E. N.	17/6–27	RH
373	E. B.	27/10–86	RH	431	J. C.	9/9–55	RH
374	K. S.	26/8–48	RH	432	L. S.	18/2–54	RH
375	G. V.	25/3–09	RH	433	E. L.	21/11–08	RH
376	V. J.	4/10–22	RH	434	M. G.	6/9–03	KH

Figure no.	Name	Born	Hospital	Figure no.	Name	Born	Hospital
435	K. G.	21/7–98	RH	480	H. A.	11/9–08	RH
436	K. G.	21/7–98	RH	481	A. H.	29/3–15	RH
437	J. P.	6/12–32	RH	482	A. S.	16/8–95	RH
438	J. P.	6/12–32	RH	483	H. A.	8/3–09	RH
439	J. N.	22/1–26	HWL	484	O. G.	6/7–01	RH
440	J. N.	22/1–26	HWL	485	G. J.	8/4–01	RH
441	S. J.	2/11–39	RH	486	H. A.	8/3–09	RH
442	J. C.	30/11–96	RH	487	H. R.	27/12–19	KH
443	K. L.	5/9–04	RH	488	P. I.	29/10–96	RH
444	L. J.	1/4–40	RH	489	L. O.	26/11–10	KH
445	J. K.	30/5–46	RH	490	K. H.	13/9–17	RH
446	J. K.	30/5–46	RH	491	G. B.	9/2–23	RH
447	P. C.	10/7–40	RH	492	G. H.	11/11–10	RH
448	P. C.	10/7–40	RH	493	K. Z.	16/8–10	RH
449	L. M.	2/2–15	RH	494	P. D.	24/6–22	KASGe
450	J. H.	8/6–19	RH	495	S. N.	15/9–65	RH
451	O. H.	26/8–10	RH	496	P. R.	20/12–62	RH
452	O. H.	26/8–10	RH	497	A. S.	23/3–65	RH
453	O. J.	12/7–27	RH	498	A. S.	23/3–65	RH
454	A. H.	7/9–14	RH	499	A. S.	23/3–65	RH
455	E. C.	26/3–11	RH	500	J. C.	9/4–53	KH
456	W. B.	19/11–50	RH	501	B. M.	5/3–44	RH
457	C. C.	2/6–01	RH	502	K. U.	8/9–45	RH
458	I. S.	16/7–04	RH	503	P. E.	11/11–42	RH
459	O. N.	6/11–32	RH	504	K. U.	8/9–45	RH
460	O. N.	6/11–32	RH	505	F. M.	3/2–38	RH
461	I. S.	16/7–04	RH	506	E. S.	15/12–33	RH
462	B. R.	5/5–29	RH	507	E. S.	15/12–33	RH
463	O. D.	18/11–15	RH	508	C. N.	28/3–45	RH
464	J. J.	28/1–32	RH	509	I. B.	8/5–50	RH
465	I. S.	16/7–04	RH	510	A. J.	30/4–38	RH
466	E. H.	26/2–11	RH	511	J. C.	10/4–47	RH
467	H. B.	1/4–15	RH	512	J. S.	15/2–44	RH
468	W. N.	16/1–25	RH	513	P. H.	11/11–25	RH
469	T. M.	29/10–08	RH	514	S. J.	6/3–37	RH
470	W. B.	8/4–02	RH	515	S. J.	6/3–37	RH
471	I. J.	23/7–55	KH	516	C. N.	28/3–45	RH
472	H. N.	2/3–99	KH	517	N. O.	12/4–22	RH
473	A. P.	18/12–25	RH	518	B. J.	28/11–41	RH
474	S. C.	25/11–54	HWL	519	B. J.	28/11–41	RH
475	A. R.	10/2–39	HWL	520	S. H.	16/5–06	KASGe
476	L. P.	7/3–23	RH	521	V. A.	4/11–20	RH
477	M. A.	29/4–36	RH	522	P. W.	20/1–26	RH
478	A. K.	25/10–29	RH	523	A. R.	4/6–89	RH
479	V. C.	15/6–07	RH				

INDEX

Numbers without parentheses refer to figure numbers.
Numbers in parentheses refer to page numbers.